ADVANCE PRAISE FOR PAUL WADE'S
CONVICT CONDITIONING 2

"Paul Wade's section on developing the sides of the body in **Convict Conditioning 2** is brilliant. Hardstyle!"
—**Pavel Tsatsouline,** author of **The Naked Warrior**

***

"The overriding principle of **Convict Conditioning 2** is 'little equipment-big rewards'. For the athlete in the throwing and fighting arts, the section on Lateral Chain Training, Capturing the Flag, is a unique and perhaps singular approach to training the obliques and the whole family of side muscles. This section stood out to me as ground breaking and well worth the time and energy by anyone to review and attempt to complete. Literally, this is a new approach to lateral chain training that is well beyond sidebends and suitcase deadlifts.

The author's review of passive stretching reflects the experience of many of us in the field. But, his solution might be the reason I am going to recommend this work for everyone: The Trifecta. This section covers what the author calls The Functional Triad and gives a series of simple progressions to three holds that promise to oil your joints. It's yoga for the strength athlete and supports the material one would find, for example, in Pavel's **Loaded Stretching**.

I didn't expect to like this book, but I come away from it practically insisting that everyone read it. It is a strongman book mixed with yoga mixed with street smarts. I wanted to hate it, but I love it."
—**Dan John,** author of **Don't Let Go** and co-author of **Easy Strength**

"Coach Paul Wade has outdone himself. His first book ***Convict Conditioning*** is to my mind THE BEST book ever written on bodyweight conditioning. Hands down. Now, with the sequel ***Convict Conditioning 2,*** Coach Wade takes us even deeper into the subtle nuances of training with the ultimate resistance tool: our bodies.

In plain English, but with an amazing understanding of anatomy, physiology, kinesiology and, go figure, psychology, Coach Wade explains very simply how to work the smaller but just as important areas of the body such as the hands and forearms, neck and calves and obliques in serious functional ways.

His minimalist approach to exercise belies the complexity of his system and the deep insight into exactly how the body works and the best way to get from A to Z in the shortest time possible.

I got the best advice on how to strengthen the hard-to-reach extensors of the hand right away from this exercise Master I have ever seen. It's so simple but so completely functional I can't believe no one else has thought of it yet. Just glad he figured it out for me.

Paul teaches us how to strengthen our bodies with the simplest of movements while at the same time balancing our structures in the same way: simple exercises that work the whole body.

And just as simply as he did with his first book. His novel approach to stretching and mobility training is brilliant and fresh as well as his take on recovery and healing from injury. Sprinkled throughout the entire book are too-many-to-count insights and advice from a man who has come to his knowledge the hard way and knows exactly of what he speaks.

This book is, as was his first, an amazing journey into the history of physical culture disguised as a book on calisthenics. But the thing that Coach Wade does better than any before him is his unbelievable progressions on EVERY EXERCISE and stretch! He breaks things down and tells us EXACTLY how to proceed to get to whatever level of strength and development we want. AND gives us the exact metrics we need to know when to go to the next level.

Adding in completely practical and immediately useful insights into nutrition and the mindset necessary to deal not only with training but with life, makes this book a classic that will stand the test of time.

Bravo Coach Wade, Bravo."
   —Mark Reifkind, Master RKC, author of ***Mastering the HardStyle Kettlebell Swing***

"I've been lifting weights for over 50 years and have trained in the martial arts since 1965. I've read voraciously on both subjects, and written dozens of magazine articles and many books on the subjects. This book and Wade's first, *Convict Conditioning,* are by far the most commonsense, information-packed, and result producing I've read. These books will truly change your life.

Paul Wade is a new and powerful voice in the strength and fitness arena, one that is commonsense, inspiring, and in your face. His approach to maximizing your body's potential is not the same old hackneyed material you find in every book and magazine piece that pictures steroid-bloated models screaming as they curl weights. Wade's stuff has been proven effective by hard men who don't tolerate fluff. It will work for you, too—guaranteed.

As an ex-cop, I've gone mano-y-mano with ex-cons that had clearly trained as Paul Wade suggests in his two *Convict Conditioning* books. While these guys didn't look like steroid-fueled bodybuilders (actually, there were a couple who did), all were incredibly lean, hard and powerful. Wade blows many commonly held beliefs about conditioning, strengthening, and eating out of the water and replaces them with result-producing information that won't cost you a dime."
—**Loren W. Christensen,** author of *Fighting the Pain Resistant Attacker,* and many other titles

"*Convict Conditioning* is one of the most influential books I ever got my hands on. *Convict Conditioning 2* took my training and outlook on
the power of bodyweight training to the 10th degree—from strengthening the smallest muscles in a maximal manner, all the way to using bodyweight training as a means of healing injuries that pile up from over 22 years of aggressive lifting.

I've used both *Convict Conditioning* and *Convict Conditioning 2* on myself and with my athletes. Without either of these books I can easily say that these boys would not be the BEASTS they are today. Without a doubt *Convict Conditioning 2* will blow you away and inspire and educate you to take bodyweight training to a whole NEW level."
—**Zach Even-Esh,** Underground Strength Coach

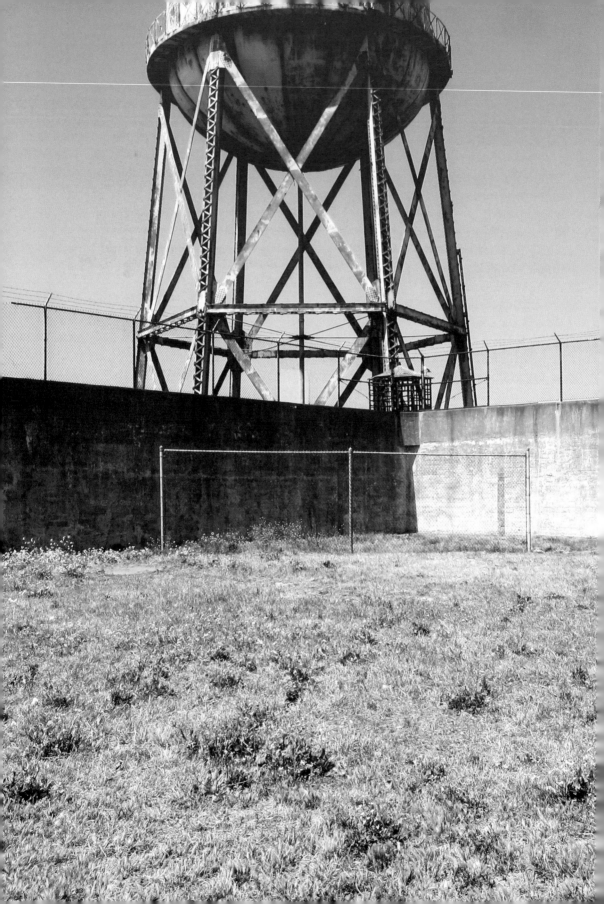

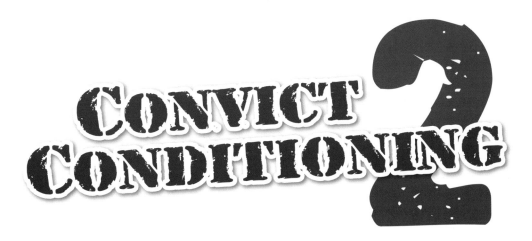

ADVANCED PRISON TRAINING TACTICS
FOR MUSCLE GAIN, FAT LOSS
AND BULLETPROOF JOINTS

BY PAUL "COACH" WADE

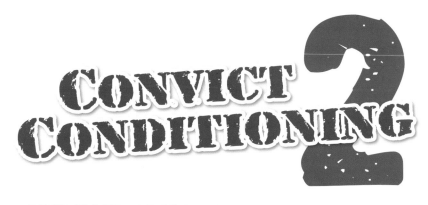

CONVICT CONDITIONING 2

ADVANCED PRISON TRAINING TACTICS FOR MUSCLE GAIN, FAT LOSS AND BULLETPROOF JOINTS

BY PAUL "COACH" WADE

Copyright ©2011 Paul "Coach" Wade
All rights under International and Pan-American Copyright conventions.

Published in the United States by:
Dragon Door Publications, Inc
5 East County Rd B, #3 • Little Canada, MN 55117
Tel: (651) 487-2180 • Fax: (651) 487-3954
Credit card orders: 1-800-899-5111
Email: support@dragondoor.com • Website: www.dragondoor.com

ISBN 10: 1-942812-14-0   ISBN 13: 978-1-942812-14-2

Second Edition, first printed in June, 2018

Printed in China

Book design, and cover by Derek Brigham
Website www.dbrigham.com • Tel/Fax: (763) 208-3069 • Email: bigd@dbrigham.com

DISCLAIMER
The author and publisher of this material are not responsible in any manner whatsoever for any injury that may occur through following the instructions contained in this material. The activities, physical and otherwise, described herein for informational purposes only, may be too strenuous or dangerous for some people and the reader(s) should consult a physician before engaging in them.

To Pete H,

You gave me a computer, edited every word I ever
wrote,and arranged an account so I could pick up
my paycheck. Back on day one, you even gave me
a pencil to write with! None of this could have
happened without you or Stella.

You really are my brother from another mother.

—DISCLAIMER!—

Fitness and strength are meaningless qualities without *health*. With correct training, these three benefits should naturally proceed hand-in-hand. In this book, every effort has been made to convey the importance of safe training technique, but despite this all individual trainees are different and needs will vary. Proceed with caution, and at your own risk. Your body is your own responsibility-look after it. All medical experts agree that you should consult your physician before initiating a training program. Be safe!

This book is intended for entertainment purposes only. This book is not biography. The names, histories and circumstances of the individuals featured in this book have accordingly been changed either partially or completely. Despite this, the author maintains that all the exercise principles within this volume-techniques, methods and ideology-are valid. Use them, and become the best.

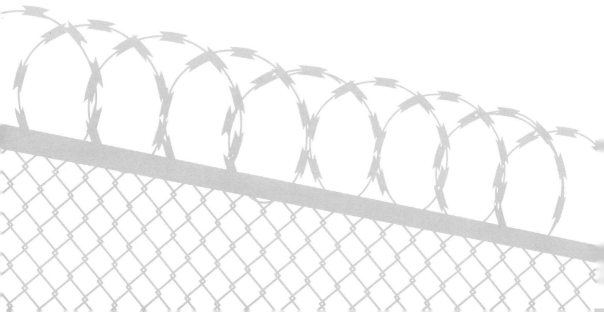

—TABLE OF CONTENTS—

PART I: SHOTGUN MUSCLE
Hands and Forearms

Lateral Chain

Neck and Calves

PART II: BULLETPROOF JOINTS

PART III: WISDOM FROM CELLBLOCK G

!BONUS CHAPTER!

FOREWORD

The Many Roads to Strength

By Brooks Kubik

A fter writing over a dozen strength training books and courses of my own, and literally hundreds of training articles, I'm finally able to take it easy and write a short foreword to someone else's book. In this case, Paul Wade did the heavy lifting (if I can use that term in the foreword to a book about old-school physical culture through advanced calisthenics), and after Paul knocked out 300-plus pages, I get to be lazy and type a few words of my own.

The fact that Paul asked me to write this foreword may surprise you – just as you may be surprised by the fact that I agreed to his request. After all, Paul is the guy who wrote *Convict Conditioning*—a book devoted to old-school calisthenics—and I'm the guy who wrote *Dinosaur Training* and other books dealing with old-school weightlifting and weight training.

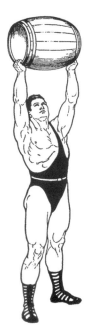

"So where's the common ground?" you might ask.

Well, I'll tell you.

Let's begin with the cover of *Dinosaur Training*. It features a simple line drawing of an old-school physical culturist lifting a heavy barrel overhead. The photo comes from an old-time forearm and grip training course written and sold by George F. Jowett, an old-school lifter, wrestler, strongman and athlete who was setting records about 100 years ago, and who wrote his courses and books way back in the 1920s. If you're familiar with his work, you know that he was one of the best and most inspiring writers in the history of Physical Culture—and you also know that a lot of people have gotten really strong over the years by following his training advice.

(Brief note: Jowett's best book is *The Key to Might and Muscle*, which is available in a high quality modern reprint edition from a very good friend of mine—Bill Hinbern at *www.superstrengthbooks.com*. Bill also carries that old George Jowett forearm and grip course I mentioned. Both are well worth reading.)

In any case, imagine my reaction when I read through the final draft of Paul's manuscript for *Convict Conditioning 2* and spotted a line drawing of an old-school physical culturist lifting a heavy barrel. It's not the same drawing that appears on the cover of *Dinosaur Training*, but it's from the same George Jowett course.

And that's a clue to why a guy who primarily writes about lifting heavy iron is writing this foreword.

The real link is an appreciation for old-school physical culture, and the training methods of old-school athletes and strongmen. As both Paul and I have noted many times in our respective books and other writing, most people who think about building strength and muscle make the HUGE mistake of thinking that the way to do it is to go to the nearest commercial gym—what I refer to as "Chrome and Fern Land" in *Dinosaur Training*— and start following the latest super program in whatever muscle comic you happen to be reading. In other words, they start doing a modern-day bodybuilding program, they train for the pump, they use the latest exercise machine knock-offs of the Nautilus machines that flooded the training world in the 1970s, they use the cardio equipment, they guzzle the supplements and follow this month's version of the super-duper muscle-building and fat-burning diet for bodybuilders, and in way too many cases they start looking for someone who can supply them with their first stack of steroids.

I'm opposed to that nonsense. I believe in building strength and muscle the old-fashioned way. I believe in things like hard work, sensible training programs, and training for lifelong strength, health and organic fitness. I believe in following the training advice of the old-time strongmen who flourished in the period I call the Golden Age of Strength—which was roughly from 1890 and the days of the French-Canadian powerhouse, Louis Cyr, and the magnificently muscled and remarkably strong German, Eugene Sandow— through the 1930s, and 1940s, and the amazing exploits of men like Tony Terlazzo, John Grimek, Steve Stanko, John Davis, and others— and into the 1950s and the era of men like Reg Park, Tommy Kono, Doug Hepburn and Paul Anderson.

And Paul seems to believe much the same thing. Interestingly, in *Convict Conditoning* and *Convict Conditioning 2* he mentions many of the men I write about in my various books and courses. I'm working off memory right now, and this isn't an exhaustive or complete list, but we both cover the strength, power and exploits of Sig Klein, John Grimek, Maxick, Doug Hepburn, Bert Assirati, George F. Jowett, Eugene Sandow, and Thomas Inch. And as Paul properly notes, each of these men—all of whom are Iron Game immortals, meaning that long before steroids, wraps and super-suits they set lifting records that very few men can match even today—were accomplished gymnasts, hand balancers, and acrobats or combined their weight training with some form of advanced calisthenics.

So that's the common thread. Both of us have turned our backs on modern-day training—which really means modern-day bodybuilding—and have turned back to old-school physical culture. We've done that because the old-school stuff works—and the modern stuff doesn't. And both of us want YOU—the reader—to do what works. We both want you to achieve great things—and to develop the type of strength and development exemplified by the legendary athletes of the Golden Age.

You hold in your hands a book that can help you build some serious strength. Use it wisely, and use it well—and grow strong!

Yours in strength,

Brooks Kubik

OPENING SALVO

"I've come here to chew bubblegum and kick ass...

...and I'm all outta bubblegum."

Roddy Piper in *They Live* (1988)

Before you dig into this pile of notes, stray ideas, and hard-worn advice that some have generously called a "book", I feel you need to be given some kinda warning.

First up: if you are looking for a basic strength or muscle-building workout, *don't pick up this book*. You'll find that stuff in the original *Convict Conditioning*. In that book, I let loose the goods on how convicts use bodyweight skills to develop maximum strength and muscle—especially the old school guys who were around before the weight piles hit the yards.

Since *Convict Conditioning* landed on the shelves, I've been asked lots of questions about stuff that go beyond the basics. Questions like:

- What about the extremities of the body? The neck, forearms and calves?
- How do I train the muscles at the sides of the body?
- What's your philosophy for building strong joints?
- How do convict-athletes get so big on the prison diet?
- Do inmates have any tricks for dealing with injuries?
- What about mental training in jail?

The answers to all those questions are in this book. If you want to know this kinda thing, pick it up. (And preferably pay for it. I got bills too, dude.)

That leads me to a second warning to potential new readers. This manual is not like the thousands of other books about strength and fitness that you can find on the internet or littering the shelves of *Barnes & Noble*. Those books are written by guys with dozens of certificates, maybe doctorates, all with their own websites and *Youtube* accounts.

That's not me.

If you want to be told s*** like:

- Lift weights
- Do three sets of ten
- Stretch
- Eat six times a day
- Consume lots of protein

Then you are wasting your time reading this book. I don't say any of that—in fact, the stuff that comes out of my mouth is, very often, the exact *opposite* of what the modern fitness scene thinks is acceptable. (That's why it works.)

I'll say it straight. I'm not certificated, I'm not officially ranked, and you won't find me on *Youtube*. I don't pretend to have degrees in nutrition or kinesiology. If you are looking for all that, you won't get it here.

I learnt what I learnt behind bars. I spent nearly twenty years total in some of the toughest prisons in America. I'm not proud of it, and I don't want to glamorize it, but there it is. I can't teach you anything about the latest exercise machines, current studies in nutrition or biochemistry, or even the new workout fashions.

I'm not claiming that I can tell you stuff "experts" and personal trainers will agree with, and I'm not trying to be contentious. I'm just trying to teach you—in the best way I can—about all the stuff I picked up on the inside.

Bear this in mind when you read this book, and don't get too hot and sweaty about the controversial stuff. I just ask that you read it. If you don't like what I have to say, don't take it too seriously. If you do like what you see in these pages, then try it, test, it, use it.

It worked for us. Who knows? It might work for you too.

Paul Wade

1: Introduction

Put Yourself Behind Bars

magine the very *best* hardcore gym in the world.

- Imagine an arena where men—there are no women—train as if their very *survival* depended upon it. A politically incorrect environment where the goal of training isn't cute little Chippendale muscles or a cheap trophy, but ungodly animal power, raw, functional athleticism and sheer brutal *toughness*.

- Imagine a "gym" where—for the vast majority of the time—there is no access to new training equipment or flashy gadgets to distract you from a brutal regime of bodyweight training...the most primitive and effective form of conditioning known to man. A place with no juice bar, no air conditioning, and no other luxuries. A place where you are literally *locked in* to sweat, struggle and strive alone—with no audience or accolades—just the power of your own muscles and mind.

- Imagine if this place was largely cut off from the here-today-gone-tomorrow fitness fads and fashions of the outside world...so that all that really counted was the kind of punishing daily training which really produces results—quickly *and* efficiently.

Just imagine what you could learn about physical training—*and what you are really made of*—from an environment like this, if such a place existed.

Well, a place like that does exist. It's called the federal and state corrections system—that's *jail* to you and me.

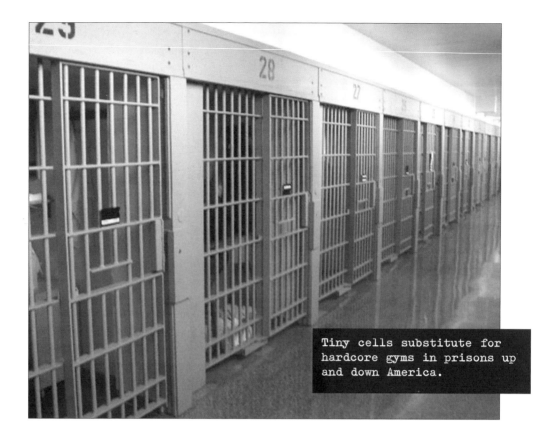

Tiny cells substitute for hardcore gyms in prisons up and down America.

The evolution of prison training methods

Many prisoner athletes—particularly those guys stuck inside for the long haul—often learn their conditioning methods from other, older convicts, who in turn learned their skills from the inmates who were locked up before them. These old time inmates rarely had access to the new forms of equipment and training fads so popular in the outside world. As a result, prisons are almost like a bubble, separated from the training world beyond the bars; prison-spawned training methods have remained, pure, functional, based on *toughness* and *results* rather than aesthetics and fashion. Stripped of training equipment or new training technologies, prisoners have traditionally been forced to turn to ancient methods, the forgotten but tried-and-tested conditioning arts and techniques that turned men into supermen centuries before steroids and other performance drugs were conceived.

Inmate athletes have had to be innovative, often inventing new methods and effective training tactics that simply don't exist on the outside. Real prison athletes—guys that have been training non-stop in their cells for decades in the search for ultimate strength and athleticism—can teach you a lot. Secrets and tricks you could never learn from a magazine or a modern personal trainer in a million years.

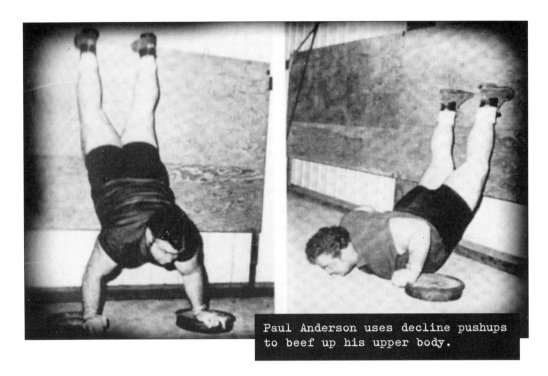

Paul Anderson uses decline pushups to beef up his upper body.

My time

I don't know much about most things, but training behind bars—especially bodyweight work—is something I know very well. I spent nearly twenty years of my life in prisons, starting in San Quentin for drug offences, and later "graduating" to a federal correctional facility for trafficking in-between prison stays. I'm not proud of it, but there it is. During that whole period I must've done a quarter of a million pushups, and about as many bodyweight squats.

Throughout my time behind bars, training my body became a passion; an obsession. It was the one thing that kept my mind sane, and—in all likelihood—my heart still beating. I learned what I did from all kinds of different people; ex-Navy SEALs, marines, karate guys. In particular I absorbed what I could from older inmates, and the former generations of cons who practiced bodyweight training in their tiny cells like it was some kind of *religion*.

Over the years I mastered the bodyweight arts that had been handed down from convict-to-convict, and I began training other inmates. My system is the most authentic (and effective) distillation of the older traditional prison calisthenics—the time-honored stuff that thrived in jails before the weights leaked into the yards. It's based on the way the very best prison athletes train: it's bodyweight, it's minimal (or no) equipment, it's progressive, and it's brutally intense. Prison training has to be this way.

The Convict Conditioning system

The approach I learnt behind bars is the reverse of what's taught on the outside. To most modern personal trainers, calisthenics is seen as an "easy" activity, or a warm up. But to prison athletes, calisthenics is based on *strength*.

That's the foundation. You can use my methods to build inhuman stamina, Olympic-level balance and agility, or even phenomenal reflex speed. But strength is the cornerstone. It has to be. This makes perfect sense if you think about it. You can't build explosive power and speed by working on clapping pushups unless you have built a solid base of tendon and muscle strength by doing regular pushups. Without strength, you can't build peak endurance, either: if you try to build stamina by doing hours of burpees, you will only injure yourself if you are not strong. That's why the most basic, most hardcore movements—the Big Six of prison strength training—form the nucleus of the entire *Convict Conditioning* system. Everything radiates outward from the Big Six (see the chart below).

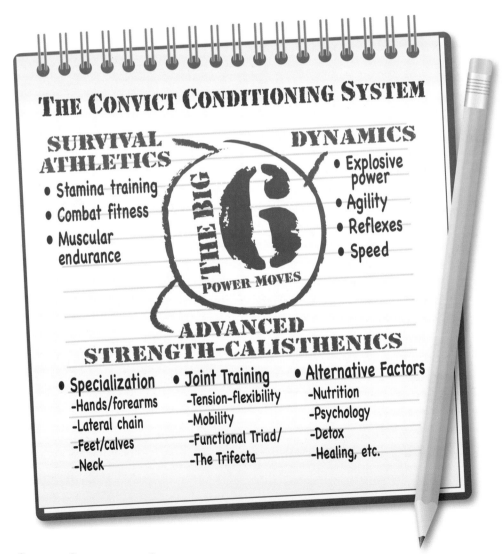

Getting bigger and stronger —the advanced info

The first volume of *Convict Conditioning* was completely dedicated to the fundamental strength system: the Big Six moves and their progressions, along with useful variant exercises. This second book follows on from that, and is devoted to advanced strength-calisthenics.*

The advanced areas of the system aren't meant to *replace* the Big Six moves—they grow out of them. Strength and muscle growth don't come from new gimmicks, complex techniques or pseudo-scientific approaches. That stuff's all snake oil. Real, total body development comes from a consistent, disciplined, progressive dedication to the basic, total body exercises you learned in the first *Convict Conditioning*. These basic movements—along with their variants—allow for a *lot* of creative training time. As you advance, you can change your rep ranges, your speed, your program, and so on. Trust me on this; there's a lifetime of productive training in that book.

Despite this fact, as athletes advance, they often have further questions. The information they need usually falls into three categories:

1. **Specialization areas** – *grip, neck, calves, side-waist, etc.*
2. **Joint training** – *tendon strength, mobility, pain elimination, etc.*
3. **Lifestyle advice** – *fat loss, recovery, psychology, etc.*

These three areas are the subject of this book.

Part One of this book is called *Shotgun Muscle*. *Convict Conditioning* contained a lot of information about working the major muscles of the body, as well as the smaller muscles. But sometimes these little muscles—in particular the forearms, side-waist, neck and calves—require specialized training for various reasons. The chapters in *Shotgun Muscle* represent a highly condensed grab bag of secret tricks, exercises and little-known techniques and equipment which will take these (usually feeble) areas and blast their development right up to "superhero" levels. These are all techniques I learned in the joint, so they stay true to the *Convict Conditioning* philosophy of *little equipment—big reward*.

One of the most underrated areas of modern physical culture is the training of the *joints*. This is especially true as you get bigger and stronger: as athletes become more advanced, the greater the load that's placed on their joints and tendons. Juiced-up bodybuilders might have big muscles, but they often have weak, painful joints; their training has given them stiff, unnatural movement and connective tissue prone to injury. This is where calisthenics scores. Old school calisthenics is built on an approach which *strengthens* the joints and tendons, building them up rather than wearing them down, over time. In Part Two of this book, *Bulletproof Joints*, I show you how to build the strongest joints possible, while eliminating those old aches and pains—forever. Along the way, I'll share with you the traditional prison attitude to stretching. This old school approach

* I originally planned on cramming the entire *Convict Conditioning* system into a single book, but it was far too big. So we tried two books. Even that was optimistic. So it made sense to keep things focused and include just the advanced strength-calisthenics material in this second manual. As for the *survival athletics* and *dynamics* parts of the system, if you guys and girls tell me you want it, they'll get their very own volumes too.

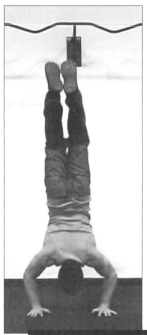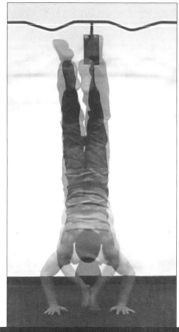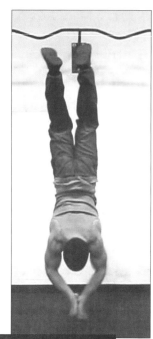

Prison training can and does generate world class athletes. Everyone knows that bodyweight can build endurance, but it can also build muscle and explosive strength. Clapping handstand pushups require ungodly power.

will strengthen your joints instead of weakening them, but beware—it's probably the *opposite* of what you've been taught on the outside. In Part Two I'll also teach you the *Trifecta*—my secret, minutes-per-day program for functional mobility and optimal joint health.

Becoming a superior athlete—whether you are interested in sports, personal development, or if you are just stuck in a cell on lockdown twenty-three hours a day—depends on a lot more than just how you exercise. Part Three, *Wisdom From Cellblock G*, looks at those areas of an athlete's life which exist *outside* the sweat and pain of training sessions. I'm not qualified to be a personal trainer or life coach, but I can teach you the lessons prisoners learn about these subjects. You'll find out about:

- The prison diet
- The value of regulated lifestyle ("living by the buzzer")
- The significance of high levels of sleep and rest
- Mental control (coping with demons)
- The benefits of the "straight edge" for an athlete (living clean)
- Healing skills (with minimum meds/professional healthcare)

The book finishes with a look at the role of the *mind* in training. The power of the mind over human life is skimmed over (or completely overlooked) in most books on fitness. I think this is probably because people living on the outside have so many things available to distract themselves from the old-fashioned practice of introspection. As a man who has been forced to spend many thousands of nights caged up alone with only my thoughts and the memories of past mistakes for company, I've learned something about the tricks the mind can play. I've also learned some of the tactics you can use to fight back. Hopefully you will find what I have to say of help in your own training.

This book also includes a bonus chapter. Since leaving prison I've been asked a lot of questions by guys who work out about the typical weight-training and bodybuilding methods convicts use, when they do have access to the heavy stuff. There seems to be a real fascination about this topic. I'm all about the older methods of calisthenics, but people are pretty insistent, so I've included an extra chapter at the end of the book. It's called *Pumpin' Iron in Prison*. It'll answer all your questions.

Lights out!

You know the biggest training mistake most wannabe tough guys make? They're fickle. They flip from one method to another; they change systems; they drop what they're doing when the next tool or technology busts out. Constantly switching goals and approaches like this is *training suicide*. Some of the most incredible athletes in the world are those inmates who train alone, in their cells. It's *not* because they are genetically gifted compared to you or me. It's *not* because the have access to world class coaching. And it's sure as hell not because they have cutting edge nutritional programs or supplements. These guys become the best because they are—literally—locked in to one method of training.

The less you chop-and-change, the less you rely on external stuff and the more you focus on basics, the better your results will be. And this is not *less* true as you become advanced—it's *more* true. As you get bigger and stronger, resist the instinct to add more elements in—weights, machines, gadgets. Look at the most basic, stripped-down way your body is meant to move, then use it that way. Your grip evolved to support your body in a tree. You want the strongest grip your genetics will allow? Throw all the grippers, special weights and spring machines in the trash, and go and actually *hang* from something. You want to get lean? Avoid the fat-loss pills, expensive supplements and complex diets, and go back to three squares a day—like a convict.

Message understood? Cool. Now lock yourself in, and let's get training.

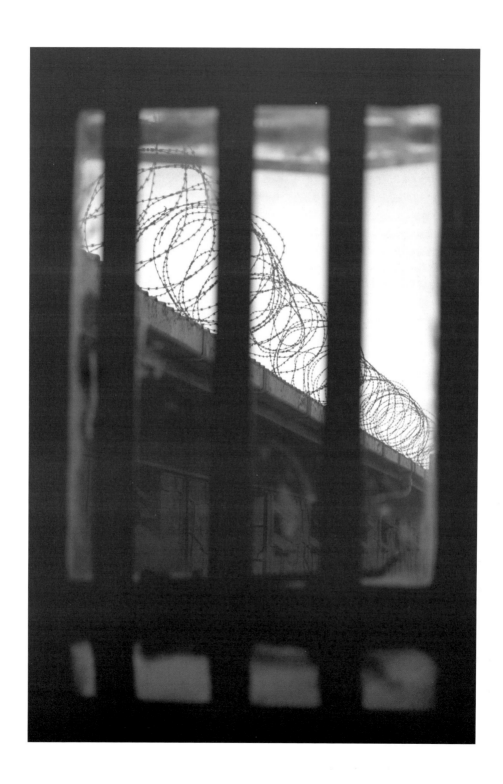

– Part I –

Shotgun Muscle

The Big Six bodyweight exercises will work all of your primary muscles-thighs, midsection, back, chest, shoulders and upper arms. This is where a man's true power lies. But sometimes the "minor" muscles at the extremities of the body need a little toughening up, too-I'm talking about often-neglected areas like the forearms, obliques, neck, and calves. These groups were often called *shotgun muscles* by the old time prison athletes, because they ride shotgun with the bigger movers.

This section is a condensed encyclopedia of prison training methods guaranteed to turn your puny little shotgun muscles into goddamn artillery cannons!

2: IRON HANDS AND FOREARMS

ULTIMATE STRENGTH— WITH JUST TWO TECHNIQUES

Hand and forearm training is often seen as being on the periphery of strength training. Many bodybuilders—even professionals—don't specifically train their forearms at all. The theory behind this is that the forearms get plenty of secondary work from exercises like rows, ground lifts and curls; and that the hands get more than enough training from just gripping the bar during heavy exercises.

I don't agree with this theory.

Any engineer will tell you that in order to know how strong a machine is—how much work it can do—you don't need to look at its strongest part, but its *weakest*. Any system—even a simple chain—is only as strong as its weakest link. The same holds true for the human body. Unfortunately, most modern men have weak hands, and this limits the strength of their bodies as a complete unit. Go into any gym and you'll see guys using wrist straps and hooks to help them hold onto the barbell during heavy pulling exercises. They may tell you that this is so that they can lift "more"—but that's not really true. Their body is capable of lifting the weight, it's just that puny hand strength has let them down. Trust me, it's a bad state of affairs if you need straps and hooks to be able to tap into your physical potential. It creates a false groove to exercises and it's very artificial. You might be able to get away with this cheating nonsense in the gym, but what about in the real world? What if you have to spend some time doing manual labor, or manhandle something heavy in an emergency? Fake gadgets and gimmicks won't be able to help you.

The old time strongmen never had this problem. In fact, a few generations ago men in general had much stronger hands than guys today. This was in the era before heavy lifting was done by hydraulic machines, when men had to roll up their sleeves to do the work we let technology do for us now. These men worked long hours in mines, in foundries, out on the farms. As a result, our forefathers had thick, callused hands with strong tendons and powerful forearms. Healthy, useful hands. When these guys went on to become strongmen, they sure as hell didn't need straps and hooks. But it seems like the most use the average guy gets out of his hands and fingers is tapping away on a computer keyboard or popping a beer.

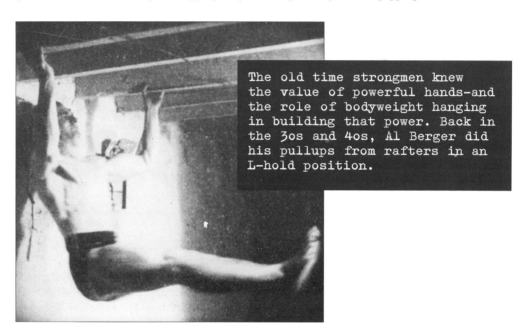

The old time strongmen knew the value of powerful hands—and the role of bodyweight hanging in building that power. Back in the 30s and 40s, Al Berger did his pullups from rafters in an L-hold position.

Strong, capable hands with massive stamina are *useful*. Everything from opening a jar to undoing a stuck screw requires strong hands and forearms. To a strength athlete, powerful hands are even more important. They are *vital!* Every time you pick up a barbell or dumbbell you use your hands. Even the best leg exercises like deadlifts and barbell hack squats require that you pick up a heavy bar with your hands. The same principle applies to calisthenics. You can't do pullups without powerful hands and forearms to support your bodyweight. Without extremely strong fingers and palms, hand-balancing is totally impossible. This is not to mention specialist techniques like fingertip pushups. Forget impressive feats on the rings or parallel bars—a gymnast with weak hands wouldn't even be able to perform the basic maneuvers taught to children. Wrestlers and martial artists require powerful hands to excel in grappling. In terms of raw strength and athletic ability, weak hands limit practically everything you do.

Modern methods? Forget them.

It's not a surprise that modern athletes are wanting when it comes to powerful hands and forearms. To find out why, just look at the kind of methods being pushed these days. The top two hand exercises in gyms today are *wrist curls* and *reverse curls*. Wrist curls can only be performed with light weights. They actually do very little for hand strength, but—on the bright side—they go a long way towards screwing up your wrists. Reverse curls primarily work the forearms at the elbow joint, bypassing the hands, wrists and fingers. Again, due to leverage factors, light weights are the order of the day. The average bodybuilder can only reverse curl about half the weight he can curl. Unless you are taking big doses of anabolic steroids, this kind of chickens*** nonsense is really not enough to add any lower arm strength and mass.

Hardly anybody in gyms today knows how to work their lower arms *properly*. This is ironic, because (with the exception of the neck), the forearms are on display more frequently than any other muscle group. This, of course, is one of the reasons that forearm training is so important to so many convicts. Big, beefed-up forearms are intimidating. It's also one of the reasons that forearms are still the number one place for tattoos.

Old school forearms

One reason many convicts—particularly of twenty or thirty years back—had such monstrous, powerful forearms was because they knew how to train them using proper *bodyweight* methods. The good news is that if you are currently investing your energy in a bodyweight strength program, you are already leagues ahead of most other athletes. Whereas most bodybuilders can get away with pumping up their muscles using machines, cables or dumbbells, calisthenics strength athletes are forced to bite the bullet and use something heavier—their bodyweight. Believe it or not, this is more than the average weak-gripped gym-built athlete's hands could cope with for long. Just hanging from the overhead bar for leg raises will strengthen the fingers and grip considerably.

Pullups kick things up a notch. Pullups are an excellent basic exercise for the lower arms. Not only do they require that you hold onto a bar, supporting your bodyweight, but the flexion of the elbows as you draw yourself up works the bulkier muscles of the forearms. The main muscles trained are the *brachioradialis* which runs along the top of the forearm, and the deep, knotty *brachialis* which lies a little further up. The brachioradialis makes up about a third of the muscle mass on the forearms, and the brachialis underlies the biceps, so you'll be pleased to know that when it's well developed it pushes the biceps out and makes the upper arms appear a lot bigger. (Arnold Schwarzenegger had exceptionally well-developed brachialis muscles.)

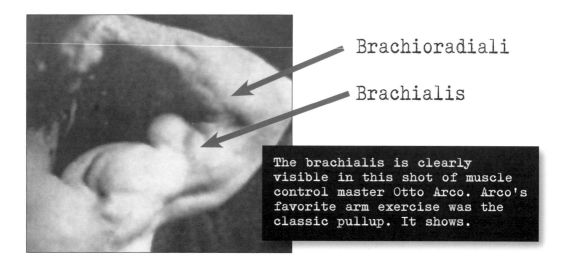

Brachioradiali

Brachialis

The brachialis is clearly visible in this shot of muscle control master Otto Arco. Arco's favorite arm exercise was the classic pullup. It shows.

Although a routine containing solid work on pullups (as described in the first volume of *Convict Conditioning*) will strengthen your hands and forearms, you'll find that with a little added work you can take your lower arm power into another league entirely. In fact, just six months of specific attention to the exercises described in this chapter will put your hand strength and health light years ahead of the average guy who works out. It'll do a lot for your forearm muscularity too. In this chapter I'm going to show you the key to building hands and forearms that aren't just *strong*, but are *superhumanly strong*—with wrists, fingers, thumbs and tendons as powerful as your genetic potential will allow. And you're going to get there by building your training around a single leading exercise—the *hang grip*.

Why just *one* core technique? Because you were born to hang, baby!

Evolution and hanging out

The hands are extraordinarily versatile tools; capable of acts as diverse as repairing the pin lever on a wristwatch to sculpting the Pietà. Without the complex manipulations the hands make possible, human beings couldn't have advanced into the dominating force we have become—even simple technology is rendered impossible without the blessings of nimble fingers and opposable thumbs.* This enormous functional capacity is mirrored by anatomy. The hands are incredibly complex instruments. Each hand is stabilized by over a hundred twenty ligaments, and controlled by well over thirty muscles. These muscles and their corresponding tendons are attached to twenty-seven distinct bones. (Some anatomists count twenty-nine. That's more than *four times* as many bones as there are in a giraffe's neck!)

---

*Although I should point out that the well-held notion of humans as being the *only* species with opposable thumbs—i.e., thumbs that can pinch with the index fingers—is a *myth*. What makes human hands so uniquely dexterous is our capacity to *rotate our ring and pinky fingers to meet the thumbs*—no other known species can do this. But numerous primates and other animals have opposable thumbs. Many zoologists consider chimpanzees to have opposable thumbs. Just thought I'd throw that out there in for any chimps reading. (Quit reading and get back to typing Shakespeare, you loafers.)

Despite this complexity, there's no need to run to the gym and perform dozens of different exercises to work all the individual muscles of the hands. Although there are dozens of muscles in the hands, all the major muscles have evolved to automatically work *together* when they need to perform a gross motor movement—in particular the chief survival function of the hands; *hanging on something*. Our species is capable of activating all our associated hand and finger muscles separately in exquisitely delicate fashions (imagine playing a piano concerto) and then, a split second later, the same diverse muscles can immediately work in perfect unison to generate unbelievable gripping power (imagine hanging onto a rope for dear life).

This phenomena of profound muscle synergy in the hands is something seen in many primates, and it probably results from a period of evolution high above the ground; hanging in trees. Primates in particular base their method of locomotion in the canopy or from tree-to-tree to find food and avoid predators. It's as if our species were born to hang on—literally. One of the most primitive instincts babies possess is called the *palmar grasp reflex*, which is a throwback to the time when the offspring of our ancestors had to grip onto their mother's fur in order to survive. As our species developed, having a strong grip from birth was a matter of life or death. The human grip becomes proportionately weaker as we age, due to disuse; but babies and infants have long been known for having notoriously strong grip capabilities, given their size. (The power of a baby's grip is even referred to in verse fifty-five of the *Tao Te Ching*, written roughly 2500 years ago.)

Even our basic anatomy is shaped by the need to hang from our hands. Our clavicles (collar bones) are a great example. Clavicles are probably a very, very ancient throwback to a time when vertebrates possessed exoskeletons. Very few mammals still retain proper clavicles, but one group that has kept them is primates, including human beings. Why? Because collar bones allow primates to hang vertically suspended, without straining the shoulders. Many forward-thinking physical culturists promote the idea that training should be based around "natural" movements to maximize progress and avoid injuries. Well bud, if any movement comes naturally to you or me, it's a hang grip.

Balancing the hands: fingertip pushups

If conventional forearms training methods are like a Crock-Pot when it comes to building hand and forearm strength, hanging grip work is like a microwave oven. It produces noticeable results, fast—and these results come not just over the short-term, but for long periods. The muscles that control the hands are capable of ferocious strength, and it can take an entire career to unlock this full potential. Many of the old school strongmen used to claim that hand strength was the "last thing to go", and I well believe it.

Hanging grip work is so effective at developing strength in the muscles and tendons that *close* the fingers, that there may be a minor risk that these areas become disproportionately strong in comparison to their antagonists—the muscles which keep the fingers *open*. These extensor muscles are relatively small in comparison to the muscles which control the grip, but in the interests of balanced strength and hand health, they need to be trained by any athlete who is looking to seriously strengthen their hands.

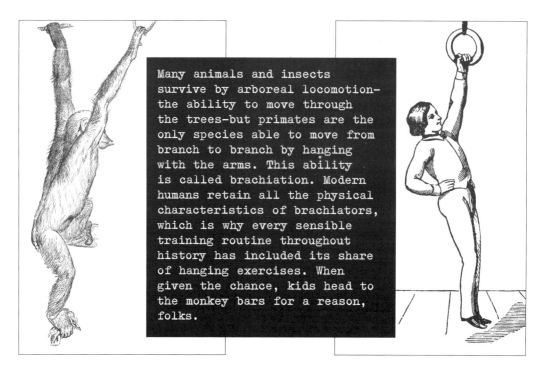

Many animals and insects survive by arboreal locomotion—the ability to move through the trees—but primates are the only species able to move from branch to branch by hanging with the arms. This ability is called brachiation. Modern humans retain all the physical characteristics of brachiators, which is why every sensible training routine throughout history has included its share of hanging exercises. When given the chance, kids head to the monkey bars for a reason, folks.

I only advise one type of training for the finger extensors: *fingertip pushups*. Fingertip pushups radically increase strength in the extensor muscles, as well as the hands and wrists, because they force you to support your weight on your digits. This pressure strengthens not only muscles and tendons in the hands but also the cartilage, and even the bones, of the fingers and thumbs. If you can't yet perform classic fingertip pushups, don't panic. I'll show you how to achieve this ability gradually.

Some athletes resort to training their extensors by wrapping elastic bands on the backs of their fingers and then opening them, but this isn't very effective and it's certainly not functional or convenient. (It's no fun, either!) Fingertip pushups are the perfect complement to grip work, because both techniques are *isometric*; that is, they don't involve movement of the target muscles. Not only is isometric work in tune with the way the hands operate, it also protects the finger joints, the vulnerable moving parts of each hand.

There you have it; the basic *Convict Conditioning* approach to working the hands and forearms. Focus on hanging work to build lower arm strength, and balance this strength out with a course of fingertip pushups. Two exercises are all you need. Anything else is overkill.

Remote control muscles and diesel forearms

Of course, many well-meaning bodybuilders perform a lot more than just two exercises for their forearms. Most of that energy is totally wasted. For example, these pumpers add various wrist curl, reverse wrist curl and leverage movements to their routines in a misguided attempt to pack more muscle mass to the forearms. The thinking behind this is that the muscles of the forearm are associated with flexing the wrist joint (the way the biceps muscle are responsible for moving the elbow joint). On the surface, this might seem like a good idea, but it's based on a misunderstanding of kinesiology. The lion's share of muscles in the forearm aren't there to flex or bend the wrists at all; the muscles which move the wrist joint are relatively few and fairly small and weak. In fact, the large, powerful muscles of the forearm (particularly those below the elbow) have just one function: they are *gripping* muscles.

It might sound strange to hear that the forearm muscles exist to move the *fingers* and not the *wrists*; particularly if you are used to the notion that muscles should be right next to the joints they operate. This is certainly true of the biceps, triceps, deltoids, etc., but it's not true of the forearm muscles. The forearm muscles (along with a few muscles in the palm) operate the fingers from a distance, almost like puppets on strings. It has to be this way, because *the fingers themselves have no muscles inside them.* None. They have to be operated from a distance, by muscles in the forearm. This makes the fingers a unique body part. All our other moving parts are pulled by muscles immediately adjacent to them. The fingers are the only part of the human body operated by "remote control".

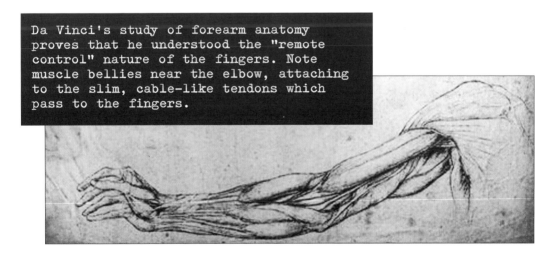

Da Vinci's study of forearm anatomy proves that he understood the "remote control" nature of the fingers. Note muscle bellies near the elbow, attaching to the slim, cable-like tendons which pass to the fingers.

What's the upshot of all this? It's this: if you want big, strong, muscular forearms, you are barking up the wrong tree by performing silly wrist joint movements like wrist curls, reverse wrist curls, leverage raises, wrist rolling, and so on. Why? *Because the big, strong muscles of the forearms don't control the wrist anyway.* They were put there to operate the fingers. So if you really want to add mass to those lower arms, forget the puny bodybuilding-type nonsense and start working hard on your grip!

Why the hang grip?

There are various approaches to grip work seen in gyms today. People use everything from barbells and leverage bells to spring-loaded grippers. If you're going to work your grip, I'm a firm believer that the natural way is best—by hanging, using nothing but bodyweight. If it's cool with you, I want to take a little bit of your time to check out different types of grip and explain exactly why I believe the hang grip is the best.

There are at least a dozen grip positions strength athletes employ. Let's look at the seven most often used and most basic ones, examining the pros and cons.

THE SUPPORT GRIP

Lifting or holding a bar upwards against gravity, with the thumb over the fingers

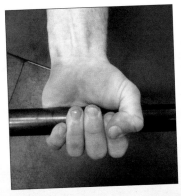 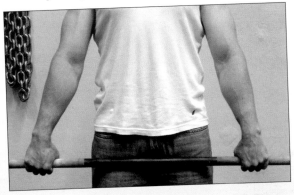

PROS: A very functional lift for weight trainers. Where heavy weights are used (e.g., one-arm deadlifts, hand-and-thigh lifts, etc.) the fingers become strengthened and forearms developed. (Look at a powerlifter's forearms.)

CONS: Heavy poundages must be utilized to exploit the strength potential of the hands, and this places huge stresses on the spine, hips and other joints. In addition, the thumb gets very little work during support gripping.

THE HOOK

Lifting or holding a bar upwards against gravity, with the fingers over the thumb

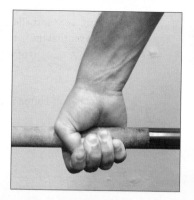 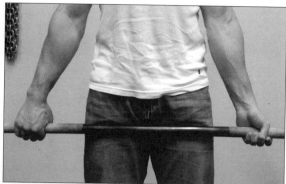

PROS: This is a little-known grip, usually used only by Olympic lifters. Wrapping the fingers over the thumb can help to keep the bar "locked" into the hands during sudden changes in velocity.

CONS: The hook grip is little more than a trick used to prevent a heavy bar flying out of the lifter's fingers during explosive movements. It also puts the thumbs in a very unnatural position. Useless outside of competition.

THE FALSE GRIP

Gripping with the bar cupped in the palm and fingers, without the thumb curled round

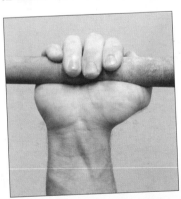 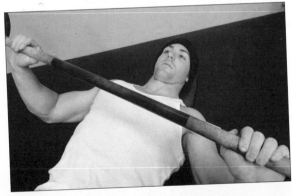

PROS: The false grip (sometimes called the "thumbless" grip) is a common type of grip found in bodybuilding. Many bodybuilders believe that pressing or pulling without the thumbs takes the forearms and arms out of a movement, throwing extra pressure instead on the pecs, delts, lats, etc.

CONS: The false grip is rarely used in grip training. It's unstable, provides no work for the thumbs, and offers little in the way of forearm benefits.

THE MONKEY GRIP

Lifting or hanging by the tips or pads of the bent fingers, without any thumb support

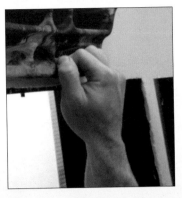 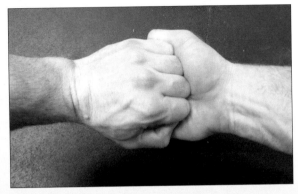

PROS: It's fun to try your pullups on doorframes using this grip, which works well to build powerful fingers. Also quite functional; resembles the hand shape used by climbers, or when lifting the edge of an unwieldy object.

CONS: Like all the grips reviewed so far, this kind of grip gives little or no work to the thumbs. Because of the finger angle, the palm muscles receive less work than during support grip lifting.

THE PINCH GRIP

Gripping a narrow object with the pads of four fingers, plus the thumb

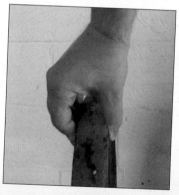 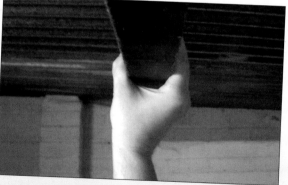

PROS: The beauty of the pinch grip is that if forces the thumbs to work hard during the movement. For this reason alone, all serious barbell grip aficionados include the pinch grip in their training.

CONS: Since most lifters perform the pinch grip with fairly straight fingers and thumbs, the leverage means that the weight lifted has to be radically reduced compared to other, much heavier gripping techniques.

THE CRUSH GRIP

Gripping by dynamically squeezing something in the hands under tension

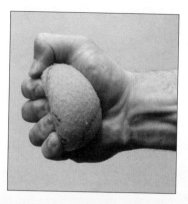 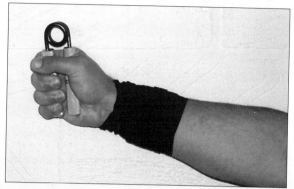

PROS: Heavy duty gripping forces the hands to actually move *isotonically*, rather than just staying isometrically static as with other kinds of gripping.

CONS: Crush gripping is notoriously hard on the finger joints and knuckles, because these areas are forced to torque under high tension. The functionality of crush gripping is also questionable; the majority of athletic movements require a good static grip, not a peak-contraction crush grip.

THE HANG GRIP

Gripping an overhead base while suspended vertically off the ground

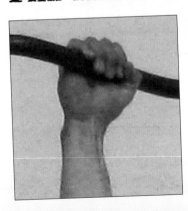 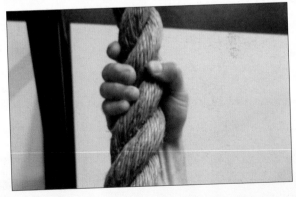

• The hang grip can be done from a horizontal bar, but the most productive (and difficult version) should be performed suspended from a vertical towel or rope.

The hang grip continued on next page

THE HANG GRIP *continued*

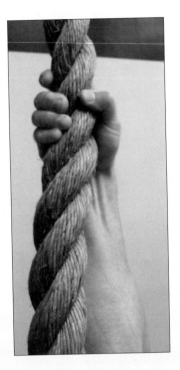

- Hanging from a bar provides excellent training for the fingers, but very little work for the thumbs. The advanced *vertical* towel or rope version forces the athlete to utilize the thumbs to hold on. Consequently, it works all the muscles of the hand to their maximal capacity.

- Unlike standard support gripping—which involves lifting a heavy weight from the ground—hang gripping places no pressure on the spine, hips or knees. This fact alone makes hang gripping superior to support gripping, even if you never get round to using a towel.

- Because the towel is cushioned (unlike a metal bar), the fingers and thumbs have to close extra tightly around it in order to maintain the hold. This delivers the same peak-contraction strength benefits as a crush gripping (for example, on heavy duty grippers) but without the injury risk associated with full-range crush gripping.

- Fans of barbell lifting will argue that barbell-based grip lifts are superior to bodyweight hanging, because progressive resistance can be easily applied as the athlete gets stronger—more weight can be added to the bar. Students of old school calisthenics will know that this is false. All bodyweight strength techniques can be divided into progressive steps applicable to anybody, no matter their level of strength and conditioning. The same is true of hang gripping.

The one-arm towel hang

The one-arm hang gripping a towel is the ultimate grip exercise. Even if you've trained yourself to hang by your hands from an overhead bar, you'll find this exercise a challenge. I've met some *incredibly* strong powerlifters who have had trouble with this variation; even guys who can pull more than six wheels on an Olympic bar have been known to falter, badly.

There are several reasons why even advanced strength athletes can struggle with this simple variation. For one thing, most gym-built lifters are used to picking up *bars*; barbells, dumbbells, machine handles, and so on. These devices are manufactured with relatively slim, cylindrical bars for one reason only—it makes them easy to hold on to. Unfortunately, "easy to hold" is the opposite of what you need if you desire a truly *monstrous* grip. A doubled-over towel, on the other hand, is much, much harder to hold onto than a cylindrical bar. Because the towel hangs vertically (rather than lying horizontally), it won't just "rest" in the cup of your palm—you gotta really *squeeze* it just to maintain a grip. This works the hell out of your palm muscles. When you pick up a heavy bar, the *fingers* get work curling around the bar, but with towel hangs your *thumbs* get a major workout too. Without strong thumbs and deep palm muscles, towel hanging is straight up impossible. This is precisely what most lifters are lacking—*complete* grip strength. Towel hangs will deliver that total power.

Lights out!

If you don't believe all this stuff I'm spouting about towel hangs, try 'em. Right now. Pick up a big towel—it can be a bath, sports or gym towel, but make sure it's the thickest one you can lay your hands on. Then go to your regular pullup bar (or a sturdy tree branch, or whatever). Loop the towel over the top of the bar, so it's double thickness, and hang from the sucker. Just one handed, mind you. If you can hold on at all, try maintaining your grip like that for a full minute.

If you can make the full sixty seconds, congrats, stud—your grip strength is already in the top one percent of the population. You are the elite. (Try hanging one-handed but with *two* towels over the bar, doubling the thickness.) If you can't hold on, welcome to the rest of the human race. In the next chapter I'll teach you how to get there.

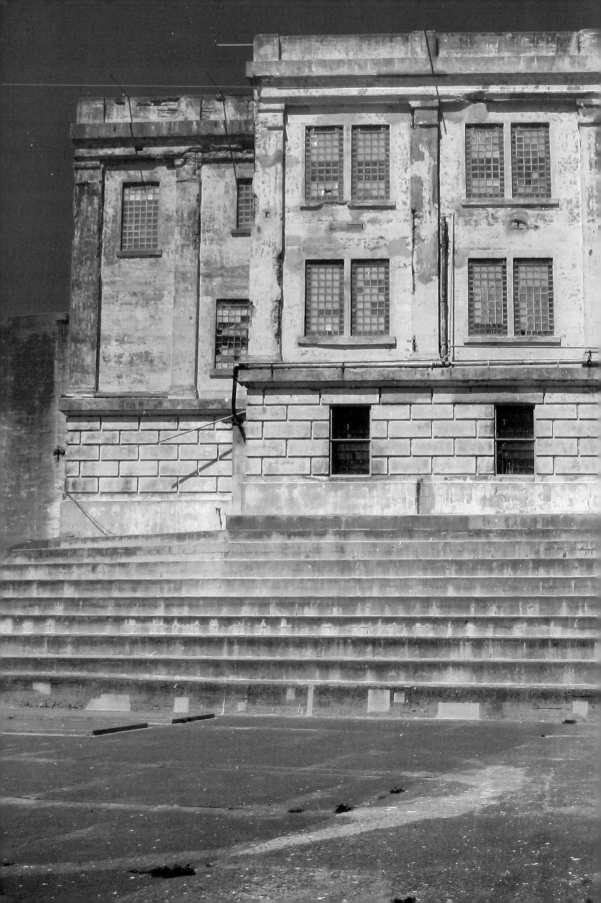

3: The Hang Progression

A Vice-Like Bodyweight Grip Course

The key to developing huge grip strength—and mastering advanced exercises like *one-arm towel hangs*—lies in working progressively towards your goal. This principle is universally true for all types of resistance training. Getting stronger gradually is easy to do if you're working with a barbell; you just slap more plates on over time. It's not so simple if you don't have access to a barbell. If—for whatever reason—the only "barbell" you regularly have access to is your own body, you need to learn how to make the same basic movements (pushups, pullups, etc.) progressively harder over time. You do this by laying out a "movement series"—a sequence of progressively harder exercises, intended to be mastered one-by-one.

Anyone who bought the first *Convict Conditioning* book will be good buddies with the idea of a "series of progressions". For those of you who picked up this book but not its big brother, I'll take a sec to explain the basic principle.

To build a good progressive movement series, you need to take a look at the tools at your disposal—your equipment, leverage and positioning factors—and work out whether they make the exercise harder or easier. From there, you manipulate them to construct a list of exercises, from easy to hard. Simple, huh? (Well, simple if you've been shown what to do.)

When it comes to hanging grip work, we have *six* of these basic factors to play with. They are:

3: Hanging from a bar – 4: Hanging from a towel: This is a great way of making your hanging easier or harder. As explained, not only is hanging from a towel harder than hanging from a bar, it also involves your whole hand, palm and thumbs as well as the fingers.

5: Regular towel – 6: Folded towel: The thicker the object you are gripping, the harder it is to keep hold of it. (This is why so many grip devotees train exclusively with thick-handled barbells and dumbbells.) Trying to hang when gripping a towel that's been doubled over is a lot harder than gripping a regular width towel.

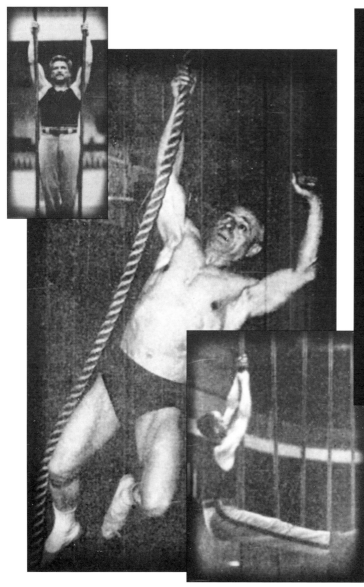

Old school bodybuilders knew the massive value of hanging grip training. Where the space permitted, many used thick ropes in place of towels. Legendary strongman Sig Klein kept broad, powerful forearms well into old age as a result of his consistent work on the rope. Military men have also practiced rope hangs. The inserts are from the 1914 US Army PT Manual. Note the twin hang (top) and L-hold (below) variations.

So, just by working with a bar, a couple of towels and bodyweight, we have at least six different, fundamental, ways to make our training harder or easier. Obviously if you want to get creative, these can be mixed and matched into even more combinations—for example, you can hang with one hand from a bar, while the other grips a towel, and so on. Our goal is to manipulate these various combinations into a progressive sequence, so we can begin with the easier exercises and condition the fingers and forearms while we *bank* strength and head towards the harder exercises. Ultimately we want to gradually gain raw power on the more advanced exercises which will allow us to attempt our ultimate goal—the *one-arm towel hang*.

Luckily for you my brothers and sisters, prison grip athletes have been working on progressive protocols for many years. The usual procedure involves starting by mastering bar work and intermittently throwing in some towel training until you eventually progress to only using the towel for your grip sets. There are several different ways to do this, but I'm going to show you my favorite sequence of progressions in the next part of this chapter.

Training tips for hanging out

Before we get to the nitty-gritty of the grip series, I want to shoot a few simple pointers at you, that'll help you along the way to making your hanging grip work a whole lot more productive:

- **The eight steps:** In the movement sequence leading up to the *one-arm towel hang*, I've included eight progressively harder exercises—*the eight steps*. There's nothing particularly special about the number ten. Some advanced bodyweight strength athletes might not need this many steps. Some more cautious trainees might want to break the exercises up and use more than eight steps. It's up to you.

- **Go slow:** Whatever your level, when you begin the series *resist the temptation to start with the hardest step you can do*. If you are new to specific grip work, begin at step one, get the most outta each exercise and work your way up. Not only will this give your joints and soft tissues time to adapt, it will also build training momentum and help you reach higher levels of strength in the long run.

- **Warm up:** Even if you are a big, strong, bull mastiff kind of a dude, the tendons of the hands and forearms are relatively small and can be irritated easily. Before your grip work, do some *fingertip pushups* (chapter five) to get the blood flowing hot through the hands and wrists. Bust out some easy hangs, and stretch out your fingers until you're happy they're good and warm. Performing work sets for grip after pullups or leg raises can also be a smart tactic.

- **Use time:** With most calisthenics techniques, you can judge your progress by counting reps. Hanging is an *isometric* exercise—you don't move, so there are no reps to count. Instead, you'll be counting seconds. Most gyms have large clocks on their walls so that clients can time their workouts. If you are training at home, I want you to set a large clock opposite you when you train—remember, the second hand has to be visible from where you hang.

- **Watch it:** If you can't train using a timepiece, you'll have to go by subjective counting (saying *one...two...three*, in your head). But be aware that an athlete's perception of time can be unreliable when the pain sets in. I've known some athletes to utilize a metronome to help regulate their counting. If you're working on unilateral hangs of course, you can just hold your watch in your non-working hand.

- **Progression standard:** Each step lists a *progression standard*. Once you can hang for the time stated in the progression standard, you can move on to the next step.

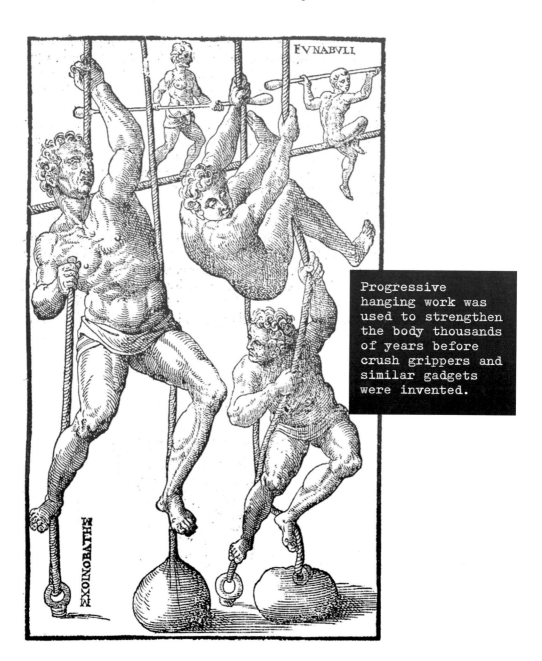

Progressive hanging work was used to strengthen the body thousands of years before crush grippers and similar gadgets were invented.

• **Progression speed:** From workout to workout, try to increase the amount of time you are able to hang, until you meet the *progression standard*. You might only add a second or two every workout—or you may add ten or twenty seconds, or more. It will vary from person-to-person. Beginners with their "virgin" grips on the early steps will progress faster than trained strength athletes working with harder steps. Whatever your level, the *speed* of progress is irrelevant—*consistent* improvement is the only thing that matters. The muscles and tendons of the hands will adapt to become very, very strong, but they will do so at their own pace—not yours.

• **Avoid failure:** When you're hanging, push yourself hard, but try not to go to "failure"—to the point where your hands just give up. This is easier said than done, I know. Just remember that suddenly crashing down from a bar isn't the safest way to travel.

• **Tight shoulders:** When you hang, you should keep your shoulders "tight" to prevent injury or joint strain. Tense your lat muscles and keep your arms pulled tight into their shoulder sockets. Never allow your shoulders to be stretched out while hanging. Stay strong and in control. (See *Convict Conditioning* page 117 for more details on maintaining "tight" shoulders.)

• **Soft elbows:** By a similar token, keep your elbows "soft" when you hang. This means keeping a slight kink in your arms—never allow them to be stretched out straight. This bend can be almost imperceptible to onlookers, but it will protect your elbow joints and the surrounding tendons from strain or hyperextension.

• **Rest between sets:** When working with multiple sets of hangs, don't feel the need to rush from set to set. Take some time to shake the acids and waste products from your hands and fingers. Many athletes stretch their hands and wrists between sets, and this certainly helps dissipate tension if you are prone to cramping. Rest as long as you need to, but don't let the lower arms get cold, either. Bear in mind that the forearms are made up of dense muscles (like the calves) and they have evolved to recover quicker from hard work than big muscles like the quads or lats. More than four minutes rest is probably overkill.

• **Weakest first:** Some of the exercises in the eight steps I'll show you are unsymmetrical, or unilateral (one-sided). Where this is the case, start your workout with your weakest side first, then use the resulting time to limit hang time on your strongest side. This is a great way to iron out strength imbalances.

• **Consistency:** Be consistent with your training tools; try to use the same bar, the same size and thickness of towel, etc. Using different bars and towels will make it difficult to gauge your progress.

• **Retain towel work:** You begin the grip series by training the fingers, and start using the towel only when you hit step three. Once you begin using the towel, you need to retain the thumb and palm strength it develops. If you progress to exercises which don't require a towel (like *one-arm bar hangs*), keep your palm and thumb conditioning by always finishing your grip workout with some towel hanging.

Okay, that's enough theory to get anyone started. Now you just need a bar to hang from, a clock or watch, and a couple of towels. Bingo—you're ready to embark on a grip training program that will not only last you a lifetime and provide a helluva lot of fun and satisfaction, but will also protect your joints and give you a functional grip like a titanium vice.

Let's check out the eight steps of the *Convict Conditioning* grip series.

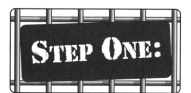 **STEP ONE:**

HORIZONTAL HANG

Performance

Get underneath a sturdy horizontal base, such as a desk or a table. Reach up and take hold of the lip with an overhand grip. Straighten your body and lift it off the floor so that your weight only goes through your fingers and heels.

Exercise X-Ray

Horizontal hangs are a great way to begin your hand training, because they work the fingers but without the need to support the entire bodyweight. If this exercise is too tough at first, try hanging from a higher base. If you want to make the exercise harder, use a lower base or raise your feet up.

Training Goals

- Beginner standard: 1 x 10 seconds
- Progression standard: 4 x 30 seconds

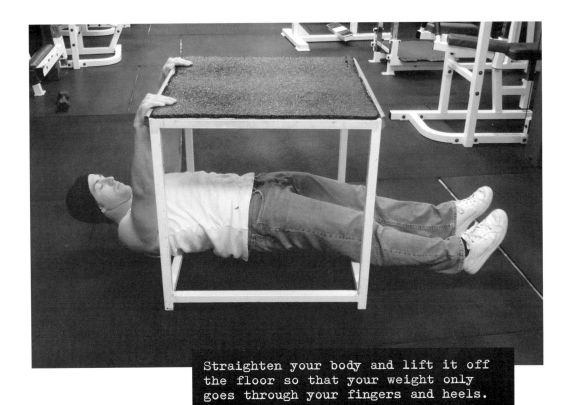

Straighten your body and lift it off the floor so that your weight only goes through your fingers and heels.

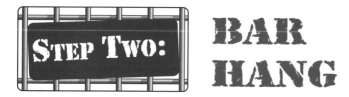

STEP TWO: BAR HANG

Performance

Jump up and grab an overhead bar with both hands. Use an overhand, shoulder-width grip, and make certain that your feet are clear of the floor. Keep your shoulders tight and your arms, trunk and legs symmetrical.

Exercise X-Ray

Bar hangs are a classic grip exercise. They continue on from where *horizontal hangs* leave off, making the athlete hold the full bodyweight with the fingers. They also increase shoulder strength and flexibility, conditioning the trainee for more intense hanging work.

Training Goals

- Beginner standard: 1 x 10 seconds
- Progression standard: 4 x 1 minute

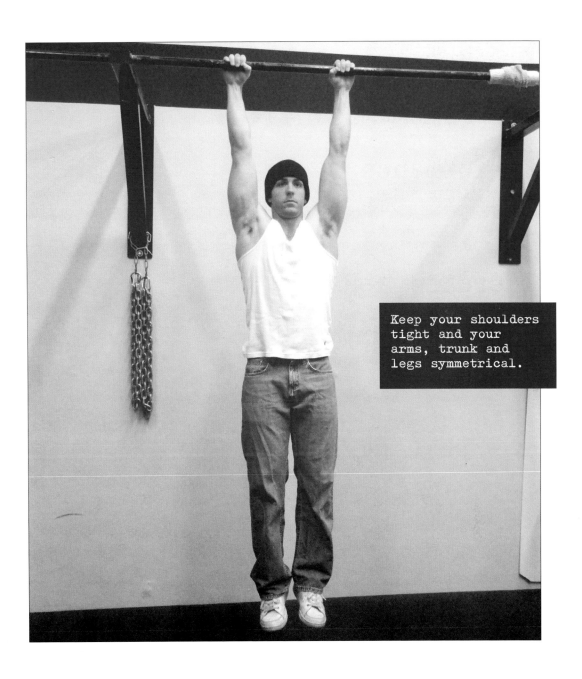

Keep your shoulders tight and your arms, trunk and legs symmetrical.

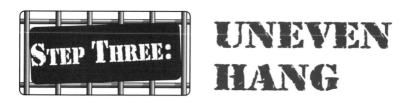

STEP THREE: UNEVEN HANG

Performance

Loop a towel around an overhead bar. Jump up and grab the bar with an overhand grip, then firmly grip the towel with your other hand. Try to distribute your weight evenly through both hands. Your hands should be about shoulder-width, your shoulders tight and your body symmetrical.

Exercise X-Ray

Once an athlete is comfortable with regular *bar hangs* for the *progression standard*, it's time to start adding some towel work to begin conditioning the thumbs. *Uneven hangs* allow you to start towel gripping without strain.

Training Goals

- **Beginner standard:**   1 x 10 seconds   (both sides)
- **Progression standard:** 3 x 1 minute   (both sides)

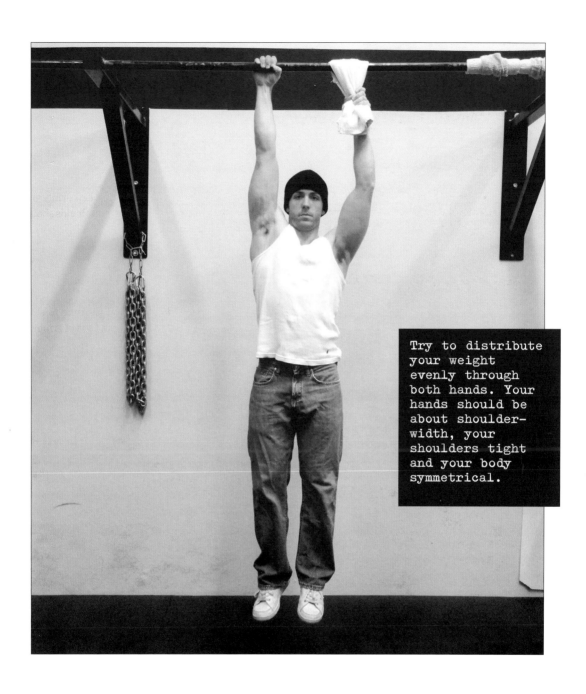

Try to distribute your weight evenly through both hands. Your hands should be about shoulder-width, your shoulders tight and your body symmetrical.

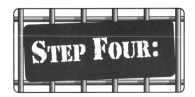

STEP FOUR:

ONE-ARM HANG

Performance

Perform the regular *bar hang* (step two) with an overhand grip. Once you feel "set", release one hand and hang by one arm. Keep your working shoulder good and tight, and place your non-working arm in a comfortable, neutral position; either out in mid-air or in the small of your back.

Exercise X-Ray

This is a crucial training stage, because it conditions the arms and shoulder girdle to full unilateral hanging. The thumbs get less work than the fingers, so follow this exercise with one or two sets of *uneven hangs* with the towel.

Training Goals

- Beginner standard: 1 x 10 seconds   (both sides)
- Progression standard: 3 x 1 minute   (both sides)

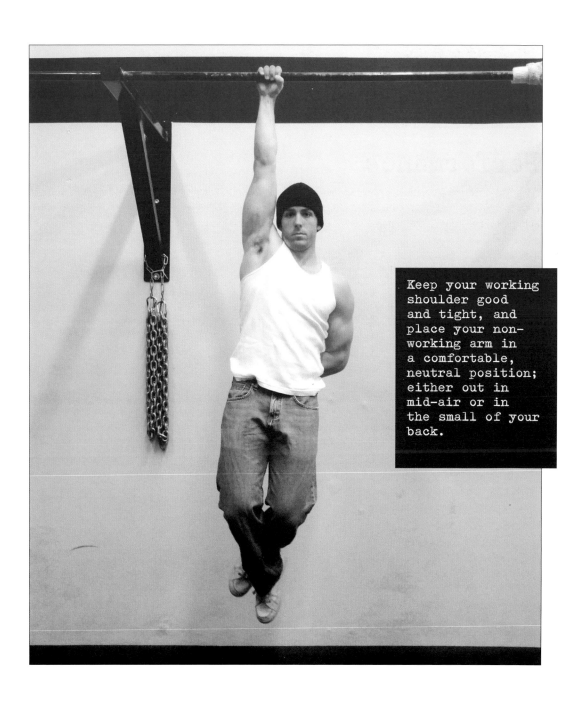

Keep your working shoulder good and tight, and place your non-working arm in a comfortable, neutral position; either out in mid-air or in the small of your back.

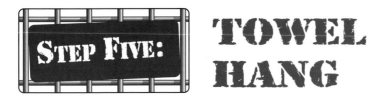

STEP FIVE: TOWEL HANG

Performance

Loop a single towel around an overhead bar. Grip each end of the towel with either hand, and allow your body to hang free. Your hands should remain fairly close, but without touching. Keep your shoulders tight.

Exercise X-Ray

During *uneven hangs* (step 3), the towel-gripping hand can potentially carry less than half the body's weight; but this exercise *forces* you to carry half of your bodyweight through each hand while gripping onto the towel. This adjustment gives the thumb and palm muscles a greater share of work.

Training Goals

- Beginner standard: 1 x 10 seconds
- Progression standard: 3 x 1 minute

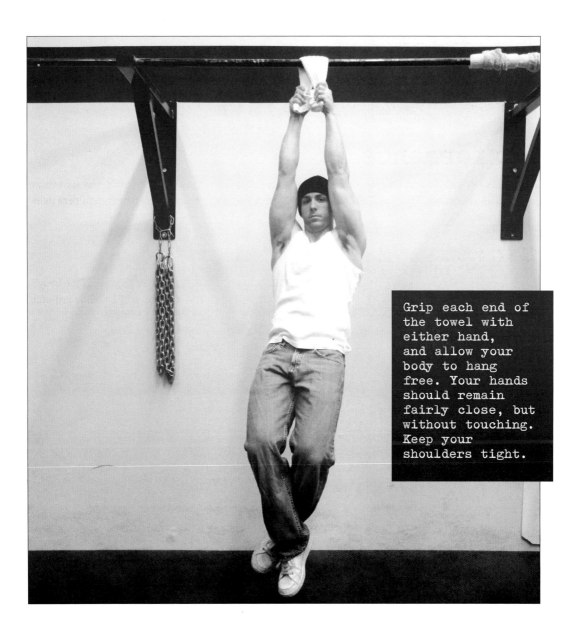

Grip each end of
the towel with
either hand,
and allow your
body to hang
free. Your hands
should remain
fairly close, but
without touching.
Keep your
shoulders tight.

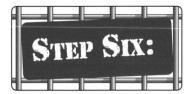

STEP SIX: TWIN TOWEL HANG

Performance

Loop two towels around an overhead bar. Grip each doubled-over towel with either hand, and allow your body to hang free. Your hands should be about shoulder-width, your shoulders tight and your body symmetrical.

Exercise X-Ray

During *towel hangs* (step 5) both your hands are gripping either end of just *one* towel. By using two towels doubled-over, you are doubling the thickness of the towel, and making the exercise correspondingly harder. This variation builds some of the total hand strength required for the later stages.

Training Goals

- **Beginner standard:**   1 x 10 seconds
- **Progression standard:**   3 x 1 minute

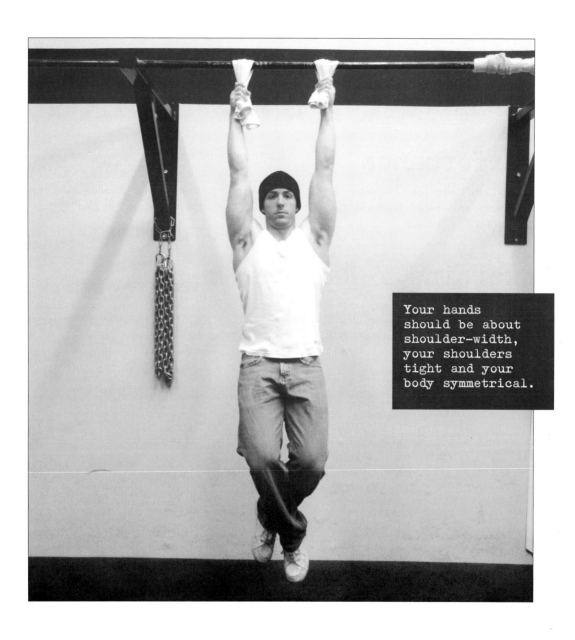

Your hands
should be about
shoulder-width,
your shoulders
tight and your
body symmetrical.

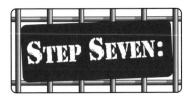

UNEVEN TOWEL HANG

Performance

Loop a single towel around an overhead bar. Grip the doubled-over towel with both hands, but place one hand above the other. (The further the distance between the hands, the tougher the exercise.) Hang free, keeping your shoulders tight.

Exercise X-Ray

By now, an athlete should be comfortable hanging symmetrically with a doubled-up towel. This step makes the grips unsymmetrical, which inevitably forces the higher hand to grip more powerfully. *Uneven towel hangs* are the ideal way to gradually advance to unilateral towel hanging.

Training Goals
- Beginner standard: 1 x 10 seconds   (both sides)
- Progression standard: 2 x 1 minute   (both sides)

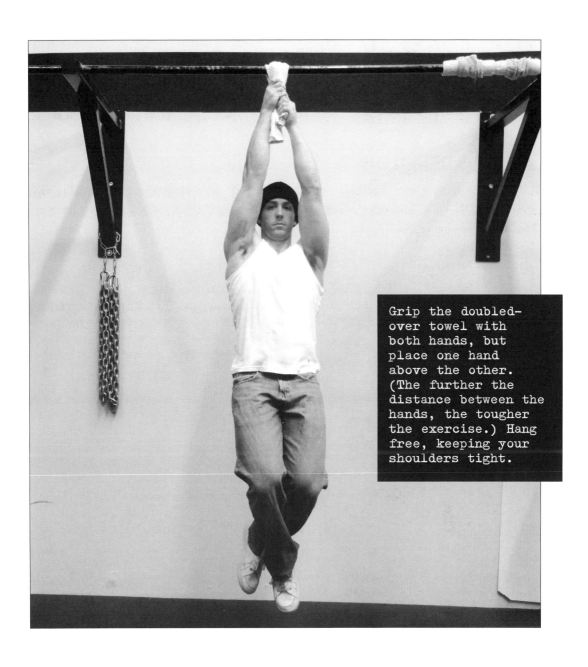

Grip the doubled-over towel with both hands, but place one hand above the other. (The further the distance between the hands, the tougher the exercise.) Hang free, keeping your shoulders tight.

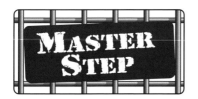

MASTER STEP

ONE-ARM TOWEL HANG

Performance

Loop a single towel around an overhead bar. Grip the doubled-over towel with one hand, and allow your body to hang free. Keep your working shoulder tight, and your non-working arm neutral.

Exercise X-Ray

The *one-arm towel hang* is the ultimate grip feat. It will turn the tendons of your fingers into something resembling tempered steel cable, and—unlike most grip feats—it will also give you thumbs like bionic pistons. Every grip athlete should master this hang for time before moving to any other exercise.

Training Goals

- Beginner standard: 1 x 10 seconds (both sides)
- Super grip: 5 minute hold (both sides)

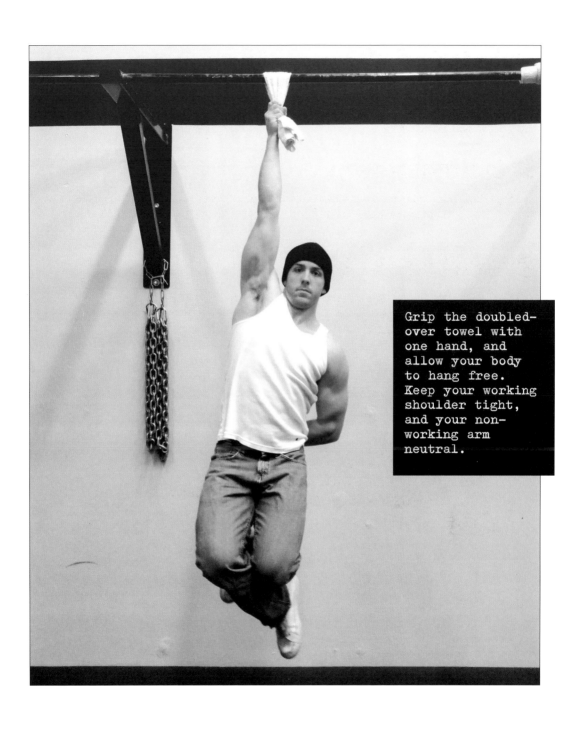

Grip the doubled-
over towel with
one hand, and
allow your body
to hang free.
Keep your working
shoulder tight,
and your non-
working arm
neutral.

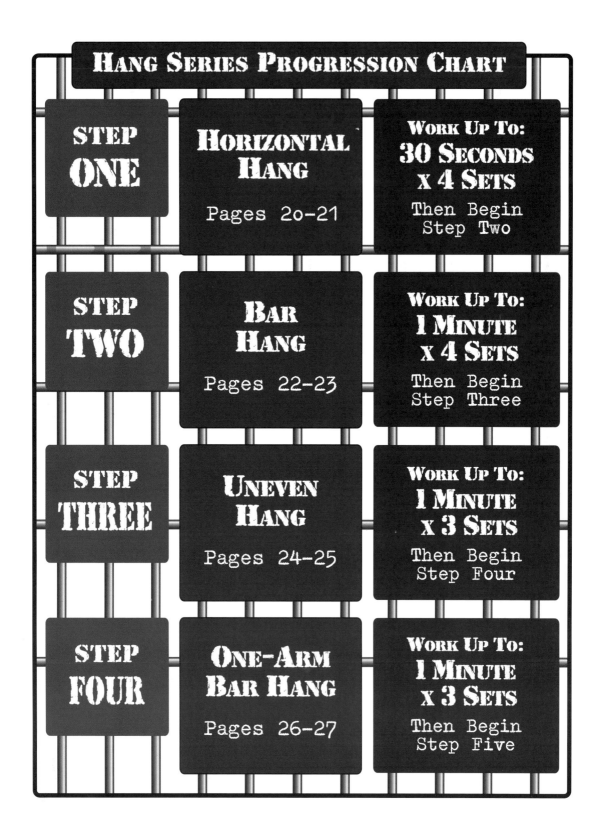

HANG SERIES PROGRESSION CHART

STEP ONE

HORIZONTAL HANG

Pages 20-21

WORK UP TO:
30 SECONDS x 4 SETS
Then Begin Step Two

STEP TWO

BAR HANG

Pages 22-23

WORK UP TO:
1 MINUTE x 4 SETS
Then Begin Step Three

STEP THREE

UNEVEN HANG

Pages 24-25

WORK UP TO:
1 MINUTE x 3 SETS
Then Begin Step Four

STEP FOUR

ONE-ARM BAR HANG

Pages 26-27

WORK UP TO:
1 MINUTE x 3 SETS
Then Begin Step Five

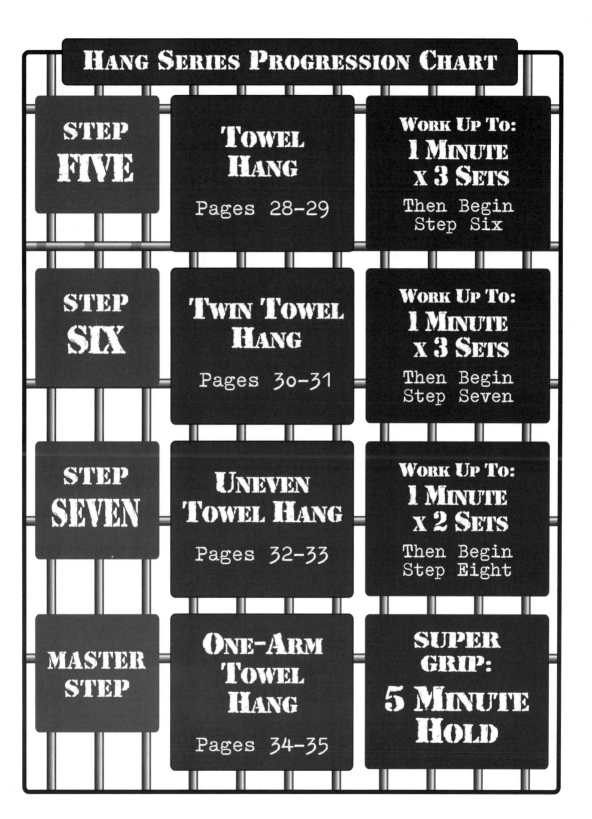

HANG SERIES PROGRESSION CHART

STEP FIVE	**TOWEL HANG** Pages 28-29	**WORK UP TO:** **1 MINUTE x 3 SETS** Then Begin Step Six
STEP SIX	**TWIN TOWEL HANG** Pages 30-31	**WORK UP TO:** **1 MINUTE x 3 SETS** Then Begin Step Seven
STEP SEVEN	**UNEVEN TOWEL HANG** Pages 32-33	**WORK UP TO:** **1 MINUTE x 2 SETS** Then Begin Step Eight
MASTER STEP	**ONE-ARM TOWEL HANG** Pages 34-35	**SUPER GRIP:** **5 MINUTE HOLD**

Lights out!

Whether you want to strengthen your fingers or jack up the belly of your forearms, forget grippers or wrist curls. Work your forearms the way they evolved to work—by hanging your bodyweight. Hanging on a regular pullup bar is great, but it doesn't work the entire hand—the thumbs and deep palm muscles hardly get any work. Some athletes get round this by pinch gripping rafters while busting out pullups. This is an impressive feat, to be sure—but in training terms, it's hard to make it *progressive* (you'd need to have access to sets of gradually thicker rafters). The simplest way to work the entire hand (including the thumb) is to hang from a vertical cylinder. A rope is good, but towels are more versatile.

Once you've built a great base of hand strength from towel hangs, what's next? Maybe nothing. Most athletes won't feel the need to progress beyond towel hangs. As part of a well-constructed total-body strength routine, it'll give you everything you want.

But if you're one of those specialists who maybe needs truly monstrous grip strength, I'll show you some more options for advanced grip training in the next chapter.

But beware—this ain't for beginners.

4: ADVANCED GRIP TORTURE

EXPLOSIVE POWER
+
TITANIUM FINGERS

In many ways, the *one-arm towel hang* is unlike a lot of other Master Steps performed in calisthenics. For one thing, it's not real flashy. In fact, unlike most strength feats, it kind of *looks* a lot easier than it really *is*. Many strong guys assume a one-arm towel hang will be easy—until they try it. A one-arm pullup will get respect in any gym in the world, but a one-arm towel hang with a doubled over towel? Most people won't even figure what you're trying to do.

Another issue is the *incredible* potential for strength your grip muscles have. Many advanced bodyweight strength techniques take years of training to master; but the towel hang can be owned much quicker. Very few untrained men can perform the one-arm towel hang for a full minute on the first time of asking, but it has been done fairly quickly by trained athletes—particularly those guys at a low bodyweight.

Once you get to the point where towel hanging with one arm is "easy" (it's never really *easy* unless you're a cyborg or something), what's next? Well, a lot of athletes will be content to stop right there. If your fingers, thumbs and palms are powerful enough to support your weight gripping a doubled-over towel, then very few exercises are gonna cause you trouble. But if you want to keep on getting stronger and stronger until your grip is goddam *bone-shattering*, then there are some options I want to put to you.

The first response most athletes will have is to add weight to the towel hang. If you can barely hang on, it might make sense to make the hold harder by grabbing a plate or a dumbbell with your free hand. I don't advise this—apart from the need to access multiple dumbbells, there is a risk of dropping the weight, or of coming down too heavily. Besides, as with all bodyweight training, there's no need to add weights to make a basic exercise harder.

Often, adding weights to an exercise—whether squats, pushups or hanging work—is the lazy man's way. If you use your brains plus a little creativity, you can always find superior ways to test your abilities, using nothing but bodyweight.

If you get to the point where you are progressing well with your towel hangs and want to add something tougher into your repertoire, what follows are a few ideas I've used or seen used behind bars. When it comes to grip training, there's a huge field of techniques and methods you can use to eke every bit of power out of those fingers. These approaches are some of the best.

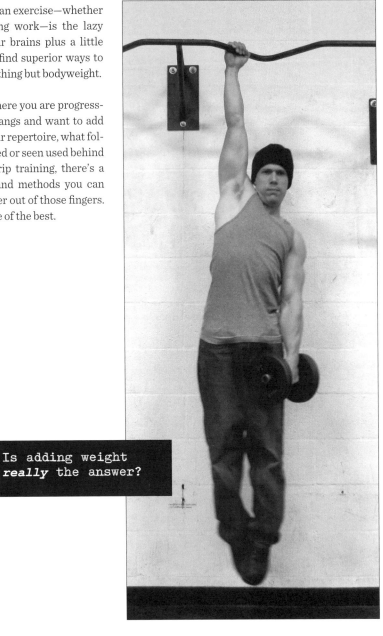

Is adding weight *really* the answer?

Advanced grip work 1: Going Beyond

If you want to make your hangs harder, the simplest way to do it is by increasing the *leverage* of the technique. On towel hangs, this is easily done by gripping something thicker—remember, the thicker the object, the harder it is to grip. But you don't need any obscure, expensive equipment to achieve this. Once you can hang from a doubled-over towel, make it thicker by adding to it. Add layers progressively. Lay over a dish towel; two dish towels; a hand towel; a hand towel and a dish towel...you get the idea. Some grip monsters can hang from two doubled-over towels! (Try it, if you want to be scared.) Can you make *three* some day?

If you want to keep adding advanced grip work—it's addictive to some of you psychos— there are two further specialist methods I advise you to try: *finger holds* and *explosive gripping*. Let's look at both of these arts.

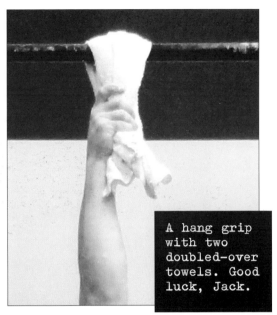

A hang grip with two doubled-over towels. Good luck, Jack.

Advanced grip work 2: Finger holds

If you enjoy hanging grip work and want to take your hand strength to the next level, you need to take a lesson from the athletes who have the strongest fingers of all—not weightlifters or bodybuilders, but *climbers.*

Why do climbers have stronger fingers than weightlifters? It all has to do with the biomechanics of the hand. When you grip a weight in the palm, you are lifting that weight, plain and simple. But when you support a weight with your *fingertips,* the force generated by the muscles which bend the fingers must be *at least four times greater* than that weight. Climbers rarely get to grip with their palms—often they have to support their hanging weight on just the tips of their fingers—maybe only two or three fingers. As a result their total hand power becomes awe-inspiring. If you ever get the chance to compare grips with an elite climber, do it. These guys have finger strength that verges on frightening. They need it to survive.

Most people don't know it, but you can buy equipment to train your finger holds. Climbers sometimes use carved fingerboards with special holes and ledges, and wall-mounted moldings for training their fingers to the max. But not all climbers use these devices and you really don't need them unless you're a specialist. If you get to the point where a *one-arm towel hang* is easy, just move over to a horizontal bar and begin working on finger holds.

Begin by hanging on both arms, but don't grip with the little fingers—only the first three digits:

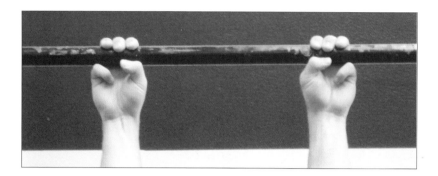

When you can manage forty seconds like this, hang from just two digits:

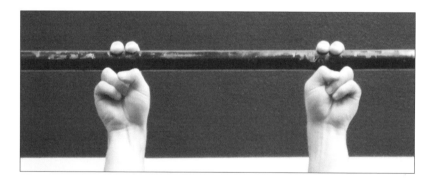

Your goal is a twenty second hang. This is hard, but a harder task still is to use your pinky finger and the finger next to it (the ring finger):

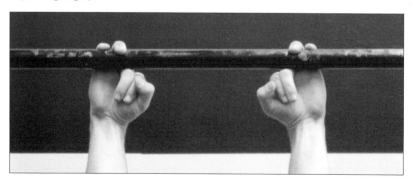

This is necessary to ensure maximum strength in all the fingers, but it's very difficult; it's only possible if the bar is quite narrow. I've seen some guys make and attach little rings to their overhead bar, just to facilitate performing finger holds. Holding bodyweight is tough on the fingers, and you might want to cushion these holds with some folded cloth or rag.

Once you get to this advanced level, you can maintain it by doing a few pullups this way every week or so. I've seen some older convicts do this—my mentor, Joe Hartigen, did finger hold pullups well into his seventies. He claimed that hand strength was the last thing to go. He was living proof—I've certainly not seen any teenagers do this.

When two-digit hangs get easy, your next option is to explore single-digit hangs, using the various fingers. Always finish your finger hold work with at least one set of *one-arm towel hangs* (per hand) to retain symmetrical finger and thumb strength.

Advanced grip work 3: Explosive grip training

Another way of really ramping up your grip training is by exploring *explosive* grip techniques. To make your hanging grip work explosive, you don't need any sophisticated apparatus. You just hang from something, lose your grip, and quickly catch hold again before you hit the ground. You can do this hanging from towels if you're advanced enough, but I prefer just using a plain old horizontal bar. It requires less technique and skill to "catch", so it's a bit safer. But either method works.

Explosive catching places sudden demands on the tendons, muscles and fascia of the hands, so it's definitely not for beginners. It can also be hard on the elbows. I wouldn't advise athletes to even *try* it until they are up to step 7 of the hanging grip series (*uneven towel hangs*). Even then, not everyone will feel the need to experiment with explosive grip work. Some athletes need to be able to catch powerfully and explosively for their sport though, and this kind of training will deliver for these folks. Examples might be:

- Martial arts requiring quick, powerful grips and locks (aikido, chin na, hapkido, etc.)
- Football plays catching and holding the ball
- Judoka rapidly grabbing the gi for a throw
- Obstacle course training (military trails require jumping and catching ropes, ledges, etc.)

To grip explosively, you need to know how to *kip* from the bar. In case you're not familiar with this term, *kipping* while hanging involves explosively throwing the knees upwards to gain some momentum. Basically, imagine cheating heavily during pullups, and you'll be able to picture what I mean.

Begin a rep by hanging from the bar. Now gain some height by kipping yourself up. Use your knees and an explosive body movement rather than pulling yourself up by your arms—this isn't a pullup, it's a grip exercise. At the very top of the momentum-movement (when you're virtually weightless) release your hands and reposition them. It's this explosive "catching" of the bar before you drop while that builds hand reflexes and a power grip. (See the examples below for various levels of difficulty.) Some athletes even like to clap before catching the bar again.

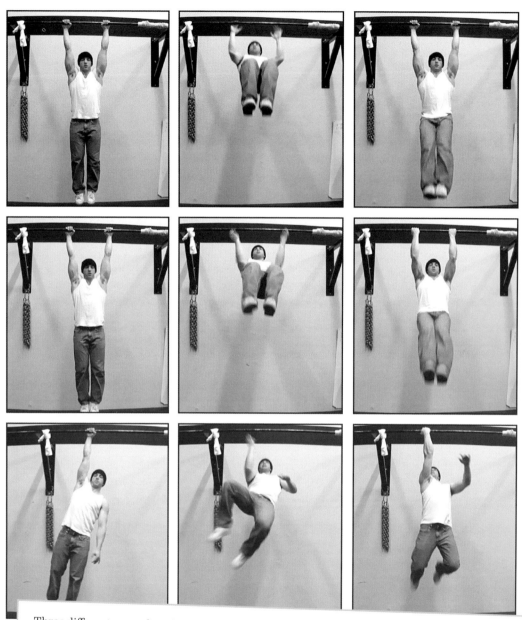

Three different examples of explosive grip work (shown above). In the top line you have the most basic level of difficulty: a double grip, kip, then catch. In the middle line you have a slightly harder version which involves going from on overhand grip to an underhand grip. On the bottom line you have an advanced technique: using just a single hand. There are too many variants to list here, but explosive gripsters should experiment with these variations, remembering that adding a clap during the kip will add difficulty, as will changing the grip type (underhand/overhand/alternate/wide). During training keep the sets and reps low and focus on sharp, clean movements.

As always, be safe and protect your body. Only do explosive grip work when your forearms are hot and warmed up. Focus on catching the bar, but always be ready in case you screw up—be prepared to land right.

Lights out!

There are probably more gadgets in the grip world than in any other area of specialist strength training. No kidding—there are grippers, special handled bars, wrist rollers, grip machines, one-arm deadlift units and much more.

Just because a huge amount of equipment is available, don't be fooled into thinking you need it. That stuff was invented by manufacturers. It was meant to be sold! Don't be tricked into believing you need weights and grippers and other stuff to build an elite grip. Truth of the matter is, men love tools—they love possessions, things they can use and play with. This is as true when it comes to strength work as for any other aspect of life. But if you want the best results, ignore the gimmicks and go back to basics. If you have a horizontal bar, two towels and your bare hands, you have everything you need to build a grip as powerful as any in the world.

An added bonus—if you need to climb a wall real quick, the bodyweight stuff sure helps in a pinch.

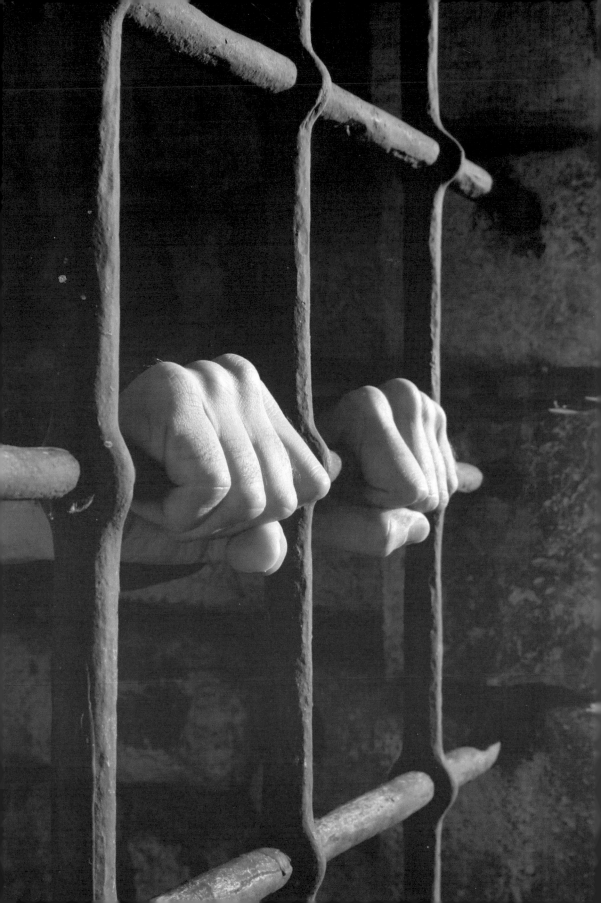

5: Fingertip Pushups

Keeping Hand Strength Balanced

In chapter two, I told you that you needed only *two* basic exercises to work your hands and forearms to the max. The first—and most important—exercise was *hang gripping*. If you've read up to this point, you are now pretty much an expert on the theory behind hang gripping; everything from the basic progressions, to advanced work like finger holds and explosive gripping. Now it's time for the second exercise, another classic in the bodyweight armory: *fingertip pushups*.

Working the opposites

The majority of lower arm muscles work by "remote control"—via the forearm muscles—to make the fingers grip. The bulk of the forearm (and palm) consists of finger *flexor* (gripping) muscles for evolutionary reasons—humans need a strong grip to hold their own bodyweight during *brachiation*. Very few non-primates have what you could call a strong grip. Hell, very few animals can "grip" with the upper extremities at all—at least in the sense that we are using the word. For this reason, any hand/forearm routine should be based around gripping exercises. The techniques already demonstrated in this chapter will give you the strongest grip—and biggest forearms—that your genetic potential will allow. But building superhuman gripping muscles without simultaneously strengthening the antagonistic muscles is asking for trouble.

There are several reasons why you should balance out a grip-based forearm program with some work for the *extensors* (the muscles which straighten the fingers). The first reason is completeness. Your hands are meant to *open* as well as *close*. If you want strong hands, you should train them open, not just closed (as in a grip). This works not only the extensors, but also all the small, neglected tissues and tendons on the backs of the hands and around the knuckles. Another reason has to do with maximizing potential. Never forget that the muscular system is a balanced entity. If you train one side of a limb without training the opposite side, the side you are training can never truly reach its maximum potential. If any machine has a weak link, the entire capacity of the machine is affected negatively. Guys who only train their finger flexors (by grip work) and neglect the extensors will, ironically, never have a grip as strong as a man whose hands are developed on both sides.

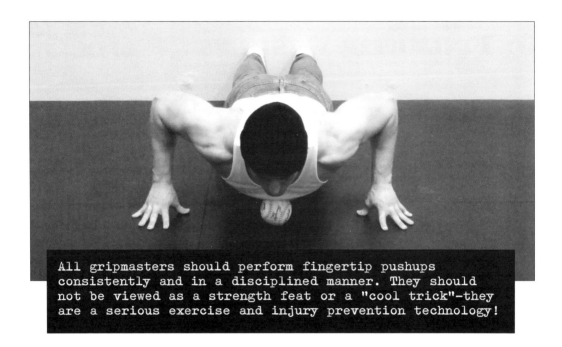

All gripmasters should perform fingertip pushups consistently and in a disciplined manner. They should not be viewed as a strength feat or a "cool trick"—they are a serious exercise and injury prevention technology!

But perhaps the biggest reason to balance out grip work with extensor work is *injury prevention*—what the kids today call "prehab". Working just one side of your forearms will make your strength unsymmetrical and give you greater potential for injury. Having a hugely developed grip when the back of your hand is weak is a bit like driving a car that's made half from steel, half from timber. When you put your foot to the floor, the thing will tear itself apart. The weaker half just can't keep up with the stronger half. This is what an unbalanced muscular system is like. It's a recipe for a constant stream of injuries.

There are numerous devices (rubber bands, cables and machines) designed to work the open hands, and most of them are complete crap. Nothing built by man has ever improved on the ancient classic *fingertip pushup*. Fingertip pushups force an athlete to keep the hands open and fingers extended in a natural position under high levels of fluctuating pressure. This not only protects and strengthens the connective tissues, it also increases hand power very efficiently. Fingertip pushups are easy to learn, they can be done progressively, and they require zero equipment.

CORRECT POSITIONING

- "Fingertip" pushups are a misnomer. Press on the pads of your fingers, not the tips.

- Keep force flowing through the fingers, thumbs, and also the wrists: your entire lower arm should be a locked unit.

- Spread your fingers to distribute your weight evenly.

- Your thumb should also be straight or slightly arched back, and placed somewhere behind your second finger.

- "Set" your fingers with high tension by pressing hard into the floor. They shouldn't move or bend during the set.

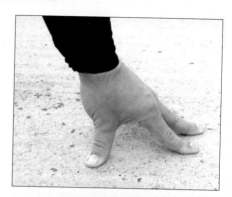

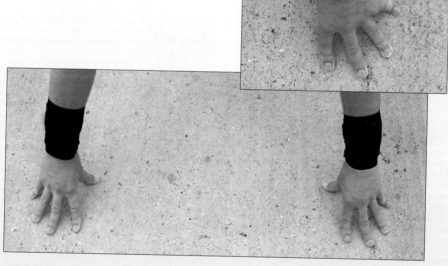

The Art of the Empty Hand

Fingertip pushups balance the hands by thoroughly working all the "open hand" muscles and tendons that "closed hand" grip work passes by. But you need to be careful from the get-go. In particular, you need to pay attention to finger extension.

During your fingertip pushups, you may notice some slight bending of your fingers. This is natural, and will vary for everybody. But you should still press *hard* through the pads of your fingers—on each and every rep—with the goal in mind of *keeping your fingers as straight as possible*. Remember, it's this straight-finger position that gives you the results you are training for; not how difficult the type of pushup is, or how many reps you can do. Whatever you do, don't allow your fingers to *bow*.

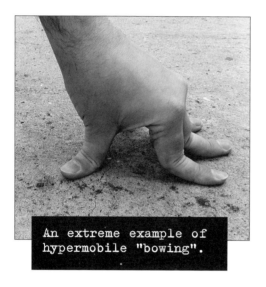

An extreme example of hypermobile "bowing".

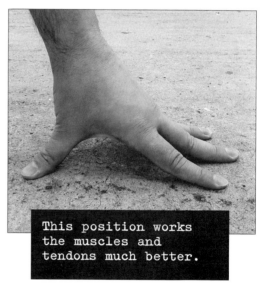

This position works the muscles and tendons much better.

Bowing your fingers may make the exercise feel like less effort, but that's only because the finger *joints* are taking your weight—it's not passing through the *muscles*. Not only is this bad for the finger and thumb joints, it also robs the muscles and tendons of the work they need to get stronger.

Some people have a helluva time stopping their thumbs and fingers from bowing, particularly those with real flexible (or even *hypermobile*) hands. For those of you who are struggling, bodyweight legend Brad Johnson has come up with the solution—*spider-ups*. I won't include the drill here, because Pavel Tsatsouline has already outlined it better than I ever could in section eight of *Beyond Bodybuilding*. (For what it's worth, that section is a *killer* treasure chest of advanced bodyweight techniques. I don't get paid a cent for saying this, but if you are serious about your calisthenics, that's a book you need to get your paws on. I'm not kidding.)

Fingertip pushups: philosophy in a nutshell

There are plenty of different ways to approach fingertip pushup work. I've found during my own training that it's best to perform this exercise *before* your hanging grip work. The fingers are fairly delicate structures compared to the rest of the body, and training grip exhausts the hands—I prefer to have my fingers reasonably fresh for fingertip pushups, so the muscles are still good and strong, for safety. Doing fingertip pushups before your grip work also seems to improve performance on the hangs. It focuses the mind and acts as a neurological warm up for the lower arms.

I also like to keep my sets and reps fairly low. Ten to fifteen reps on a warm up set is fine, but for your work sets five reps should be your maximum, and anything over two serious sets is a waste of time and energy. Remember, fingertip pushups are about benefiting from the *extended finger position* more than the *pushup movement*—high reps on this exercise will only drain your chest, shoulders and arms and compromise your regular pushup workouts. Besides, you're not looking to add mass or stamina to the extensor tendons and muscles; this is all about balancing strength. So let's make this a strength exercise.

Your hands work hard during pullups, hanging leg raises, and even get activity during exercises like pushups and bridges. If you add hard grip work on top of this, that's a hefty old workload for small areas like the phalanges *(finger bones)* to handle. So don't do what a lot of trainees do and over-train your hands by working fingertip pushups every day. A short, focused, progressive session performed twice per week beats the hell out of extended daily hand workouts that go nowhere fast and irritate the tendons. (If you're a new fish, pressed for time, or you work with your hands frequently, just one fingertip pushup workout a week is also an option.)

Your fingers *want* to be strong. They weren't designed to tap at a keyboard or text bulls*** on a stupid cell phone. They were meant to be *dangerous weapons* on the hands of a caveman! Work your hands fresh, keep your reps low, keep your form perfect, keep your finger tension and your concentration high and remember to let your hands rest when they need it. Follow these rules and trust me—you'll start noticing real-life strength increases *fast*.

Progressive strength

Just like all bodyweight training, fingertip pushups need to be done *progressively* if you want to get anywhere. You need to keep finding increasingly difficult versions of the fingertip pushup, or your strength will stagnate. As your grip strength progresses, so should your fingertip pushup work—albeit more slowly, because the extensor muscles are smaller than the grip muscles.

If you picked up a copy of the first *Convict Conditioning* book, you'll know all about the science of progressive pushups. In chapter five I laid out the perfect prison-based progressive pushup series. I'd advise all athletes new to fingertip pushups to use this ten step pushup series as a template for their fingertip pushup work. You begin at the beginning—doing fingertip pushups against a wall—then move, step by step, to harder variations like the regular fingertip pushup. This gradual progress not only ensures consistent strength gain, it also allows the joints and soft tissues to adapt at the same speed as the surrounding muscles. This is a particularly important point when it comes to training the fingers, which are small and potentially prone to injury. It also allows newer (or heavier) athletes a chance to begin training if they can't do regular fingertip pushups just yet. For those athletes who wish to maximize their fingertip strength, the series will eventually lead you to the ability to perform *one-arm fingertip pushups*. Do them right, and your fingers and thumbs will be more like solid titanium piping than the flimsy, helpless digits most modern men have.

READY FOR ACTION

Never launch into fingertip pushups "cold". You want a healthy supply of hot blood circulating in your fingers, wrists and forearms before fingertip pushups. Here are some warm up tactics I've found helpful:

1. It's a great idea to perform fingertip pushups *after* another upper-body exercise (maybe pullups) so your lower arms have already had some work.

2. From there, do some freestyle shoulder, elbow and wrist circling (for a minute or so) to get the fluids in the cartilage moving in these joints.

3. Before you perform even one fingertip pushup, amplify this warm up by doing *eagle claws*. Form your hands into tight fists, and gradually open your fingers/thumbs joint-by-joint, slowly and deliberately and under maximum isometric tension. Once your (trembling!) hands are stretched open to the max, reverse the process back into a hard fist. That's one rep. Give yourself two sets of ten reps, shaking your hands loose after each set.

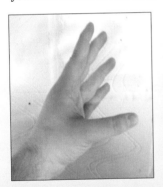 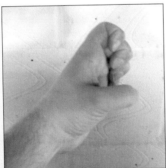 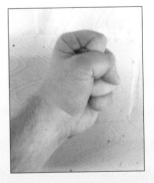

4. Finally, always perform one set of easy fingertip pushups before you get to your "work" sets. Choose an exercise lower down the series than the point you've reached. One set of 5-10 reps will activate your nervous system and tell your finger muscles and tendons that trouble's a-comin'. From here on in, you're ready for the real work.

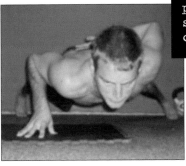

One-arm fingertip pushups are only possible when you have paid your dues strengthening your finger joints and connective tissues.

I'm not going to take up space in this book repeating all the technical instructions for each step of the pushup series, but I've summarized the steps in a simple table (see below). This will get you started. If you need more details on general pushup form, refer to the first book.

FINGERTIP PUSHUP SERIES

1.	**WALL FINGERTIP PUSHUPS:**	Perform your pushups standing, with your fingers against a wall.
2.	**INCLINE FINGERTIP PUSHUPS:**	Perform your pushups while leaning diagonally, fingers on a desk/table.
3.	**KNEELING FINGERTIP PUSHUPS:**	Perform your pushups while kneeling, your fingers on the floor.
4.	**HALF FINGERTIP PUSHUPS:**	Perform regular fingertip pushups, but only go halfway down.
5.	**FULL FINGERTIP PUSHUPS:**	Just like classic full pushups, but on the fingers instead of the palms.
6.	**CLOSE FINGERTIP PUSHUPS:**	Perform *full fingertip pushups*, but with the hands close together.
7.	**UNEVEN FINGERTIP PUSHUPS:**	Perform pushups with one palm on a basketball below you, and the fingers of the other hand on the floor.
8.	**ONE-ARM FINGERTIP PUSHUPS:**	Perform *one-arm fingertip pushups*, but only go halfway down.
9.	**LEVER FINGERTIP PUSHUPS:**	Perform pushups with one palm on a basketball out to your side, and the fingers of the other hand on the floor.
10.	**ONE-ARM FINGERTIP PUSHUPS:**	Perform your fingertip pushups with one arm behind your back. (It's okay to spread your feet and keep your working arm out to the side here: keeping your feet together will work the shoulders harder, not the fingers.)

How To Progress

For many bodyweight movements, it's a good idea to progress to the harder techniques once you've met a predetermined target rep range (10 reps, 20 reps, and so on). With fingertip pushups, you don't need to do this. Pushing too hard to meet a target isn't a good idea where such small joints are concerned. Instead:

• Keep your rep range at around five whenever you train.

• Work up the steps until you find an exercise that is moderately difficult.

• Once the exercise becomes fairly easy, then experiment with harder steps.

• Never train to "failure" on this exercise. Stay in control at all times!

• Keep your cadence regular during the pushups—never be explosive. Avoid variations like "clapping" fingertip pushups at all costs.

• Once you can perform *one-arm fingertip pushups* easily, you can try variations using fewer fingers, or explore handstand variations.

Once unilateral fingertip pushups become child's play, you've got the option of moving to handstand pushup variations where the fingers support the entire bodyweight. Only experienced trainees like Justin P need apply!

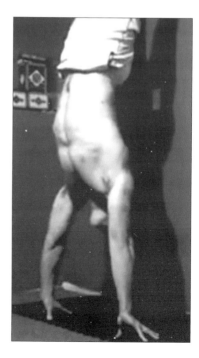

Lights out!

Fingertip pushups are seen as more of a "trick" than a genuine strength exercise. This is totally wrong. Done right, fingertip pushups are the safest, most effective way to strengthen the extensor muscles on the top of the lower arm. For athletes seriously working their grip muscles—the flexors on the meaty underside of the forearm—fingertip pushups are invaluable. They stop your hand strength from becoming unbalanced, prevent injuries, and round out hand and finger strength perfectly.

If you are performing serious grip work, begin taking fingertip pushups seriously, and treat them like you would any other bodyweight strength movement. Warm up well, start slow with easier versions of the movement, train hard but with perfect form and control, and build to harder variations over time.

6: Forearms into Firearms

Hand Strength: A Summary And A Challenge

he last four chapters of grip, finger and forearm training have been pretty dense and complex. I've thrown a lot of words and ideas at you. If you're considering working some forearm training into your current program template, now's probably a good time to summarize all the stuff I've said so far:

• To maximize your hand and forearm strength, you only need two main exercises: bodyweight *hang gripping* and *fingertip pushups*.

• When hang gripping, it's okay to hang from a horizontal bar. But this only really works the fingers. For the entire hand to be involved, you should work towards *vertical hanging*. You can use a rope, but a towel is a more versatile grip-builder.

• It's a good idea to perform your hand training after an upper body workout, when the forearms are already warm.

• Begin a hand workout with fingertip pushups—but don't forget to warm your hands up first (see page 52).

• For fingertip pushups, keep your work sets to two or three (no more) and use low reps. Two sets of five is great.

• Work your fingertip pushups progressively (see page 53), but don't push to failure, and only try harder exercises when the techniques you are using get too easy.

• It's a good idea to work your grip *after* fingertip pushups. (*Never* work your grip before hanging exercises like pullups or hanging leg raises).

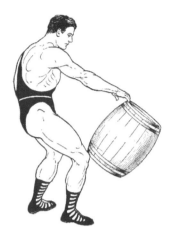

All the old school strongmen knew that grip "tricks" can be learned fairly quickly, but giant forearms cannot be built overnight. You will only reach your genetic potential through a lot of pain, consistency and intelligent progression!

- Work your grip hard, but don't overdo the number of sets you perform. This will tire out your hands, but won't get you stronger any quicker. Anything more than four sets of hangs (per hand) is overkill.

- Rest as long as you need to between sets. Don't rush, but don't screw around so long your forearms get cold.

- The length of time you hang before moving to harder techniques can vary, but anything more than a minute per set and you're building more stamina than strength.

- Your hands get plenty of work during most upper body exercises, so avoid excessive hand training. Once per week will get the job done. Twice a week is better. Three times if (and only if) you're a recovery machine.

Program template

If you apply the above tips, you'll be able to program your own forearm training—which is a good thing, coz being your own coach is just as important for training independence as being able to train without a gym.

But for those of you who want to get started right away, the following sample workout program is a good way to begin. Warm up well, be strict, focus on hang gripping (but throw some fingertip pushups in to balance the opposites) and be progressive. That's a forearm workout—prison style.

You can't go wrong, I tells ya.

SAMPLE WORKOUT

Here's what a good bodyweight forearm workout should look like:

Following an upper-body session

Joint circling—1 minute

1.	EAGLE CLAWS:	SET 1: 10 REPS Shake the hands out SET 2: 10 REPS Shake the hands out
2.	FINGERTIP PUSHUPS:	SET 1: 5-10 REPS (warm up) SET 2: 5 REPS (work set) SET 3: 5 REPS (work set)
3.	HANGING EXERCISE:	SET 1: 25 SECONDS (warm up) SET 2: 1 MINUTE MAX (work set) SET 3: 1 MINUTE MAX (work set) SET 4: 1 MINUTE MAX (work set)

- Remember that the exercise used for the warm up sets should feel pretty easy compared to the exercise you use for your work sets.

- This template can be tailored to pretty much any strength level—if you are stronger, just use proportionately harder exercises.

The CC "Iron Gauntlet"

I know many gripmeisters out there prefer to work their hands with weights. I've heard a lot of these guys tell me that calisthenic hand techniques are too "light" or "easy" to get a decent workout with. *How hard can bodyweight hand exercises be?* they tell me.

Hey, if you want to work your hands with weights, that's fine by this old lug. I'm not putting down that method. A lot of guys just love to feel the steel—I totally get it. But when someone tells me that bodyweight strength work for the hands is *too easy*...I challenge them to put their money where their big mouth is.

I'm going to share this challenge with you. I call it the *Convict Conditioning Iron Gauntlet,* and it consists of four—yeah, just four—exercises. If you've read the last few chapters and you still think bodyweight hand work is too "easy", try performing the following feats. They must be performed in sequence, without resting more than five minutes between techniques.

1. Triple towel hang: one-handed x 60 seconds

Throw three (fairly thick) hand towels over an overhead pullup bar. They should be layered, one on top of another. Wrap your hand around the ends of the hanging towels—or as far round as you can get. (You'll be grabbing the equivalent of six towels, since the three towels will be doubled over the bar. It's unlikely your fingers will meet your thumb.) Squeeze hard, and hang down, so you are hanging by just one hand. Hold your bodyweight like this for 60 seconds. Then swap and hang for 60 seconds the same way but from the other hand.

2. Index finger pullups: 10 reps

Perform ten full pullups—hanging only by your two index fingers. (You can hang from the bar, but you can also use rings, or special straps/hoops if the bar is too thick for your fingers.)

3. One-arm fingertip pushups: 5 reps

Get down on the floor, and perform five deep one-arm pushups on the four fingers and thumb. The palm must not touch the floor. The feet can be splayed apart. Repeat with the other hand.

4. Grip-and-switch: 10 times per hand

Hang from an overhead bar with one hand. Use an overhand grip. Kip up, and reverse the grip mid-air, catching the bar with the same hand, but in an underhand grip. Pause at the bottom, before kipping and reversing again. Perform ten reversals, then repeat with the other hand.

Sound tough? Well, the towel hangs are murder, but I promise you, there's *nothing* impossible about this challenge. The strongman Sandow could do one-arm pullups *with any one finger*—including the pinky and the thumb! He was also a fan of explosive grip work, and could "hop" up an angled ladder using just one hand, by kipping and catching. Many martial artists understand the value of bodyweight work and do pushups on just their two index fingers and thumbs. So the challenge above is by no means an *elite* workout.

Despite this, most men—very powerful men—who work their hands with weights, get *slayed* by this challenge. They get the shock of their lives. They think their hands and fingers are powerful as hell from weight training and spring grip work, but they discover that even simple bodyweight hand strength exercises are too much.

Here's the quick rundown:

If you've attempted this challenge and defeated it, I bow down to you. You are a Jedi Master of calisthenic hand strength. Go lift weights for your hands if you like. Train with true grip legends like Adam T. Glass, John Brookfield, or Samuelsson.

But if you *can't* beat the Iron Gauntlet, I don't want to hear you saying that the bodyweight stuff is easy. You can still gain a lot from the basics.

Lights out!

Nothing is a sign of truly great strength as much as a powerful pair of hands. Hands so strong that they can bend metal, burst open a can of cola with the pull tab still intact, or tear tree roots up out of the ground are far scarier than big biceps or wide shoulders. Strong hands are both impressive and useful, but most modern forms of hand training are a waste of time in my honest opinion.

If you really want forearms as powerful as they are big, forget modern methods and go old school—work with your bodyweight. The best exercise to beef up the top of your forearms (the *brachioradialis* and *brachialis* muscles) isn't hammer curls or reverse curls. These moves are puny compared to good old pullups, which work the forearms and elbows from the most powerful angles possible.

As for the belly, the underside, of your lower arms, forget weights (or any other type of equipment) if you want maximal results. Follow the example of nature—and thousands of years of advanced athletes and warriors—and work your forearms by hanging. Hanging from a horizontal bar is a phenomenal basic exercise, but eventually build to vertical hanging, from a rope or towel. This will build thumb strength that bar work can't.

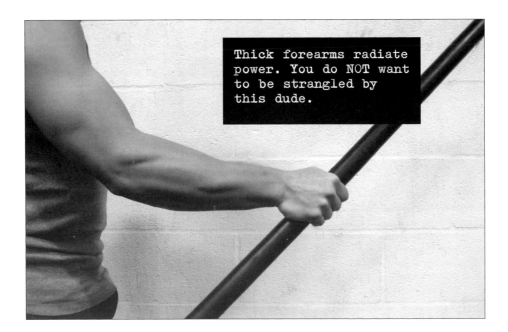

Thick forearms radiate power. You do NOT want to be strangled by this dude.

To a select group of guys in the joint, grip and forearm training is more than just important. It's like a religion to them, the way pushups are to a lot of the other cell trainers. They hang from their cell doors from one or two fingers for long periods until their whole body is racked with cramp; they do fingertip pushups until their digits are like steel rods. A lot of them train throughout the day, everyday, until after lights out when their hands are slippery with blood from calluses and torn blisters. You can recognize a member of this rare breed, instantly. Their gigantic, tattooed forearms look like cybernetic implants, undulating with massive clumps of powerful muscle tissue and decorated with thick veins.

These guys are the extreme—which is one of the reasons they probably wound up in prison in the first place. I'm not suggesting you train like them. But if you just add a little of the work detailed in this chapter to your routine, your "Popeye" forearms will be busting out of your shirt sleeves in six months time.

7: LATERAL CHAIN TRAINING

CAPTURING THE FLAG

Seems like everyone these days wants to train "obliques". Those cord-like muscles running up the sides of the abdomen are the subject of some kind of gold rush—at least if you buy into the fitness media. It's impossible to pick up a magazine, skim a training book or watch an ab-gadget infomercial without being beaten around the head with the term *obliques*. It's like some kind of ab-training buzzword...like a cake just ain't complete without frosting, your abs aren't complete until you've worked those obliques.

If you're anything like me, you find this excessive focus on developing such a minor body part in isolation for purely aesthetic reasons pretty sickening. It reminds us of the *narcissism* of our species; plus our amazing capacity to waste precious time and energy on insignificant crap. And if the idea itself isn't bad enough, checking out modern training methods for working the obliques will surely make you to make you want to hurl or put a gun to your skull. The bulk of techniques applied by coaches and personal trainers consist of *side crunches, twisting crunches, side cable crunches* and similar silly garbage.

This group of popular techniques are both misguided and ineffective. They are *misguided*, because they attempt to train a small muscle with *isolation* movements, when that muscle evolved to function as a link in a larger chain. They are *ineffective* because movements like the crunch aren't *strength exercises*—they are *low-resistance tension exercises*. They make it *feel* like you're working, while you are actually producing zero results. (Stop and "tense" your quads for three sets of twenty reps, three times a week. Will they get any bigger? Nope. Any stronger? Nope. It kinda *feels* like work, but your quads won't actually change at all, unless you actually bend those knees and start squatting.)

If you *really* want to strengthen and harden your obliques, you need to work them following the same four tried-and-true principles you would use to effectively work any muscle group. You need to:

- *Use bodyweight as resistance*
- *Apply techniques which integrate the body as a total unit*
- *Work hard*
- *Keep moving on to progressively tougher techniques*

Use this as a basis for your strength training philosophy, and you *will* get great results, no matter what muscle group you want to work. Don't be afraid of getting strong!

The modern obliques myth

This warning—*don't be afraid of getting strong*—isn't nearly as dumb as it might sound. Believe it or not, there are guys and girls in gyms all over the world scared to death of training their obliques hard, for fear that it will thicken their waists, detract from their "V taper" and spoil the symmetry of their physiques. Only one response to that attitude—bulls***!

There are only two things which will bloat out your waistline and give you chunky "love handles". One is excess body fat. The other is steroid and growth hormone abuse, which will cause *all* your muscles to gain water and expand the size of your internal organs, swelling your overall midsection. Functional strength training won't affect your waist size—unless it causes you to lose body fat and become slimmer.

The obliques are small, dense muscles, and naturally working them to maximum strength will cause them to become powerful and sculpted, but it won't stretch the tape much. Just look at elite martial artists and gymnasts. These men and women need *incredibly* powerful obliques for their respective disciplines; but take a look at their waists and you'll see that they are slim, tight, and hard as iron.

Modern gym-rats could take a lesson from these athletes. If you have been brainwashed into doing light, pointless exercises for your obliques, don't panic, partner. In this chapter I'm going to show you how to get a waist that's Bruce Lee-strong; no side crunches, cables, rubber bands or ab-gadgets required.

Do you need to work your obliques?

Before we get started, it might be helpful to ask a simple question: *do you really need to start performing specific oblique work at all?*

If you read the ab-training articles in modern muscle rags, you'll assume the answer is obviously "yes". But wait. Hold your horses. Don't forget that all the muscles of the midsection work together, a bit like a big, muscular girdle. When one of these muscles fires hard, they all have to fire—even if only isometrically. This anatomical reality also applies to the obliques. Your obliques fire when you do bridges, and when you squat—and the harder you work on these exercises, the harder your obliques have to work to keep up.

This effect is enhanced if you perform specific work for the abdomen—particularly leg raises. If a tight, powerful midsection is what you're looking for, strict hanging leg raises will get the job done. Not only do leg raises work the hell out of your anterior chain, the obliques get a great workout just holding the hips in place. In *Convict Conditioning*, I also included *twisting leg raises* as a supplemental variant exercise for those athletes who wanted to amplify the effects of leg raises for their obliques.

In reality, if you are working hard on leg raises and the rest of the Big Six movements detailed in *Convict Conditioning*, you may not feel the need to give your obliques any specific ancillary work at all. Truth is, they're already getting a workout from what you are doing.

That said, there will always be sportspeople who need to give their obliques extra specific training for their chosen sport. The muscles of the flank (including the obliques) are responsible for bringing the side of the ribcage and hips closer together, so optimal obliques are essential for any sport that involves kicking or lifting the legs out to the side. Acrobats, skaters and dancers are examples of athletes who need beyond-normal oblique strength. There will also be some hardcore bodyweight athletes for whom mastering leg raises is just not enough—they have to master *everything*. These brutes will also want to know how to work their obliques right.

Plus, the moves I'm gonna teach ya in this chapter are badass...as cold as ice. They are satisfying as hell to master, and goddam impressive to show off to others. A lot of bodyweight athletes will want to experiment with oblique training for these reasons.

And why not? You pay taxes too, right?

The ultimate lateral chain movement: the flag

Bridges work the *back* of your body: hamstrings, glutes, spinal muscles, traps—*the posterior chain*. Leg raises work the *front* of your body: abs, hips, deep thigh muscles—*the anterior chain*. If you are looking for an exercise to work the muscles of the *side* of your body—*the lateral chain*—look no further than the human flag.

There are many variations of the flag, but the hardest versions all involve maintaining a straight body out from a vertical base. From this position you look like a flag standing out in the wind—hence the most common name of the exercise. (Though you should know that the term "flag" is not a universal one. Some call it a *side* or *horizontal lever*. The athlete who taught me the movement called it the *side plank*, and I didn't hear of it referred to as anything else until years later.)

The flag is a wonderful example of a total body exercise. Maintaining this position works the entire lateral chain—not just the obliques, but also the *lats* under the armpits, the *serratus* of the ribcage, the *intercostals*, the *hip abductors*, and the *tensors* on the outside of the thigh. The spine and trunk muscles need to be steely to lock everything in place safely. Because the lower leg has to be held up against gravity, the *adductor* muscles of the inner thigh also get trained by this hold. It also works the upper body hard, because the athlete has to hold onto the base with the arms. For sure, the flag can leave the side of your waist sore for days after you do it, but *every muscle in your body* has to be strong if you want to have a hope of holding the flag.

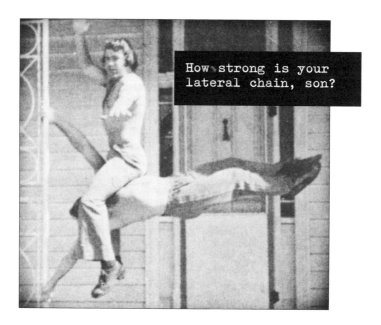

How strong is your lateral chain, son?

LATERAL MUSCLED WORKED BY ALL FLAG TECHNIQUES

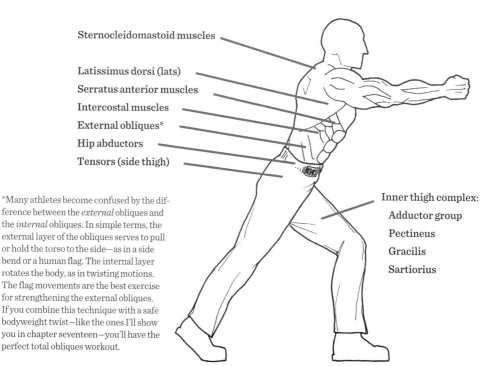

Sternocleidomastoid muscles

Latissimus dorsi (lats)

Serratus anterior muscles

Intercostal muscles

External obliques*

Hip abductors

Tensors (side thigh)

Inner thigh complex:

Adductor group

Pectineus

Gracilis

Sartiorius

*Many athletes become confused by the difference between the *external* obliques and the *internal* obliques. In simple terms, the external layer of the obliques serves to pull or hold the torso to the side—as in a side bend or a human flag. The internal layer rotates the body, as in twisting motions. The flag movements are the best exercise for strengthening the external obliques. If you combine this technique with a safe bodyweight twist—like the ones I'll show you in chapter seventeen—you'll have the perfect total obliques workout.

The flag is not drawn from modern gymnastics—there are no vertical bases in modern gymnastics, only horizontal bases (think of the floor, vaulting horses, beams and rings, rather than upright poles). The flag is an ancient exercise, and is still seen in disciplines which require a vertical base; Indian pole training (*mallakhamb*), Chinese pole exercise and circus rope acrobatics are examples where flag progressions are still formally taught. I learnt how to do the human flag where I learnt the rest of my skills—in jail. There are plenty of rails, bars, and fence posts in prison.

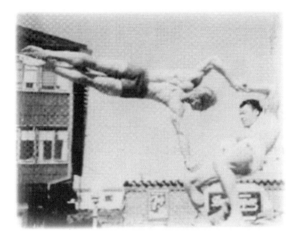
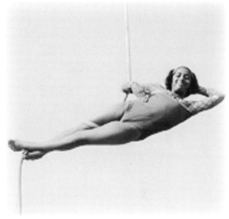
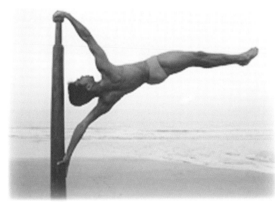
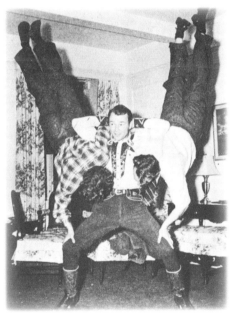

Assorted forms of lateral chain training. From top left: partner calisthenics; rope acrobatics; traditional mallakhamb training; and a circus stunt. (That's the great Roy Rogers supporting a couple of pals.)

Wherever and whenever you learn the flag, one fact remains true—it's an incredible strength feat. It needs to be treated with respect. If you don't approach it progressively, you won't have a prayer of mastering it properly.

Two types of flag

There are two major variations of the human flag hold. One is called the *clutch flag*, the other is called the *press flag*. In the clutch flag, you clutch the vertical base—a pole, staff, slim tree trunk, whatever—to your chest, hence the name. In the press flag, you press your body out from the vertical base using straight arms.

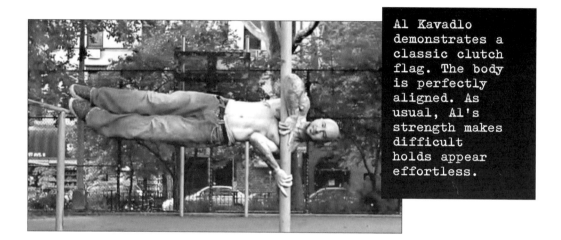

Al Kavadlo demonstrates a classic clutch flag. The body is perfectly aligned. As usual, Al's strength makes difficult holds appear effortless.

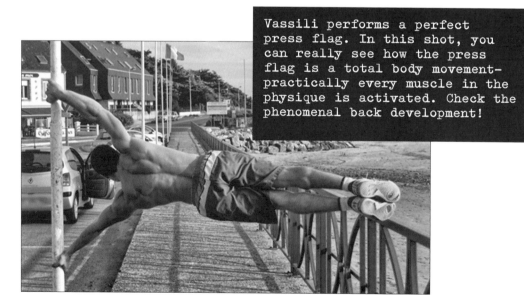

Vassili performs a perfect press flag. In this shot, you can really see how the press flag is a total body movement—practically every muscle in the physique is activated. Check the phenomenal back development!

I'm going to show you a series of progressions to help you learn *both* these variations of the flag hold. The clutch flag is a significantly less demanding version because of the reduced leverage. This makes the clutch flag easier and quicker to learn, but ultimately the press flag delivers greater benefits in terms of lateral chain and total body strength.

Because of the difference in difficulty between these two forms of the flag, I always advise my students to master the clutch flag progressions first—before they try to take on the press flag. This rule of thumb is particularly true for athletes who aren't used to full body holds (like the regular *plank*, or *elbow lever*). Becoming proficient in the clutch flag first will not only systematically strengthen your body and give you a radically reduced chance of injury, it will also make your progression towards the press flag that much quicker if you decide to give it a shot.

Lights out!

True strength is born of the ability to use your body as a *unit;* and fast muscle growth comes from using the best strength exercises possible. This is why modern training of the "flanks"—or the side waist musculature—is so ass-backwards. Modern exercises focus on isolating the obliques to the maximum degree possible.

Wrong.

You want a powerful, sculpted waist like the ones you see in classical statues? Those statues were carved millennia before the *side crunch* was dreamt up by whatever idiot was to blame. You know my rallying cry by now, cuz. Ignore modern methods. Find a vertical base and learn the flag instead. With side crunches, you *might* feel a teeny burn *somewhere* in your waist. But bust out a flag variation and you *will* feel *all* the muscles along the side of your body—neck to lats to ribs to obliques to hips and thighs—clenching like nothing on earth. You'll know those muscles and tendons are being stimulated, strengthened, and tightened. They won't have a choice!

If you want to develop your lateral chain muscles to their limit, you'll need to learn the press flag. But, as always in strength training, learn to walk before you can run. Master the clutch flag first. I'll show you how to do it in the next chapter.

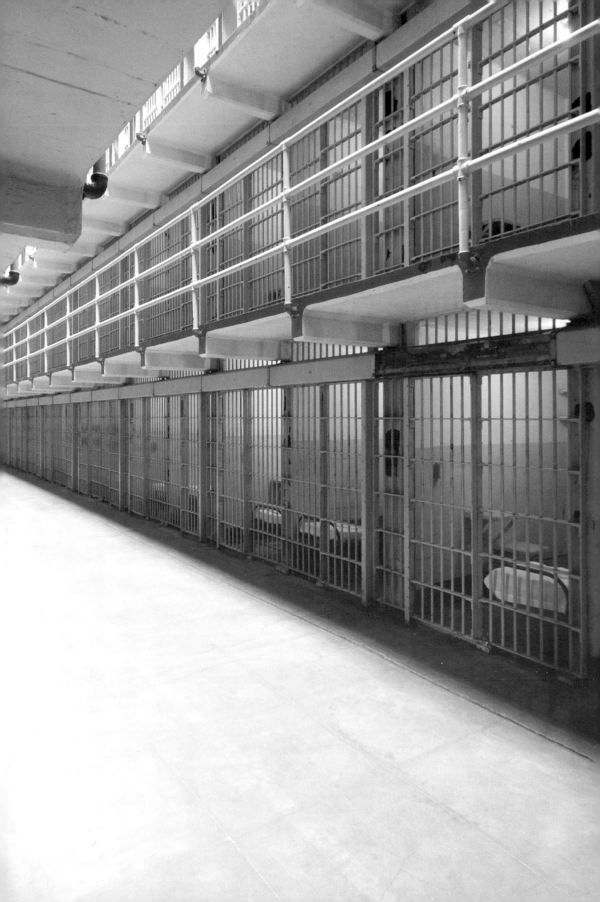

8: The Clutch Flag

In Eight
Easy Steps

Serious training for the side of the body—especially the side of the waist—is nothing new. Check out statues of ancient Greek or Roman heroes and you'll notice that they all had impressive, cut up obliques and side-waists. These statues were based on athletes and warriors—those men needed powerful lateral chains, for throwing the discus and javelin. They were originally battlefield weapons, remember. To the ancients, athleticism and fighting power were the same thing. A tiny, underdeveloped waist was the opposite of what the Greeks admired. If you didn't have strong-looking obliques, you just weren't a man.

Writers often talk about the "Greek ideal" of a physique—wide shoulders with a tiny waist—but the concept of the petite waist as masculine was never a Western idea at all. It's found in ancient *Egyptian* art, but that's only because—to the Egyptians—their pharaohs and gods were not warriors or athletes. They were rulers. They didn't sully themselves with something so mortal as actual battlefield combat. They didn't *need* strong waists.

Strong sides are not just crucial for warriors. Trunks which are muscular and strong around their *entire* circumference are essential for high levels of real-world strength. Some men can seem incredibly strong in the gym because they hoist huge weights, but when you ask them to help you move house, they have trouble picking up a fridge or TV that's a fraction of the weight. Why is this? Because the weights in the gym— whether on machines or barbells—are symmetrical. Balanced. Real life objects like desks and human beings are impossible to pick up "evenly". One side is always heavier, often in a random or fluctuating way. The big gym guy's front and back muscles are strong, but his side muscles are the weak link.

Old time strongmen understood this real well. They didn't shy away from training the muscles along the side of their waists and hips, like modern lifters. Their staples were lifts like the bent press and one-arm deadlift, movements which built incredibly powerful side-waists. Over a century back, the legendary strongman Arthur Saxon bent pressed 370 lbs under official conditions—although he did 385 unofficially. Can you imagine how strong his hips and flanks were? These days, you'd be lucky to find an elite-level lifter who can lift *half* that amount! One thing's for sure—Saxon didn't need any help moving house.

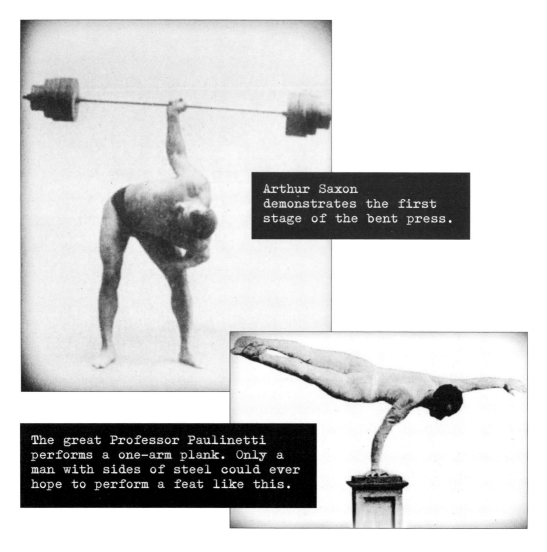

Arthur Saxon
demonstrates the first
stage of the bent press.

The great Professor Paulinetti
performs a one-arm plank. Only a
man with sides of steel could ever
hope to perform a feat like this.

Strong side muscles are also essential for bodyweight strength feats. Look at an acrobat performing tricks, or observe a gymnast on the pommel horse. Whenever the legs are swung out or supported to the side, all the muscles of the hips and waist come into play. Due to the length and weight of the legs, this means powerful side-waist muscles are essential.

If you want to reach this high level of bodyweight strength and control, I can show you how to do it. It starts with the *clutch flag*.

Where to train?

Before you get going on the clutch flag, you need to find a vertical base to train on. Ideally, you need a sturdy, smooth cylinder of a regular thickness. As for "how thick?", I'd say at least the diameter of your palm, although even thicker is usually easier to hold. Here are some ideas:

- Light poles
- Signposts
- House beams
- Slim pillars
- Smaller trees
- Park equipment (pullup columns, etc.)

These objects are all around us—they're just invisible most of the time, because we're not looking for them. If you want to get good at the flags, you need to think like a parkour athlete and start viewing every-day architecture in a new way. You'll soon discover that, in fact, there are training tools all around you. Ironically, the one place you're not likely to find a good base for clutch exercises is in the *gym*. This is no bad thing. Getting your ass away from the gym is probably the number one thing you can do to start kicking your gains up a notch.

Whatever vertical base you choose, make sure it is stable and strong enough to take your weight, and check that it has no shiver or jagged edges to catch on. You're my buddy, and I don't want you hurting your-self. (See how I got your back? Next, I'll set you up with my sister...)

Clutch flag training concepts

Before we get to the clutch flag progressions, I want you to review a few training ideas first. These will help you advance more efficiently.

- **Hold it:** The clutch flag works better as a static, isometric technique than an isotonic, moving tech-nique (a "hold" as opposed to a "move" as we said in prison). You pop up into the position shown as best you can, then *hold*. If you're used to moving calisthenics, be aware that this change of pace requires a different psychology. The hold is brief and the set up is technical, with less room for error than is true for most moving sets. Think *focus* and *awareness*.

- **Holistic strength:** You can learn to perform flag holds as part of any training routine, and it will strengthen your lateral chain and boost your ability to use your body as an integrated unit. But results will come faster if you are already training in the Big Six exercises I described in *Convict Conditioning*. Not only will the basic calisthenics moves teach you better coordination skills, they will also increase your posterior and anterior chain strength, and this will really give you a head start if you are looking to master the flag.

• **Skipping steps:** In this tutorial, I've included an eight step series of progressions for the clutch flag. I like giving multiple progressions, because it allows for plenty of wiggle room. It also helps athletes visualize the path to success, something that's *crucial* for fostering self-belief and motivation. But remember, there's nothing magic about the number eight. It's great to experiment with every step and see how useful it is, but not every athlete will need all eight steps. If you can handle a step easily (holding it for at least ten seconds) and the next step is within your power then feel free to move on up to the next step. (This applies more to isometric holds like the flag than it does to regular exercises like the Big Six.)

For some helpful rules of thumb on how to program clutch flags into your current training, check out the table below.

How To Progress

HOW LONG?

If you are going to use progressions on holds like the clutch flag, the progression standard can be flexible. For most stages a hold of **ten seconds** is about right. Once you can hold the position shown (perfectly) for that long, try the next step.

HOW MUCH?

When you go to practise the flag, hold your best position until it starts to drop, or deteriorate. Then take a brief break (a couple minutes) and try again. Do this **five or six times** each session.

HOW OFTEN?

Flag training works your muscles hard, and can leave you sore for days. Training can be done on **three non-consecutive days per week**. If you are in great shape and motivated to master the flag, alternate day training is an option. Never train while still sore from last time, though—it's pointless.

Now you know the score. Hopefully you've got some ideas about *where* to train; and you now know *how* to program clutch flag workouts. But before you can start progressing through the steps I'll show you, you have to master the most fundamental element of this type of flag—the best technique for holding onto the base. That's up next.

Ready for a side-waist designed by Ferrari and built by Smith & Wesson? On to the training.

The basic clutch hold

Before I show you the progressions, let's look at the most basic element of the clutch flag—the *clutch hold*. There are four basic steps to getting this:

1. Approach your vertical base (whether a column, pole, post, beam or whatever). With your right arm extended, place your armpit/upper lat firmly into the base. This will help give you your initial positioning.

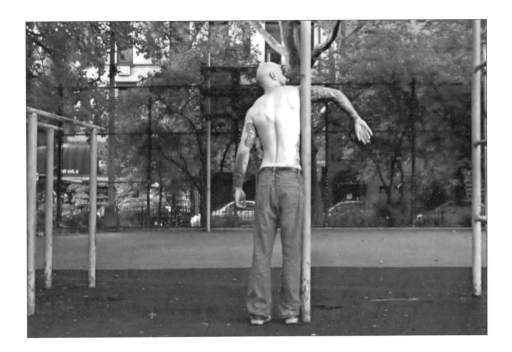

2. Curl your right arm back and round the base, bending the elbow and placing your hand firmly on the base. Your index finger should point down, but the other fingers can hug the base if it's the right shape for that. However your place your fingers, the palm-heel should be solidly against the base.

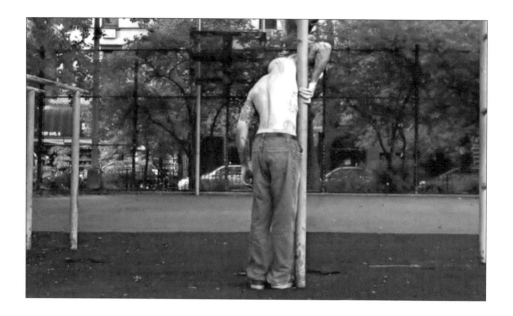

3. Place your left hand against the base. It should be at approximately hip level, with the elbow bent. Push really hard against the base, with as much tension as you can generate. This will be the hand that stops you falling later on, so it *has* to be tight.

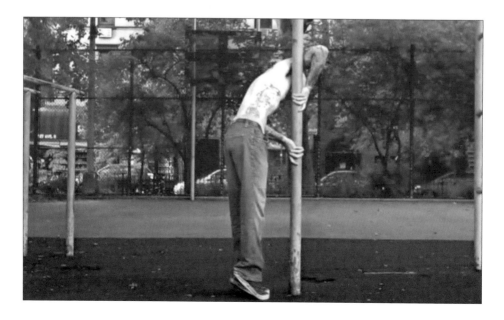

4. Position yourself back slightly by taking a mini-step back and/or bending at the waist. This is to give you space to position your left elbow firmly into your waist, a little above the left hip. At this point, your left forearm should be close to diagonal. Now brace everything for take-off!

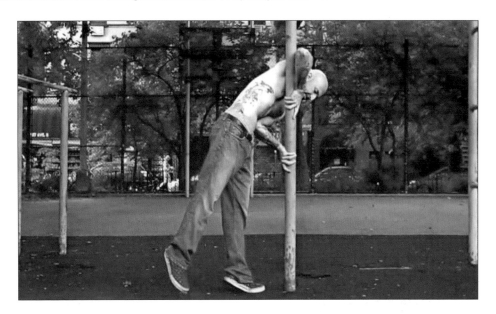

There you go—this is the basic clutch hold you'll need for all the following steps. (For a clutch hold on the opposite side, just substitute "left" for "right" and so on.) Over time you'll find that these four separate motions become one fluid movement. As you progress, you'll also find your hold technique varies slightly from what I've laid out. That's fine—diff'rent strokes, baby.

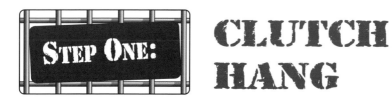

STEP ONE: CLUTCH HANG

OVERVIEW

Approach your vertical base, and begin to get into the basic *clutch hold* (pages 75 to 77). Hug the base strongly, pushing in as hard as you can with your hands, and using the elbow in your waist like a lever. Once you feel you've generated enough tension, slowly lift your feet off the floor—one at a time at first. Don't try to lift your legs out to the side just yet. Relax your lower body, and let your legs hang straight down, with your knees bent. The objective of this step is to help the athlete gain enough strength and confidence to support the body's full weight in the clutch hold.

TIPS

Lift your feet off the ground by *bending* your knees and lifting your feet slightly behind you, rather than by *raising* your knees up at the hips. This first step is meant to be an upper body exercise, not an abdominal exercise.

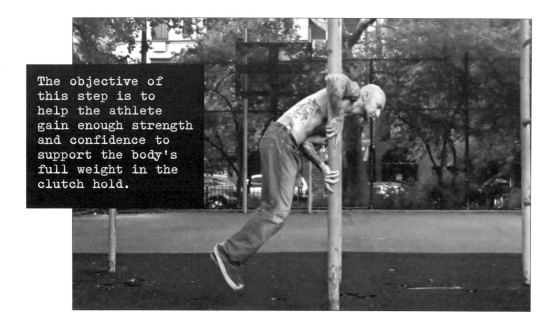

The objective of this step is to help the athlete gain enough strength and confidence to support the body's full weight in the clutch hold.

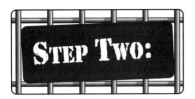

DIAGONAL SPLIT HANG

OVERVIEW

Approach your vertical base, and get into the basic *clutch hold* (pages 75 to 77). Your elbow should be securely positioned in your waist above the hip. This elbow position will push your hips off-center and out to the side a little. From here, hop out to the side as you bend the knee of your right leg and draw it up as high as possible. Simultaneously, straighten out your lower leg. Try to control the alignment of your body, so that your trunk and lower leg form a diagonal line. Hold the position, breathing normally.

TIPS

Keeping your upper leg in a tuck position makes aligning your body diagonally easier, but some will find that the body still droops. This is entirely due to weakness in the lateral chain—most people, even athletes, aren't used to testing their lateral chain strength. Keep trying.

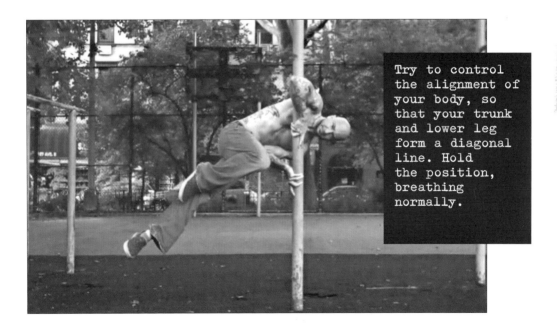

Try to control the alignment of your body, so that your trunk and lower leg form a diagonal line. Hold the position, breathing normally.

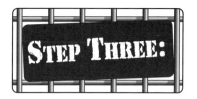

DIAGONAL TUCK CLUTCH

OVERVIEW

Approach your vertical base, and get into the basic *clutch hold* (pages 75 to 77). From here, get into a *diagonal split clutch* (step 2). Once your right leg is tucked as close to your trunk as possible, draw up your left leg so that it's next to your upper leg. Both legs should now be in a mild tuck position, and your trunk and shins should form a diagonal line. Hold the position, breathing normally.

TIPS

If you have been working on the diagonal split clutch, this maneuver won't prove to be too much of a strain on your waist. But it's an important technical stepping stone on the path to the *horizontal tuck clutch*. If you find the knees-in tuck difficult, some work on *knee tucks* (see *Convict Conditioning*) will help you master this.

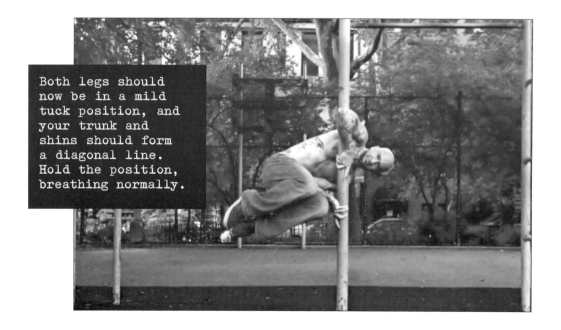

Both legs should now be in a mild tuck position, and your trunk and shins should form a diagonal line. Hold the position, breathing normally.

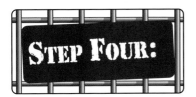
DIAGONAL CLUTCH

OVERVIEW

Approach your vertical base, and get into the basic *clutch hold* (pages 75 to 77). From here, get into a *diagonal tuck clutch* (step 3). Once you are in position, keep your trunk diagonal and extend both legs outwards until they are perfectly straight. At this point, your trunk and straight legs should form a diagonal line. Hold the position, breathing normally. This step is a useful way to begin working to the *clutch flag*, because the less strenuous diagonal position can often be held well by athletes even if they don't yet have the strength to hold the full clutch flag with a horizontal body.

TIPS

This is a key step and it's one you shouldn't skip. If the diagonal clutch is too tough to hold at first, approach it gradually; begin holding for ten seconds with both legs bent, and straighten them out as you get stronger.

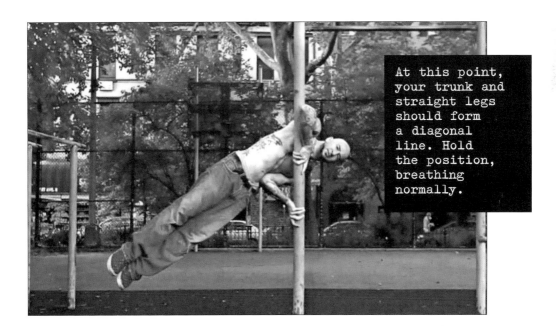

At this point, your trunk and straight legs should form a diagonal line. Hold the position, breathing normally.

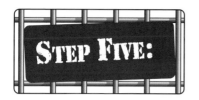

STEP FIVE:

HORIZONTAL TUCK CLUTCH

OVERVIEW

Approach your vertical base, and get into the basic *clutch hold* (pages 75 to 77). Brace yourself and hop up onto your lower forearm, simultaneously bringing your knees up opposite your hips (the *tuck* position). At this point, your trunk and shins should form a horizontal line. Hold the position, breathing normally. This step represents a big achievement; the first time an athlete holds a *horizontal* clutch position. We're getting somewhere!

TIPS

This is a crucial step for learning the correct upper body positioning required for the harder horizontal holds. So far in this series, the forearm of your lowest arm has acted like a lever. For this step, you'll notice that it's more like an angled strut jammed into the side of your waist. The upper forearm should be flat against the base, pressing hard to take your weight.

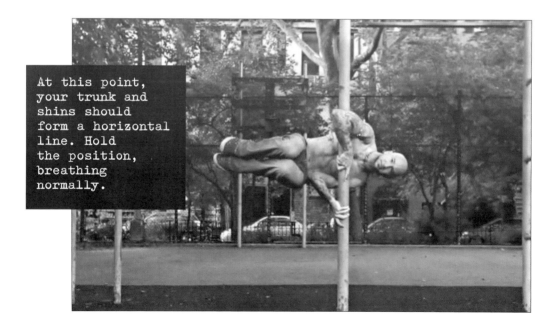

At this point, your trunk and shins should form a horizontal line. Hold the position, breathing normally.

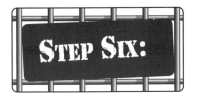

HORIZONTAL SPLIT CLUTCH

OVERVIEW

Approach your vertical base, and get into the basic *clutch hold* (pages 75 to 77). Initiate the hold by getting into a *horizontal tuck clutch* (step 5). Keep the knee of your upper leg bent and opposite your hips. Simultaneously, straighten out your lower leg. Retain the alignment of your body, so that your trunk and lower leg form a horizontal line. Hold the position, breathing normally.

TIPS

Now that an athlete can perform a horizontal clutch in the tuck position all that remains to achieve the full *clutch flag* is to extend both legs. Steps 6 and 7 represent the most gradual way to do this. In many cases, where a good horizontal split clutch has been attained, the athlete can get to the Master Step fairly rapidly. Most of the core work has been done by now.

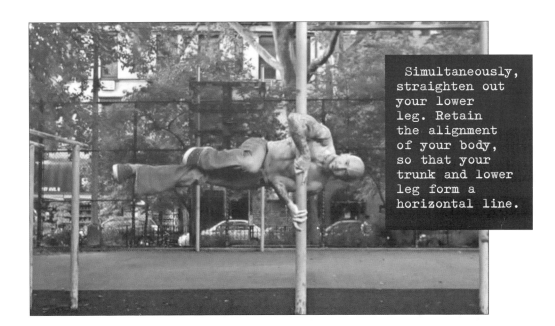

Simultaneously, straighten out your lower leg. Retain the alignment of your body, so that your trunk and lower leg form a horizontal line.

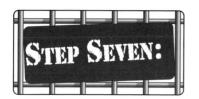

STEP SEVEN: BENT LEG CLUTCH FLAG

OVERVIEW

Approach your vertical base, and get into the basic *clutch hold* (pages 75 to 77). From here, get into a *horizontal split clutch* (step 6). Once your position is fixed, slowly draw in the lower leg by bending at the knees and hips. Simultaneously extend your bent right leg until both feet meet. At this point, the legs should be extended about half straight, or less. Although the joints bend, the body line (trunk and legs) should remain completely horizontal. Hold the position, breathing normally.

TIPS

Extending the leg's mass away from your centre-point increases the difficulty level of all flag movements, which makes this kind of hold very useful. It's also real easy to adjust the intensity of this hold; more bend in the legs makes the leverage easier, straighter legs makes the exercise tougher.

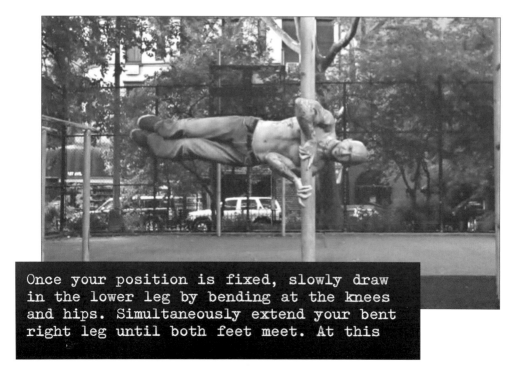

Once your position is fixed, slowly draw in the lower leg by bending at the knees and hips. Simultaneously extend your bent right leg until both feet meet. At this

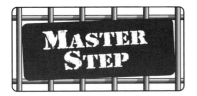

MASTER STEP

CLUTCH FLAG

OVERVIEW

Approach your vertical base, and get into the basic *clutch hold* (pages 75 to 77). From here, get into a *horizontal tuck clutch* (step 5). Once your position is fixed, smoothly extend the legs outwards until they are locked out. At this point, your trunk and body should form a perfectly straight horizontal line, with no sagging. Hold the position, breathing normally.

TIPS

During the full *clutch flag,* your gut should face outwards—not up. If your stomach turns up, towards the sky, it means that your lateral chain is weak, and your abs (anterior chain) are trying to compensate. Stay side on. As you become more comfortable in this hold, you'll find you don't need to get into a tuck clutch before straightening out into the flag; you'll be able to start with straight legs, and slowly lever them up using pure lateral chain power.

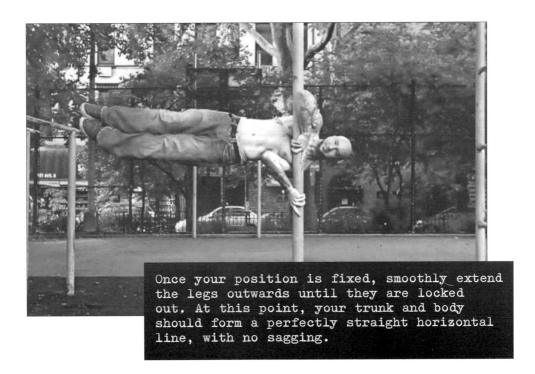

Once your position is fixed, smoothly extend the legs outwards until they are locked out. At this point, your trunk and body should form a perfectly straight horizontal line, with no sagging.

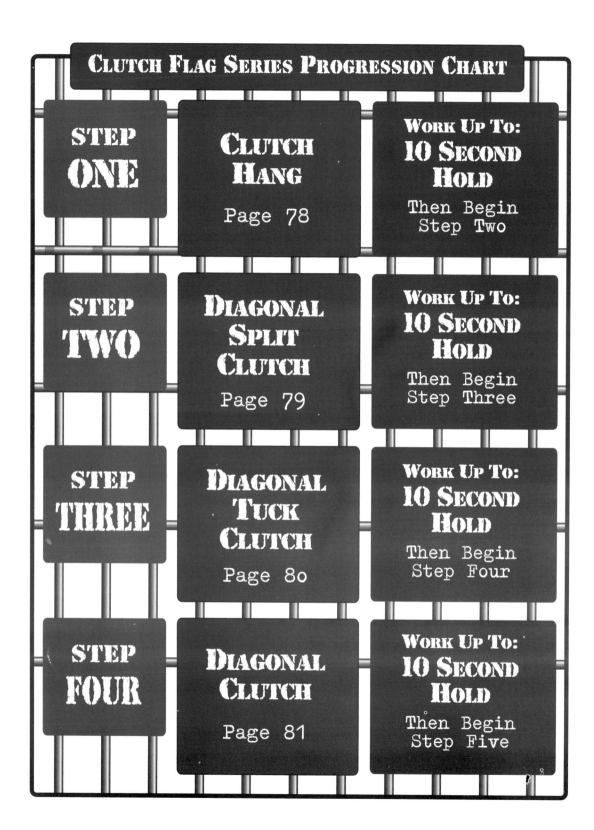

CLUTCH FLAG SERIES PROGRESSION CHART

STEP ONE

CLUTCH HANG

Page 78

WORK UP TO: 10 SECOND HOLD

Then Begin Step Two

STEP TWO

DIAGONAL SPLIT CLUTCH

Page 79

WORK UP TO: 10 SECOND HOLD

Then Begin Step Three

STEP THREE

DIAGONAL TUCK CLUTCH

Page 80

WORK UP TO: 10 SECOND HOLD

Then Begin Step Four

STEP FOUR

DIAGONAL CLUTCH

Page 81

WORK UP TO: 10 SECOND HOLD

Then Begin Step Five

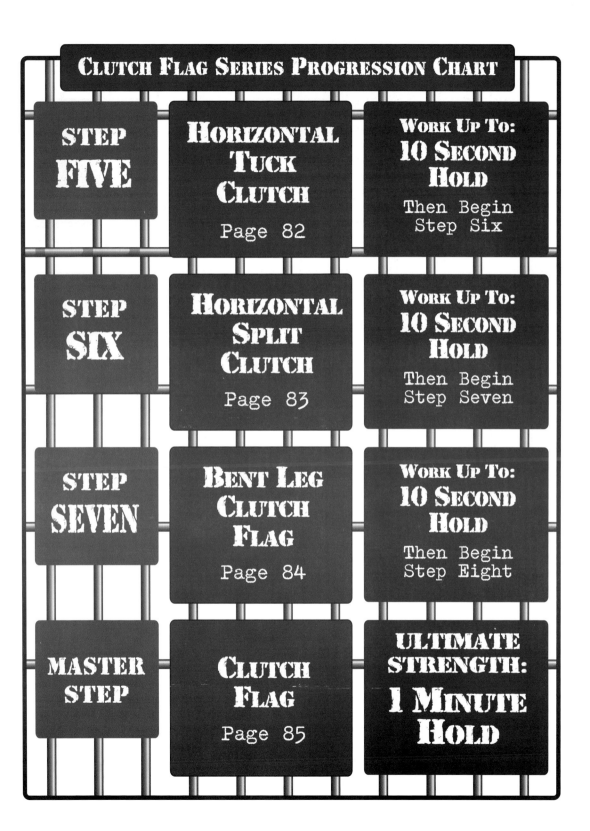

CLUTCH FLAG SERIES PROGRESSION CHART

STEP FIVE	**HORIZONTAL TUCK CLUTCH** Page 82	**WORK UP TO: 10 SECOND HOLD** Then Begin Step Six
STEP SIX	**HORIZONTAL SPLIT CLUTCH** Page 83	**WORK UP TO: 10 SECOND HOLD** Then Begin Step Seven
STEP SEVEN	**BENT LEG CLUTCH FLAG** Page 84	**WORK UP TO: 10 SECOND HOLD** Then Begin Step Eight
MASTER STEP	**CLUTCH FLAG** Page 85	**ULTIMATE STRENGTH: 1 MINUTE HOLD**

Lights out!

REALITY CHECK: thousands of reps of side crunches won't do jack for your overall strength and appearance. An athlete fed on a diet of crunches and similarly useless modern midsection nonsense would get the shock of his life if he tried the clutch flag—a hold which requires *genuine* strength and athletic ability.

Despite this, the clutch flag will be relatively easy to learn for most athletes, provided they are committed, sensible, and not too overweight. Begin by mastering a good, tight clutch hold. From there, explore the progressions I've laid out. Many of you won't need all eight—no problem. Some of you will experiment and invent your own progressions and pass them on to others—even better!

Once you get to the point where you can perform a strong clutch flag, you can be sure you have no weak links in your lateral chain. Perform the hold two or three times a week—perhaps as part of your regular training sessions—and you'll find your side-waist tightening up a hundred times faster than on a course of daily crunches.

For many, that'll be enough. That's fine—you can do something most bodybuilders can't. For those who want to join the ranks of the bodyweight elite, there's a further option—the press flag. If you've got the balls, I'll show you how next.

9: The Press Flag

In Eight Not-So-Easy Steps

Some athletes will be satisfied with their development once they master the clutch flag. Others will want to attempt the legendary *press flag*.

This version of the flag is the *ultimate* test of lateral chain strength. Forget your side crunches and broomstick twists: this feat of strength is in another league entirely—a league of its own, brother. Serious weightlifters (the ones who are even *aware* of the lateral chain—most aren't) might perform side bends with dumbbells or suitcase deadlifts with heavy weights, but even these movements can't come close to approximating the side-body strength benefits of the press flag.

Not only does mastery of the press flag bring better balance and coordination benefits than pulling heavier weights, it's also a hell of a lot safer. When you bend to the side with heavy weights, you open your discs under pressure and risk spine or hip injury. But with press flags, all the tension is held with the body straight—the spine is aligned, just like Mother Nature intended.

The bottom line? If you want athletic lateral chain power that blows away your competition, this is where it's at. If you are looking to build strong, hard obliques with plenty of "detail" muscles, look no further.

Upper body variations

There are three basic ways to place the hands during a press flag:

1. **Vertical grip:** Place the upper hand around the base in an overhand grip, and the lower hand in an underhand, or side-on grip with the fingers down. This is best done with a solid pole but the super-strong (read: "circus acrobats") can pull this kind of grip off on a rope.

2. **Horizontal grip:** Grip two horizontal bars (one high, one low); the grip of the higher arm can be overhand or underhand, but the lower grip should be underhand.

3. **Grip-to-grip:** This is a variation used by acrobats sometimes. Instead of a solid inanimate base, you hold onto a training partner's hands.

These are just the three *basic* grip variations—remember you can mix and match if the equipment allows: the upper hand can be vertical, the lower horizontal, and so on. Ultimately, whichever form you choose depends upon your personal disposition, as well as your access to equipment. Good options for the vertical grip might be signposts, thick railings, and even a light pole if your fingers are strong enough (the thicker the cylinder, the harder it is to grip). For the horizontal grip a jungle gym or some monkey bars in the park might be a good call, but look around—you might be surprised at what you can use. Check out the following pages for some ideas.

For the illustrations in this book, a vertical grip is used, but the principles taught (as well as the progressions) can be applied to any type of grip you like. Whichever version you favor, it's important to try to be consistent with that version while you are mastering the press flag.

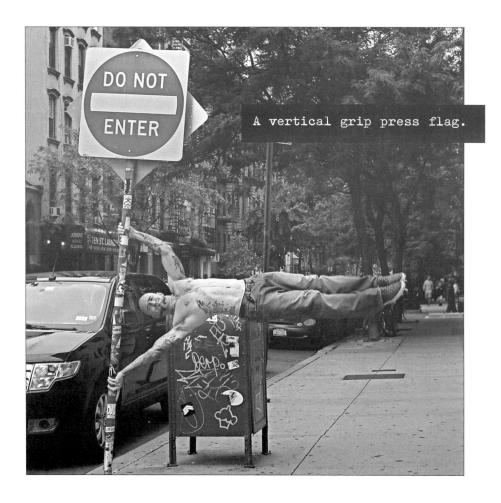

A vertical grip press flag.

Al Kavadlo performs
his signature
horizontal grip
press flag.

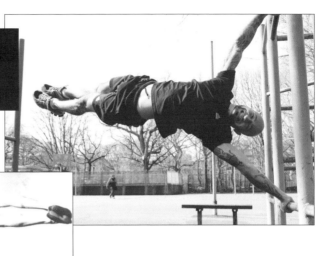

A classic shot of a grip-to-grip
press flag. Like all press flags,
the partner version requires great
balance, plus the ability to pull hard
with the top arm, while pushing with
the bottom arm.

Stuck in the city without
a gym? No problem. Super-
athlete Danny Kavadlo shows
us that New York City is
his gym! He demonstrates
the same basic press flag,
but with a variety of
improvised grips. (See how
he combines a diagonal grip
with a flat palm on the
phone booth. Genius.)

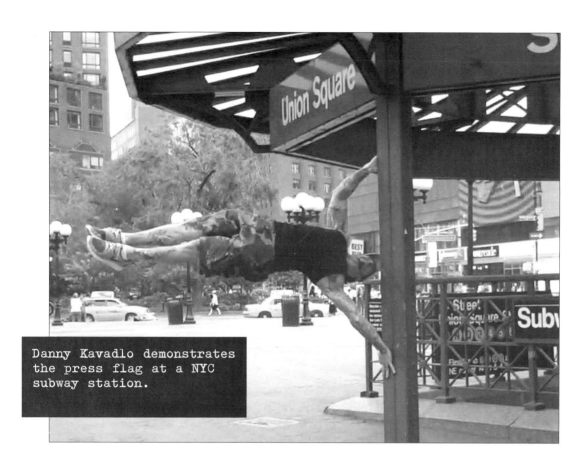

Danny Kavadlo demonstrates the press flag at a NYC subway station.

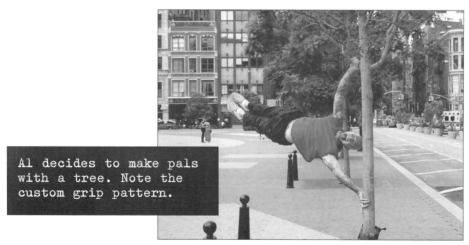

Al decides to make pals with a tree. Note the custom grip pattern.

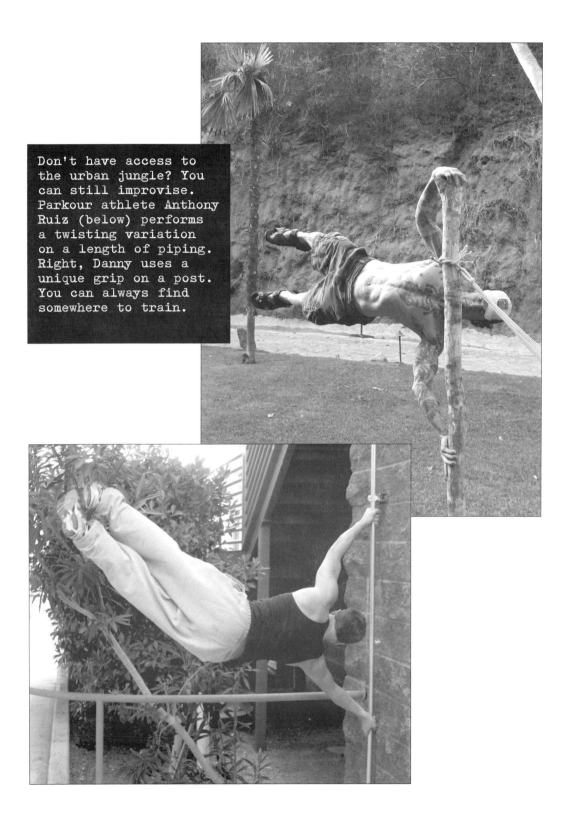

Don't have access to
the urban jungle? You
can still improvise.
Parkour athlete Anthony
Ruiz (below) performs
a twisting variation
on a length of piping.
Right, Danny uses a
unique grip on a post.
You can always find
somewhere to train.

Understanding the press hold

The clutch flag is relatively easy to start learning. This has little to do with lateral chain strength; it's simply because the upper body demands of the clutch flag aren't as great as for the press flag. The clutch flag requires mainly strength in the chest and biceps to maintain the weight of the hips and legs; and these areas are powerful enough on most athletes to do the job, with a little training. The press flag, however, requires *huge* strength in the shoulders and arms to perform correctly. In part, this is because of leverage—the entire body projects outwards, not just the hips and legs. But the real challenge when holding a press flag—as anyone who's tried it will tell you—is that it's such an *asymmetrical* hold. With the clutch flag, both arms take a good share of the load, but with the press flag, the bottom arm is forced to support the bodyweight, magnified as it is through the leverage involved.

It's pointless trying to tell you just how weird and tough this hold is on the upper body. Needless to say, if you can't hold yourself up on just one locked arm, your lower arm will fail. Likewise, if you can't hang your bodyweight with one hand, your upper arm will fail. Luckily you can quickly build strength in both these areas. Following a good handstand pushup progression will generate maximum shoulder pressing power, and some simple hanging work will do wonders to enhance your grip. If you are a little behind in these areas, now's the time to get jacked up.

Neural blasting: the up-down trick

When I was learning the flag in San Quentin, I mastered the clutch flag kind of easy (this isn't a boast; I'd earned my "stripes" doing lots of one-arm planks into one-arm handstands, and this built my lateral chain strength to a good level). Despite my success with the clutch flag, the press flag was a totally different matter. I tried to smoothly raise my body parallel to the ground, but I just couldn't seem to get the hang of it; my body would inevitably slope and droop down.

One day another con approached me in the yard and showed me a trick that proved to be the solution to the problem—it cured my crummy press flags pretty much straight away. The "secret" was the *vertical flag*. Instead of slowly lifting my straight body up into the flag, I was taught to explosively kick my bent legs up into an upwards slanted chamber position (see page 102-103). From there, I straightened my body out, with my feet pointed up into the air (pag3 104). This upwards slanting position is called a vertical flag, and it's much easier to maintain than a standard, horizontal flag. From this position, I smoothly lowered my body *down* into the classic *horizontal press flag* (page 107). Bingo—after weeks of effort I got a fairly acceptable press flag the first time I tried this.

How come I was able to lower my body into the correct horizontal flag position, when I couldn't lift it up into that position? Several reasons. The most obvious is that it's easier to control a weight you're lowering than a weight you're raising, because you aren't fighting gravity. (Imagine lowering a very heavy weight you're curling, and holding it parallel to the ground; then compare this to trying to lift that weight up, strictly, from a straight arm position.) I'm also convinced that explosively kicking up into the vertical flag activates the nerve braches in the lateral chain, "hacking" into your nervous system and automatically enhancing strength.

Whatever the reason, this sneaky trick of kicking right up into a vertical flag before lowering down into the horizontal flag really works like magic once you're advanced enough to use it. I've included it as part of the press flag progression series in the second half of this chapter.

Press flag training tactics

Okay, you now know the theory. Before you get training, I'm gonna pitch some quick tips at you that will help along the road:

- Don't even begin working on the press flag unless you can do the clutch flag (page 85) well. Trying the press flag first is just ass-backwards—it's like trying to bench press 300 before you can bench 150. Pointless!

- The early steps of the press flag are based on building a good hold more than generating maximum lateral chain power. For this reason, after your press flag training you should always finish with one or two stays in the clutch flag to retain everything you've built. Do this until at least step 5.

- Your body weight is magnified during the press flag. I've never seen a fat man do this feat. Some athletes who are stuck on a step find that losing as little as five to ten pounds of lard "magically" kick starts their progress again.

- The press flag is a totally uneven hold; it works both sides of the body very differently. This is why it highlights weakness in the chain so well, and it's also why most guys can only do press flags one way up. Don't fall into this trap. Practice the flag on *both* sides of the pole each workout, starting with your *weakest* side.

- Once you've mastered the arm positioning, you will find that balancing the outstretched body in the press flag is much harder than for the clutch flag. In particular, if the abs are weak or not contracted, or if the pole is not perfectly upright, the body can swing backwards. Be ready to compensate for this!

- Safety is a key feature of all bodyweight training. From the very first time you attempt the press hold, learn to get down safely. Cultivate control—never let yourself just *drop*.

• The press flag is tough. It takes time for a new fish to get there. Results may come in adding just one second to the hold every week or two. That's a great achievement! Your side chain is getting stronger, while all those guys doing side crunches are just getting bad backs.

How To Progress

HOW LONG?

As with the clutch flag, the progression standard with the press flag can be flexible. I advise:

- For steps 1 and 2, you should be aiming at a hold of approximately **ten seconds.**

- For steps 4-7 a *perfect* hold of **five seconds** is sufficient to move on to the next step. Once you can hold the position shown perfectly for five seconds, try the next step.

HOW MUCH?

When you go to practise the flag, hold your best position until it starts to drop, or deteriorate. Then take a brief break (a couple minutes) and try again. Do this **five or six times each session.**

HOW OFTEN?

The press flag is more demanding than the clutch flag, and your training frequency should reflect this:

- For steps 1-5 training sessions can be performed on up to **three non-consecutive days per week.**

The basic press hold

Just getting into a basic press hold requires some practice, so let's do what we did with the *clutch hold* (pages 75 to 77) and take a sec to get this basic element straight, before we launch into working the steps.

1. Initial distancing is important. Remember, at least one of your arms is locked during the press flag, so if you approach your base much closer than arm's length, you'll have to *push* your bodyweight out. Don't make it so tough, man. Stand about three-quarters of arm's length away.

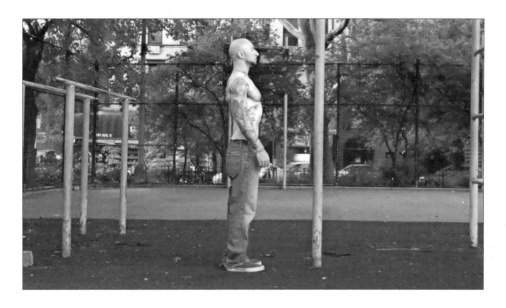

2. With your left arm, reach down and grip the base at a point about level with your hip/upper thigh. Your palm heel should point up, with your index finger pointing down. Lock your arm straight.

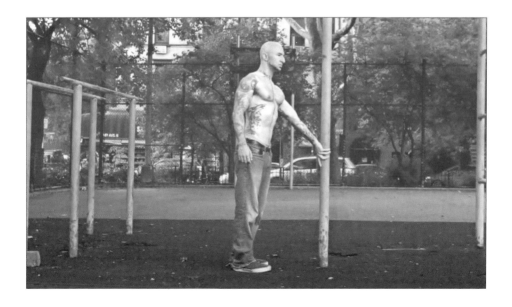

3. Now stretch up and grip the pole with your right hand, at a point somewhere above your head. Your thumb should be below your palm, and you can use either a thumbless grip, or wrap your thumb around the pole; whatever feels most natural (this will depend upon the nature of the base).

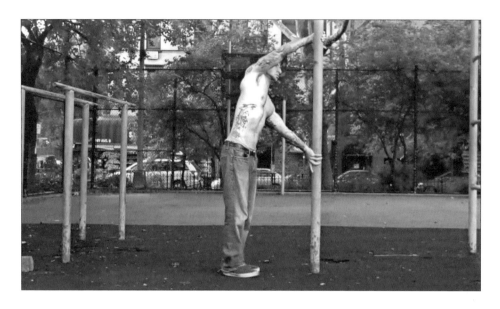

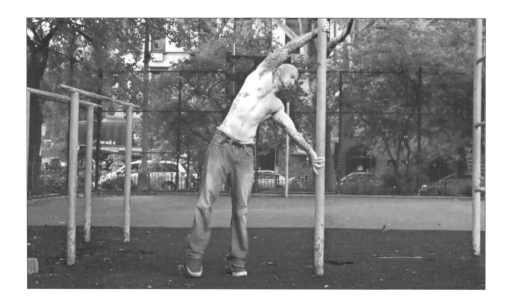

I've left these instructions desirably loose. This is because individual technique will vary with individual proportions. The key lies in experimentation. As you put in hard, thoughtful work on the steps, you'll naturally develop your own unique positioning. The direction you approach the pole in is also up to you; to reverse things, substitute "left" for "right".

Cool, let's hit the steps of the press flag series.

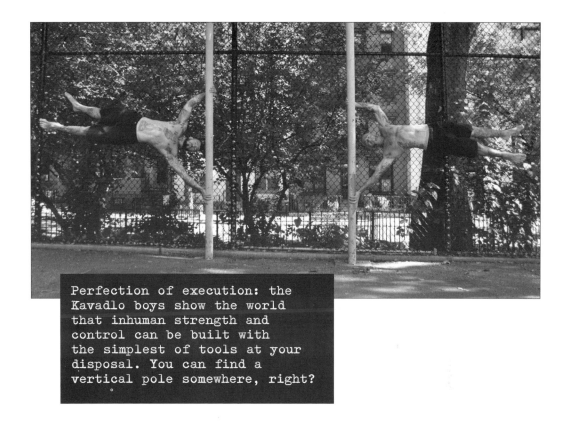

Perfection of execution: the Kavadlo boys show the world that inhuman strength and control can be built with the simplest of tools at your disposal. You can find a vertical pole somewhere, right?

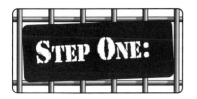

SUPPORT PRESS

OVERVIEW

The *support press* is a preliminary exercise for the *press flag*. It will allow athletes to begin gaining (or testing) their upper body strength before attempting the basic *press hang*, which is the foundation of all press flag training. For this exercise, you'll need a high horizontal bar bordered by walls or any kind of vertical supports; the overhead bar used for pullups is a good option. Hang next to the wall using an overhand grip. Take one hand (the hand nearest the vertical surface) away from the bar and place it flat on the vertical surface. Extend that arm until it is locked straight, and your body is pushed outwards. Keep your body aligned, and breathe normally.

TIPS

To make this hold progressive, inch your hanging hand in the direction of your opposite hand. When they are nearly in line, it's time to progress.

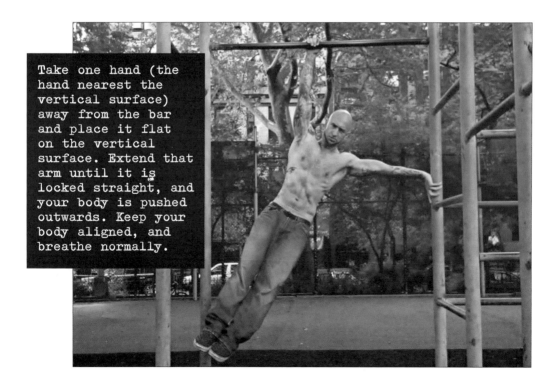

Take one hand (the hand nearest the vertical surface) away from the bar and place it flat on the vertical surface. Extend that arm until it is locked straight, and your body is pushed outwards. Keep your body aligned, and breathe normally.

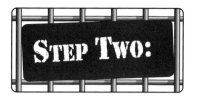

STEP TWO:

PRESS HANG

OVERVIEW

Approach your vertical base, and get into the basic *press hold* (pages 96 to 99). Brace your upper body by pulling with your higher arm, and pressing with your lower arm. For this step, your pulling arm should be braced. Once you feel you've generated enough tension, hop your legs slightly out to the side and try to hold your feet clear of the floor. You can bend your knees a little if it helps. Let your lower body hang down. Hold the position, breathing normally.

TIPS

The objective of this step is to generate enough tension in the press to hold your weight. You're not trying to go horizontal yet, so fight the urge to kick your legs out to the side, or straighten your body; for now, just transmit all your energy towards the upper body.

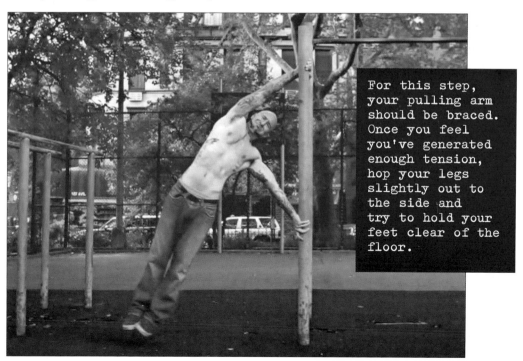

For this step, your pulling arm should be braced. Once you feel you've generated enough tension, hop your legs slightly out to the side and try to hold your feet clear of the floor.

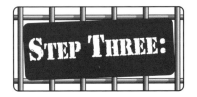

STEP THREE: KICK PRESS

OVERVIEW

Approach your vertical base, and get into the basic *press hold* (pages 96 to 99). Your hip will be out to the side, and your feet apart. Kick down hard through your leg nearest the base and explode the other leg up to the side (A). Pull with your upper (bent) arm and start pushing through your lower arm. Your jump needs to elevate your trunk up above horizontal (B). At the top of the jump, rotate your hips so that they face up. Your ultimate goal is to learn to bring your knees up over your torso (C). This is the only purely explosive move in the entire series, so I don't expect you to *hold* at the top—the point of this drill is to learn the explosive movement pattern. Just try to get the knees up high, powerfully but under control. When you can do this ten times you'll be ready to try holding at the top, which is the next step.

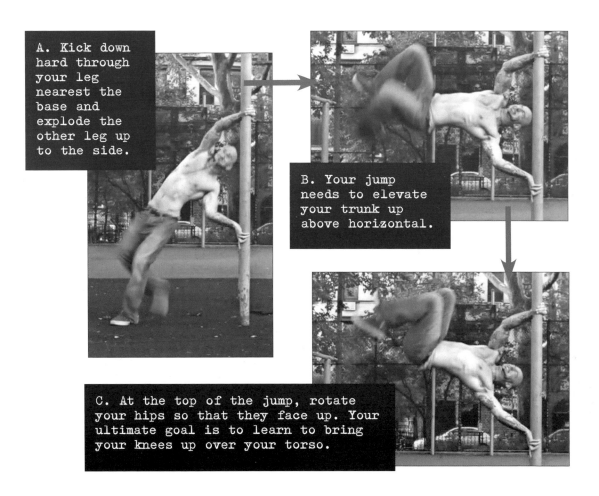

A. Kick down hard through your leg nearest the base and explode the other leg up to the side.

B. Your jump needs to elevate your trunk up above horizontal.

C. At the top of the jump, rotate your hips so that they face up. Your ultimate goal is to learn to bring your knees up over your torso.

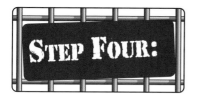

VERTICAL CHAMBER PRESS

OVERVIEW

Once you have mastered the *kick press*, it's time to try and turn that explosive *move* into a *hold*. You're about to begin the *vertical press* positions which will allow you to lower yourself into the full horizontal *press flag*. Approach your vertical base, and get into the basic *press hold* (pages 96 to 99). From here, kick up using the kick press technique, but try to hold the top position, with *both* the knees next to the highest elbow. Hold the position, breathing normally.

TIPS

This position is the chamber (i.e., "ready") position for the *vertical press* (step 5). It's not a full tuck— you don't need to draw the knees close to the trunk, they just have to be bent. Your body doesn't need to be entirely vertical, either. The correct position is out at an angle from the base, as in the photo.

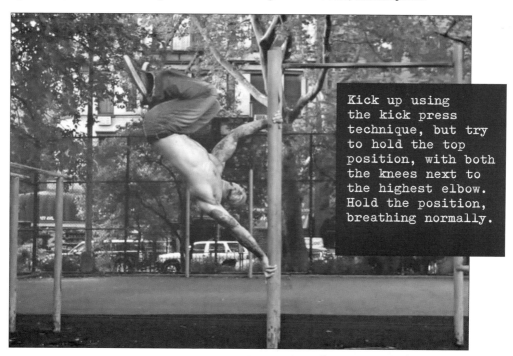

Kick up using the kick press technique, but try to hold the top position, with both the knees next to the highest elbow. Hold the position, breathing normally.

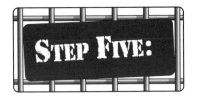

VERTICAL PRESS

OVERVIEW

Approach your vertical base, and get into the basic *press hold* (pages 96 to 99). From here, kick up into a *vertical chamber press* (step 4). Once your position is fixed, smoothly extend the legs upwards until they are locked out. At this point, your trunk and body should form an approximately straight horizontal line, with no sagging. The body won't be totally vertical, but maintaining hold will be easier if you can get an angle that's at least above an upwards diagonal. Hold the position, breathing normally.

TIPS

If you find it too difficult to move from the *vertical chamber press* to the *vertical press* in one step, you can get there gradually, by first extending just one leg (the *vertical split press*). Once you can hold this position, work on extending the second leg over time. This will give you a full vertical press.

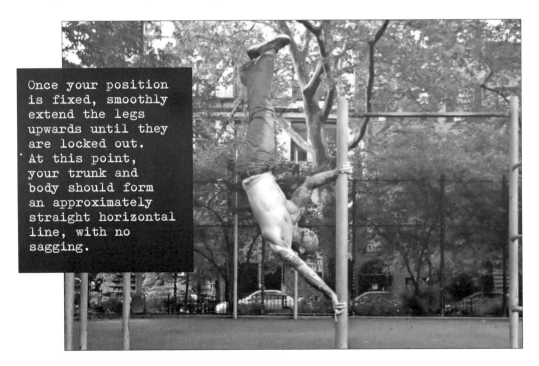

Once your position is fixed, smoothly extend the legs upwards until they are locked out. At this point, your trunk and body should form an approximately straight horizontal line, with no sagging.

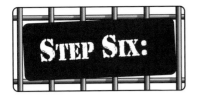

STEP SIX:

SPLIT PRESS FLAG

OVERVIEW

Now that you've mastered the *vertical press*, it's time to experiment with lowering yourself down to horizontal positions. Approach your vertical base, and get into the basic *press hold* (pages 96 to 99). From here, kick up into a vertical press (step 5). Now bend the leg closest to the base until it's at about 90 degrees (a right angle). Do this by bending the leg while bringing that knee forward a little (A). Once your position is fixed, smoothly lower your body to horizontal. Your trunk and lowest leg should form a perfectly straight horizontal line, with no sagging (B). Hold the position (even if just for a split second) breathing normally.

A. Bend the leg closest to the base until it's at about 90 degrees (a right angle). Do this by bending the leg while bringing that knee forward a little.

B. Once your position is fixed, smoothly lower your body to horizontal. Your trunk and lowest leg should form a perfectly straight horizontal line, with no sagging.

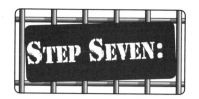

BENT LEG PRESS FLAG

OVERVIEW

Approach your vertical base, and get into the basic *press hold* (pages 96 to 99). From here, kick up into a *vertical press* (step 5). Once your position is fixed, smoothly lower your body to horizontal while you bend your legs. You can bend the knees, or the knees and hips; either method is fine, but beware that moving your legs forwards or back can affect your balance and make you spin. Your trunk and bent legs should form a perfectly straight horizontal line, with no sagging. Hold the position, breathing normally.

TIPS

When lowering yourself into a horizontal position from a *vertical press* (step 5), it's helpful to assume the correct lower body positioning *before* lowering yourself down. Doing this will build strength faster than positioning your legs at the last moment.

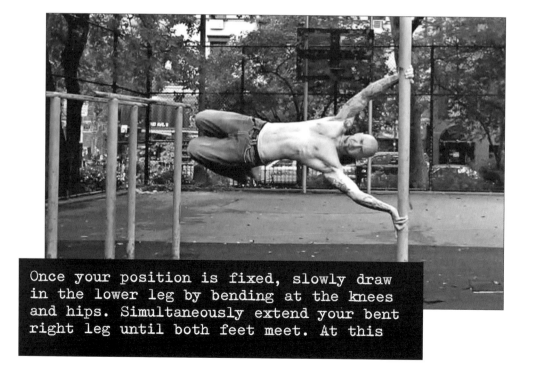

Once your position is fixed, slowly draw in the lower leg by bending at the knees and hips. Simultaneously extend your bent right leg until both feet meet. At this

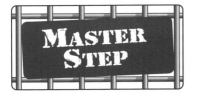

PRESS FLAG

OVERVIEW

Approach your vertical base, and get into the basic *press hold* (pages 96 to 99). From here, kick up into a *vertical press* (step 5). Ensure that your legs are locked out straight. Once your position is fixed, smoothly lower your body to horizontal. Your trunk and bent legs should be aligned to form a perfectly straight horizontal line, with no sagging. Hold the position for as long as possible, breathing normally.

TIPS

Bodyweight experts who can perform a good flag are surprisingly few in number. Good luck finding a bodybuilder who can pull this off! It shouldn't be this way. Every able-bodied athlete under seventy can achieve this strength feat—provided they have the right progressions. Some won't need all the steps I've laid out; that's great. Take what you need, brother.

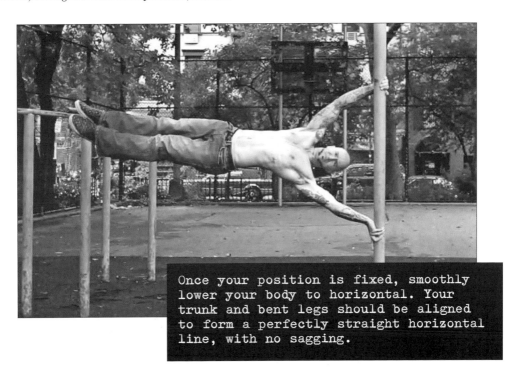

Once your position is fixed, smoothly lower your body to horizontal. Your trunk and bent legs should be aligned to form a perfectly straight horizontal line, with no sagging.

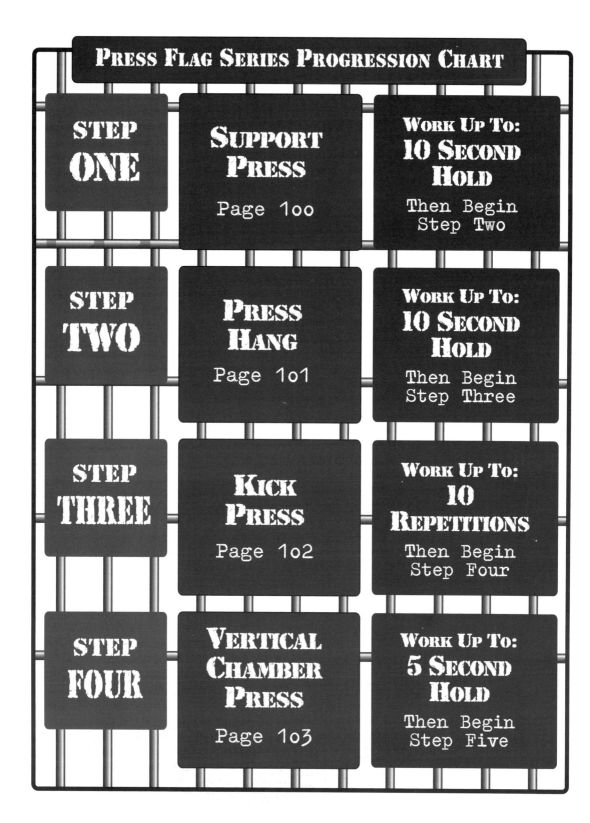

PRESS FLAG SERIES PROGRESSION CHART

STEP ONE	SUPPORT PRESS Page 100	WORK UP TO: 10 SECOND HOLD Then Begin Step Two
STEP TWO	PRESS HANG Page 101	WORK UP TO: 10 SECOND HOLD Then Begin Step Three
STEP THREE	KICK PRESS Page 102	WORK UP TO: 10 REPETITIONS Then Begin Step Four
STEP FOUR	VERTICAL CHAMBER PRESS Page 103	WORK UP TO: 5 SECOND HOLD Then Begin Step Five

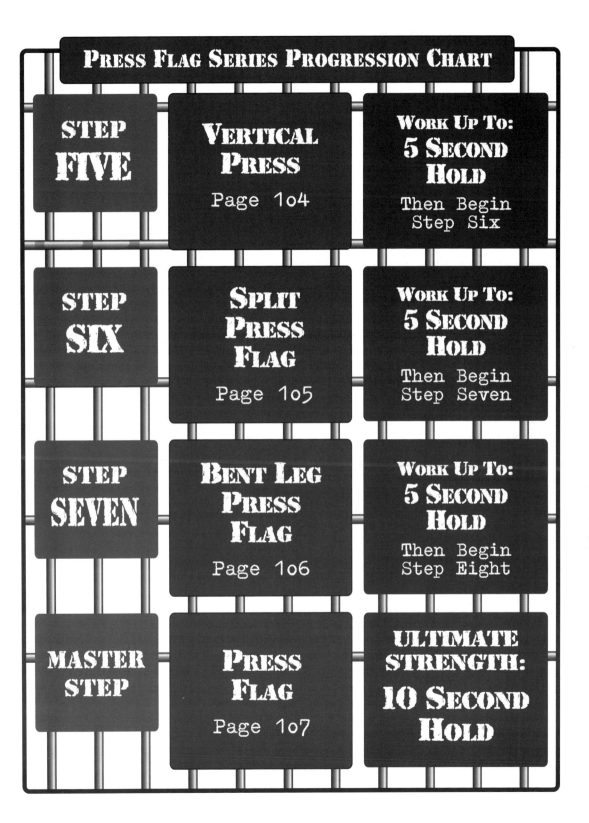

PRESS FLAG SERIES PROGRESSION CHART

STEP FIVE	VERTICAL PRESS Page 104	WORK UP TO: 5 SECOND HOLD Then Begin Step Six
STEP SIX	SPLIT PRESS FLAG Page 105	WORK UP TO: 5 SECOND HOLD Then Begin Step Seven
STEP SEVEN	BENT LEG PRESS FLAG Page 106	WORK UP TO: 5 SECOND HOLD Then Begin Step Eight
MASTER STEP	PRESS FLAG Page 107	ULTIMATE STRENGTH: 10 SECOND HOLD

Going beyond

When you get to the point that you can hold a press flag for a few seconds, congrats—not only have you achieved a strength feat that very few athletes ever get close to, you now have a lateral chain more like a titanium chain. What's next?

Just like every Master Step, there are ways you can move forward to even more unbelievable levels of strength. Once you hit your first flag press, make sure you consolidate your success. Keep training; make certain that your form is absolutely perfect. Keep it tight, horizontal, with no drooping and minimum shaking or swaying. Once you can do this for two or three seconds, see if you can improve on that. If you can hold a good press flag for ten seconds, you can certainly be called an expert in the movement—amongst any company in the world.

At this point, a lot of athletes will be pretty happy with their lateral chain strength, and be content to level out by just adding the press flag into their workouts methodically. This is understandable. Most cons would certainly rather commit more energy to building mass and strength with pullups, pushups and handstand pushups rather than focusing too hard on lateral chain work. I'm sure a lot of guys on the outside feel the same. If this sounds like you, you could do a lot worse than adding in a couple of static flag press holds after your leg raises. The leg raises warm up your core, as well as the upper limbs (if you are hanging). This sets the stage perfectly for press flags. After finishing the leg raises, gently stretch your waist for three or four minutes to help you relax, then hit the flags. Two holds at not quite maximum effort will easily retain all the side-waist power you've worked so hard to build.

1. Leg Raises:	2-3 sets (warm up) 2-3 sets (work sets)
3-4 minutes hip rolling/light stretching	
2. Press flags:	2-3 holds per side (not quite max)

This is how I worked the flag for a long time after learning it, and it's a *great* way to train. Mind-blowingly efficient. In under twenty-five minutes you can get a better waist workout than by *hours* doing sit-ups, crunches, or working all those crappy abs machines in the gym. Alternatively, if you are new to press flags and the leg raises exhaust you too much, you can always perform the flags on a separate session.

But what if you're not happy with this? What if you get hooked on the flag and want to get stronger and stronger?

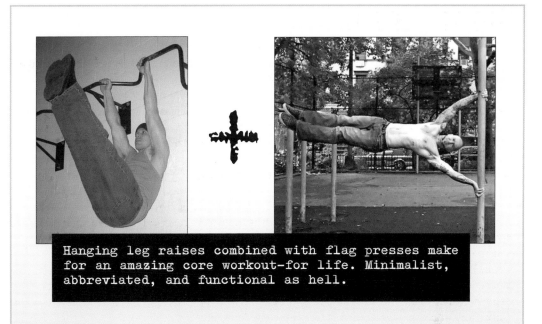

Hanging leg raises combined with flag presses make for an amazing core workout-for life. Minimalist, abbreviated, and functional as hell.

One option is to continue improving the amount of time you can hold the press flag. I tried this myself, and didn't find it real satisfying; for one thing, increasing the length of time in the hold improves endurance, but not strength. Also, after about ten seconds, it's *incredibly* hard to hold a flag. It may take *months* of training just to add a few seconds. Seriously! That's how tough the flag is. (The Guinness World Record for a press flag hold is only thirty-nine seconds, set by the *superhuman* Dominic Lacasse.)

If you want to build a *stronger* press flag, the next step is to learn to lever your straight body *up* from the floor into the horizontal position, instead of dropping *down* into a horizontal flag from a vertical flag. Once you master this—and it's tougher than it sounds—you can begin working on the flag as a *moving* exercise. You can start thinking in terms of *sets* and *reps*. Lever your straight body up and out to the side, pausing for a second at the top before descending back to the floor. That's one rep. Aim for two sets of three reps, and build up from there. Try to eliminate as much momentum as possible, over time. If you are going to follow this route, don't train the flag in the same sessions as leg raises—it's too much to ask. Train your flags fresh, on a different day.

Approaching the flag as a "move" rather than a "hold" requires great ability, but the payback in pure body-power will be incredible. It also seriously increases muscle density—anyone performing flags this way will have a waist that can break a baseball bat.

Lights out!

Bodybuilders are famous for their patchwork methods of training, dividing up the body into individual sections. Their waist training methods reflect this idea, as they hopelessly try to get results by isolating the midsection muscles using pathetic, pointless movements.

Strength athletes know better. They understand that the body was meant to work as a system—even if you are only looking to specialize on a *part* of that system. Good coaches don't work the "low back"—they think in terms of the entire *posterior chain*. Some superior strength ideologists now also talk about the *anterior chain* of muscles, along the front of the body. But how many experts do you hear talking about the *lateral chain*? The neglected muscles running up the side of the body?

Not many—if any even do. But convicts have known the key to building a flexible steel side-waist, and they've known it for generations. The secret doesn't lie in any new, super-scientific approach. It lies in a very ancient exercise: *the flag series of movements.*

Now you have the secrets too. Go use them.

10: Bulldog Neck

Bulletproof Your Weakest Link

No minor muscle group is as important and rewarding to train as the neck. A thick, strong-looking neck gives off an immediate aura of power. When we want to check out how muscular another guy is, we instinctively look towards his neck to tell us. Sheer body size can be misleading—sometimes skinny guys can look bulky in clothing, particularly if they have a boxy frame. But a powerful, bulldog neck rarely lies. Convicts who are proud of their impressive necks will often get a little tattoo on their throat or to the side of the neck, to draw attention to the area. Besides, the neck is the only muscular body part that's on public display all year round. In a shirt or sweater forearms can be completely covered, but the neck still shows above the collar. Given this, it's always amazed me that bodybuilders hardly ever include neck training in their programs. This body part is usually ignored altogether.

A sturdy, well-trained neck has greater benefits than just looking intimidating. The neck forms the cervical portion of the upper spine, and if the muscles supporting these smaller vertebrae are good and strong an athlete will have a reduced chance of injury to this crucial area. The cervical spine supports the skull and the brain, and a robust neck acts as a shock absorber to the head, protecting the brain from concussion (or worse) during trauma. This is why all boxers train their necks hard; powerful neck muscles will keep the head stable when it gets punched, and this stops the brain rattling around inside. Fight commentators often talk about a "glass jaw", but the chin and jaw actually have little to do in determining your ability to take a heavy punch and come back smiling. Neck power is far more important. This is another good reason to invest some time in neck training if you're in the joint. Should you be blindsided with a haymaker to the jaw, your brain will thank you.

Unfortunately the knowledge of how to train your neck properly is a dying art, restricted to a few special circles. No personal trainer can teach you how to train this area productively. Bodybuilding writers—at a loss for what to suggest—usually recommend silly high-rep exercises while holding tiny weights to your head.

These pitiful techniques will do zero to produce a powerful neck. In a few gyms you might see a neck harness to attach some decent weights to, but strapping heavy weights around your head area isn't always a great idea; neck harnesses are notorious for causing headaches and nagging neck pain. Neck training machines do exist, but most of them look like they were designed to decapitate you rather than build a healthy upper spine. Steer well clear of them.

The best necks in the business

I was lucky enough to learn my neck training skills from a real expert—not a bodybuilder or even a boxer, but a *wrestler*. The man in question was a damn good amateur grappler in college before his lifestyle led him down the wrong path. He wound up in Angola Pen, and it was there that I was lucky enough to spend some time with him. Nobody understands neck training like wrestlers, and it shows. If you ever get the chance to see a really good wrestler—either a freestyle wrestler or Greco-Roman style—you'll notice that they inevitably have thick, brawny necks that look like they've been carved out of granite. The Olympic Freestyle gold medalist Kurt Angle has had his neck measured at over twenty inches! In the late nineties, Angle (who is all of five eleven) became a pro with the WWE, and was often dwarfed by the hulking athletes he starred with. He appeared alongside guys with gigantic chests, tree-trunk thighs and arms like beer kegs, but nobody who stepped in the ring with him had a neck anywhere near as impressive as he did. Years of wrestling gave him this elite level of development.

There is a good reason for the incredible neck development wrestlers possess. In freestyle wrestling, your arms are usually taken up in countering your opponent during close grappling, and because of this the head has to act as a third arm to position the opponent's head and torso. This requires phenomenal neck strength. Good wrestlers automatically tie up each other's limbs, and as a result many throws have to be done holding onto the torso, and landing like this sends phenomenal forces through the neck and upper spine. If you have ever seen a *suplex*, you'll know what I mean; you basically land on your upper shoulders and neck, with the weight of your opponent slamming right on top of you. Without a neck forged from steel, such a throw would be unthinkable—it could even kill you. But wrestlers can do this dozens of times during a match without the slightest problem. This is because the art of neck training has survived in the curricula of wrestling schools.

Secret weapons

What is the "secret weapon" of a serious wrestler's neck training armory? Well, like all the best exercises, it doesn't require special equipment like machines or weights. Just the human body moving as nature intended. The ultimate program consists of two fairly simple calisthenics exercises—the *wrestler's bridge* and the *front bridge*.

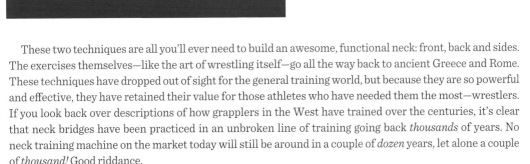

The famous "God of Wrestling" Karl Gotch, performs a perfect suplex, where the opponent is thrown backwards from standing. His mastery of the belly-to-back suplex was so great it became known as the "German" suplex in his honor. You can see the importance of the neck bridge in training to survive this move. Gotch himself was a major proponent of calisthenics, and believed that weight-training made wrestlers slower.

These two techniques are all you'll ever need to build an awesome, functional neck: front, back and sides. The exercises themselves—like the art of wrestling itself—go all the way back to ancient Greece and Rome. These techniques have dropped out of sight for the general training world, but because they are so powerful and effective, they have retained their value for those athletes who have needed them the most—wrestlers. If you look back over descriptions of how grapplers in the West have trained over the centuries, it's clear that neck bridges have been practiced in an unbroken line of training going back *thousands* of years. No neck training machine on the market today will still be around in a couple of *dozen* years, let alone a couple of *thousand!* Good riddance.

Neck specialization—health benefits

Neck training isn't necessarily essential. As long as you practice the Big Six—particularly the bridging series—your neck will get a fine workout and remain healthy and strong for life. But if you are involved in disciplines like combat sports or football that require an ultra-strong upper spine—or if you just want a cool neck that looks like pythons are crawling out of your collar—give the workout in this chapter a try. The benefits easily outweigh the investment in time and energy. In fact, the benefits of all the neck bridging techniques described in this chapter are enormous.

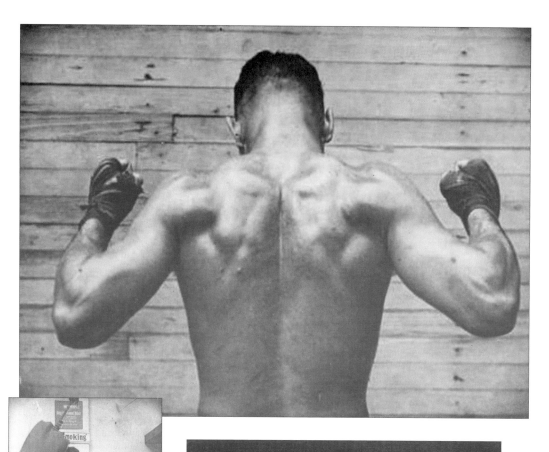

The "Manassa Mauler" Jack Dempsey
didn't have huge biceps or shredded
abs like modern fighters, but he
did build a muscular neck and upper
back because of his dedication
to neck bridges. He believed that
the exercise-combined with chewing
wood, to build up his jaw-made him
un-knockoutable. In over eighty fights
he was KO'd only once, and the smart
money says that fight was a fix.

Aside from the athletic payback, having a strong neck will save you a lot of pain. Six out of ten people experience neck problems of some kind. Is it any wonder? Our necks evolved while we were hunter-gatherers, running through the forests as we constantly looked around for predators or prey. This was a great neck workout. These days the average worker slouches over a desk, a production line or a laptop. They get home exhausted and fall down on the couch staring at the tube for a few more hours. In all these activities, the gaze is fixed in one direction, and as a result the neck is voluntarily paralyzed. It's inevitable that the pillar of muscles supporting the skull become atrophied and stiff. Combine this with the fact that the neck automatically accumulates tension when we are stressed—a throwback to the days when we had to hunch for combat when trouble hit—and the end result is chronic and acute neck and upper back pain. A genuine pain in the neck.

Mastering neck bridges will help virtually every neck problem and will cure the vast majority of them outright. A strong, balanced neck is more resilient to repetitive strain; neck calisthenics radically improve the circulation, easing old injuries and eliminating aches and pains. Practicing these exercises every so often will instantly remove any stress-based tension in the neck and shoulders that has been subconsciously building up. When your neck is strong, your posture is automatically improved, and you look and feel better as a result.

The old school neck program

Neck bridging techniques can be quite difficult, especially if you have allowed your neck to grow weak. As a result, it may take some time to be able to perform them properly. The *wrestler's bridge* requires some basic spinal power to even attempt—you need to be able to do basic back bridging as a prerequisite. If you lack the strength to perform back bridges, refer to the first *Convict Conditioning* book for a complete course of instruction. The *front bridge* has its own difficulties, largely because it requires a moderate degree of flexibility. Don't worry about these issues at this stage. First I'll introduce you to the techniques you'll be using to build your neck, starting with wrestler's bridges, followed by front bridges. Then, I'll show you exactly how to progress in your neck training. I'll finish the chapter with some important neck training ideas to keep you on the straight and narrow.

Okay, enough talk. If I haven't converted you yet, I probably never will. Let's move on to a description of the exercises you'll be using.

WRESTLER'S BRIDGES
PRELIMINARY VERSION

This is the preliminary version of the wrestler's bridge. Because the arms help with the movement, the exercise requires significantly less power than full wrestler's bridges (page 119).

Performance:

I. Lie on your back with the soles of your feet on the floor, and your palms on either side of your head with the fingers pointing towards the feet. Now push the body off the floor until your hips are high and your trunk and limbs form an arch. No part of your body save your feet and hands should be in contact with the floor. This position is called a *bridge hold.*

II. Keeping your trunk and legs braced, lower yourself slowly by bending your elbows, until the crown of your head makes contact with the floor. It will help to rest your head on a towel or slim pillow. This is the start position (image 1).

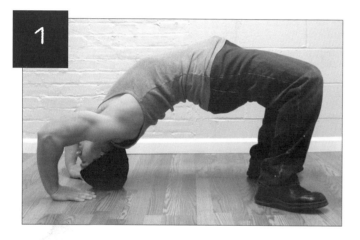

III. Keeping your palms and skull in contact with the floor, slowly bend your head forwards. This will lower your upper body slightly. At no point should your head come away from the floor. When your neck and upper shoulders rest on the floor, stop descending. This is the finish position (image 2).

IV. Slowly and smoothly press back up to the start position using the combined power of your arms and neck. Pause for a moment, and repeat.

Continued next page.

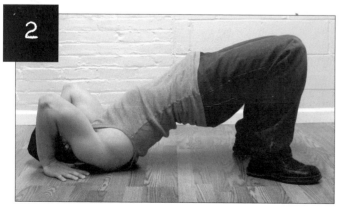

WRESTLER'S BRIDGES
FULL VERSION

This is the hard version of the wrestler's bridge. Because the arms are not involved, the muscles of the neck alone are required to move the torso. This forces them to grow rapidly in size and strength.

Performance:

I. Lie on your back with the soles of your feet on the floor, and your palms on either side of your head with the fingers pointing towards the feet. Now push the body off the floor until your hips are high and your trunk and limbs form an arch. No part of your body save your feet and hands should be in contact with the floor. This position is called a *bridge hold*.

II. Keeping your trunk and legs braced, lower yourself slowly by bending your elbows, until the crown of your head makes contact with the floor. Using a towel or slim pillow will help cushion your head. Gradually take the pressure off your palms, until only the crown of your head and your feet are supporting the body. Cross the arms upon your chest or rest the palms on the stomach. This is the start position (image 3).

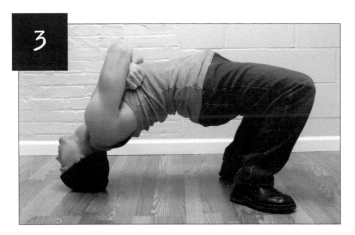

III. Slowly bend your head forwards. This will cause your torso to descend slightly. When your neck and upper shoulders rest on the floor, stop descending. This is the finish position (image 4).

IV. Slowly and smoothly press back up to the start using power of your neck muscles alone. Pause for a moment, and repeat.

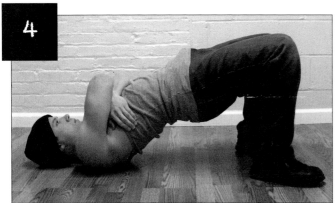

FRONT BRIDGES
PRELIMINARY VERSION

This is the preliminary version of the front bridge. Because of the kneeling position, less of the body's weight is transmitted through the neck, and the exercise can be made easier by shifting the trunk backwards and forwards using the legs. The four-way movement hits all the muscles of the front and sides of the neck. This version is much easier than the full front bridge (page 122).

Performance:

I. Kneel on the floor with your knees wide apart.

II. Straighten up, then bend over forwards. Place the palms on the ground, and lower the crown of your head between them. Rest your head on a towel or slim pillow to cushion your head.

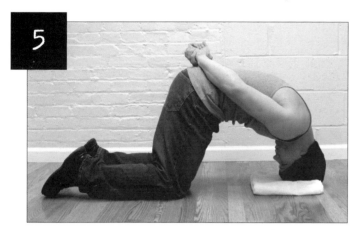

III. Take the pressure off your hands until the force of your weight is going through your knees, shins and feet, as well as the crown of your head. Place your hands behind your back to keep them out of the exercise. This is the neutral position (image 5).

IV. Under full control, allow your head to pivot back until your nose gently makes contact with the floor (image 6).

Continued next page.

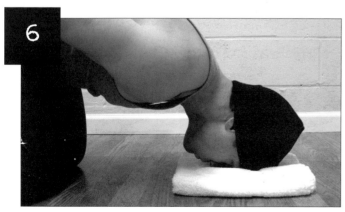

FRONT BRIDGES
PRELIMINARY VERSION cont.

Performance:

V. Return to the neutral position (image 7) using the power of your frontal neck muscles, then allow your head to pivot to the right (image 8).

VI. Return to the neutral position (image 7) using the power of your lateral neck muscles, then allow your head to pivot to the left (image 9).

VII. Return to the neutral position (image 7) using the power of your lateral neck muscles. You have just completed one full repetition. Return to step IV, and repeat.

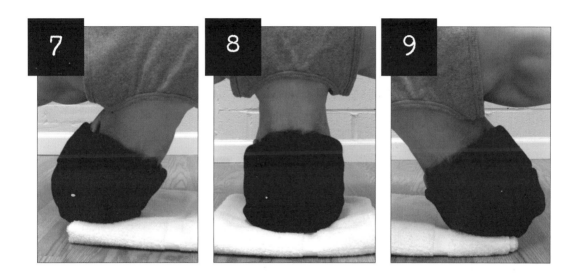

FRONT BRIDGES
FULL VERSION

This is the hard version of the front bridge. Due to the higher position of the body, a much larger amount of bodyweight is passed through the neck and head. This technique moves through four basic positions to hit all areas of the throat and sides of the neck. The forward bend also increases flexibility in the spine, hips and legs.

Performance:

I. Get into a wide stance. The feet should more than shoulder width apart.

II. Bend forwards at the hips, keeping the legs straight or nearly so. Place the palms on the ground, and lower the crown of your head between them. Rest your head on a towel or slim pillow to cushion your head.

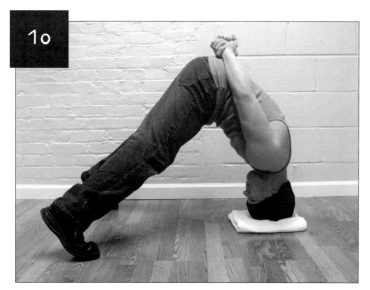

III. Take the pressure off your hands until the force of your weight is going through both feet and the crown of your head. Place your hands behind your back to keep them out of the exercise. This is the neutral position (image 10).

Continued next page.

FRONT BRIDGES
FULL VERSION cont.

Performance:

IV. Under full control, allow your head to pivot back until your nose gently makes contact with the floor (image 11).

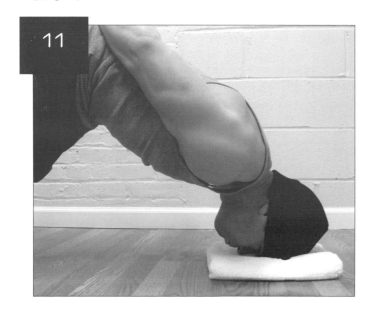

V. Return to the neutral position (image 12) using the power of your frontal neck muscles, then allow your head to pivot to the right (image 13).

VI. Return to the neutral position (image 12) using the power of your lateral neck muscles, then allow your head to pivot to the left (image 14).

VII. Return to the neutral position (image 12) using the power of your lateral neck muscles. You have just completed one full repetition. Return to step IV, and repeat.

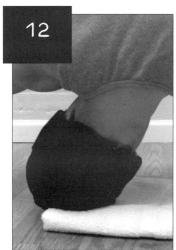

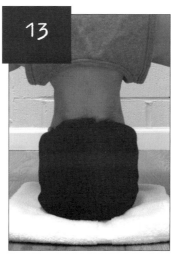

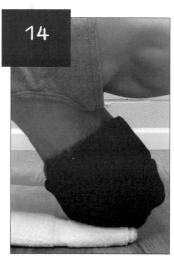

How to progress

Wrestler's bridges and front bridges are intense exercises, and they require a strong spine. Don't even attempt them unless you can do a basic *full bridge*. If you can't do full bridges, work through the bridging series in the first *Convict Conditioning* book until you can. Specialized neck training can wait until your whole spine is strong and flexible.

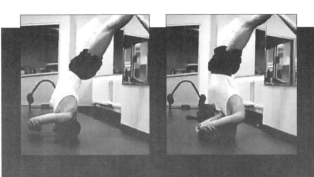

Many coaches—who should know better—dismiss calisthenics training because it's "too light" compared to the weights. Not so. If you know what you are doing, there are always methods to make bodyweight training "harder". This is as true for neck training as anything else. In the shots above, a calisthenics expert trains his neck with "inverse bridges"—he gets into a wall headstand, and rolls onto his forehead and back. All hands free. You complete the inverse bridges by rolling onto each temple and the nape of your neck, to work all the neck muscles equally. Advanced guys only, please. Don't try this at home folks.

Once you have mastered the basic full bridge, you're ready to attempt the preliminary versions of both the wrestler's bridge and the front bridge. You should always pay equal attention to all the muscles of the neck, so practice both exercises together, preferably alternated during the same training session. Once you've gotten the hang of the basic technique for both these exercises, begin building up your reps. Two sets of twenty reps per exercise is the goal you're shooting for, but the neck is a small area so don't rush the process. Begin with only one set per exercise and build up by adding a rep every week or two. Eventually you'll get to a point where you are doing intermediate workouts that look like this:

SET 1. Preliminary wrestler's bridges:	1 x 20
SET 2. Preliminary front bridges:	1 x 20
SET 3. Preliminary wrestler's bridges:	1 x 20
SET 4. Preliminary front bridges:	1 x 20

You need to master basic active flexibility exercises—i.e., the full bridge—before you qualify to attempt the full version of wrestler's bridges, and the same holds true for full front bridges. The full front bridge also requires a moderate level of flexibility in the back and hamstrings to perform, and often guys don't have this—even guys who train. If you aren't very supple, don't panic. The period while you are bringing up your reps in the preliminary exercises is an excellent time to gain the flexibility you'll need later on. If you can't bend over with straight legs and rest your head on the floor (image 10), you'll need to get to work now. If you are still lacking the flexibility you need, don't fret—you're not alone. I'll show you how to get it over the next few pages.

Flexibility stages for the front bridge

To perform the front bridge correctly, there are four postural stages to progress through that'll get you where you need to be:

STAGE 1. Get into as wide a stance as is comfortable, and bend over at the hips until you feel a stretch. Bend your knees if you really need to, and support your torso a little by placing your palms on your thighs or knees. Build up to holding this position for a full minute. This will gradually condition the muscles and ligaments of your back, hips and thighs to forwards stretching techniques. Once you get comfortable with this position, move to stage 2.

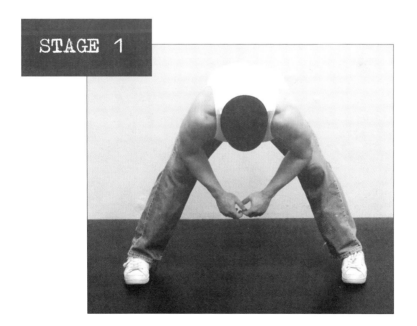

STAGE 1

STAGE 2. Get into a wide stance again. By now your feet should be able to go a little wider—at least twice shoulder width. Lock the legs straight at the knees. Now bend at the waist and touch the floor below you. At first you may not be able to touch the floor. This will be especially true if you are the average stiff-as-a-board guy. Keep trying. Eventually you will be able to touch the floor with your fingertips. Then with bent fingers. As the weeks pass your back and hamstrings will loosen and you'll be able to touch your knuckles to the floor. Finally, you'll be able to rest your palms on the floor. When you can rest your palms on the floor for a full minute, move to stage 3.

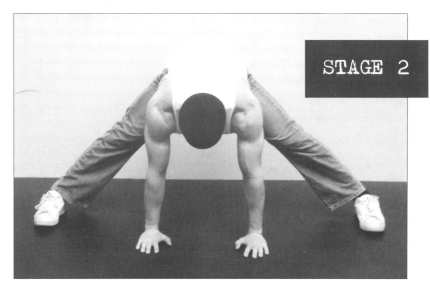

STAGE 3. Once you are have mastered the palms on floor position from a wide stance, begin bringing your torso even closer to the floor by bending your arms. This may take some time, but eventually you will be loose enough to rest your forearms and elbows on the floor for a few seconds. Build up over the weeks until you can hold this forearms-on-floor position for a full minute, then move to stage 4.

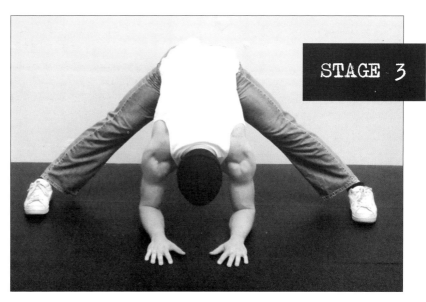

STAGE 4. While resting your forearms on the floor, continue stretching forwards—still with the legs fairly straight at the knee—until your forehead touches the ground, however gently. When you can do this, place your palms on the floor again, and try placing the crown of your skull on the floor between your hands. When you can do this, build up to holding the position for a minute. Once you have mastered stage 4, you'll be supple enough to try the basic *front bridge* position (image 10).

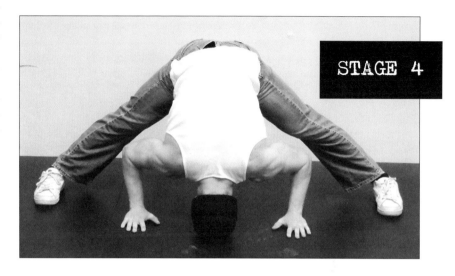

Work on these techniques for a short while after your neck training sessions—and perhaps on a second day during the week—and by the time your neck muscles are ready for full front bridges your back and legs will be more than supple enough to allow you to tackle this brilliant exercise.

Programming for the neck

Once you have got to the stage where you can do two sets of twenty on the *preliminary wrestler's bridge* and the *preliminary front bridge*, you'll have a stronger, healthier neck than almost any athlete you ever meet. Now it's time to move to the next level, and attempt the full versions of both exercises. These are advanced techniques, and if you have trouble at first, don't worry. There are lots of ways you can ease yourself into the exercises. If full wrestler's bridges are too hard, just go back to the assisted version, but using one hand. (Vary which hand you use for symmetrical development.) Over time, apply less pressure through the hand, and before long you'll be able to do the exercise as it was intended—hands free.

The front bridge is a severe exercise and requires a powerful throat and neck. If you can do the preliminary front bridge easily, but the full front bridge is just too much, use your hands for support. Gradually use less pressure through your hands week by week until you can do full bridges using nothing but pure neck power. (Look ma—no hands!)

You only have one neck, so always take things slowly and *always* apply the assistance techniques I've described if you can't do your reps smoothly and safely. Jerking and yanking your neck around is a really bad way to get strong, but a really good way to screw up your neck. Once you can do these exercises, make them the focus of your neck workouts. Reduce the preliminary wrestler's bridges and preliminary front bridges to one set of twenty each, as a warm up. Then follow with one set of full wrestlers bridges and one set of full front bridges for one set each for a handful of reps each. As you get stronger, add reps. Again, do this slowly. Take all the time you need for your neck to build in power and strength. Build up to two sets of twenty work sets per full exercise. By this stage, your neck training will be very advanced, and the workout should look something like this:

SET 1. Preliminary wrestler's bridges:	1 x 20
SET 2. Preliminary front bridges:	1 x 20
SET 3. Full wrestler's bridges:	1 x 20
SET 4. Full front bridges:	1 x 20
SET 5. Full wrestler's bridges:	1 x 20
SET 6. Full front bridges:	1 x 20

Don't underestimate this workout just because it's relatively brief. Despite the fact that it should take less than a quarter of an hour, this is an expert neck training workout. Remember, muscle and strength are built by intensity—constantly getting *better*—rather than volume—constantly training *longer*.

This kind of workout will take care of you for a long time. As you become stronger and higher reps get easier, resist the urge to add weight by holding onto a dumbbell or weight plate as you practice. Instead, strive to increase your range of motion. Adding external loads will only expand the possibility of injury, but increasing your range of motion will progressively strengthen the deeper muscles of the neck and render the vertebrae powerfully flexible. If you get to this stage—not many athletes do—reserve your final sets (i.e., set 5 and 6) for attempting range of motion increases. This will ensure that your neck muscles are red hot before you test them so severely.

Increasing your range of motion for wrestler's bridges will take a long time, and should only be attempted once you can do the above workout relatively easily. At the beginning you will only be able to rest the crown of your skull of the floor during the start position, but with practice and persistence you will find that your muscles develop the contractile strength to rotate your head further and further back-wards during the wrestler's bridge. Ultimately, you'll be able to rotate your head back until your *forehead* is resting on the floor, carrying the weight. This is a highly advanced position, but you can get there if you are dedicated and prepared to put in a lot of effort.

Increasing your range of motion for front bridges is not quite so hard. When you begin, your torso will be more or less directly over your head. As you become stronger over time, gradually increase the distance between your head and your feet. This will shift more emphasis onto the neck and force the throat muscles to work harder throughout all positions of the exercise. Go easy at first, and use your hands for support if you have to. By the time your head is about two thirds of your height away from your feet, the muscles running up the sides of your collar will be like thick steel rods, and your throat will be practically armor-plated with healthy muscle. Master both these advanced positions for reps, and your neck will be damn near superhuman.

Don't forget to keep all your muscles balanced by increasing your lateral range (when your roll your head side-to-side) over time. Begin with the angles shown in the photos and improve gradually. When I roll my head to the side in front bridges, I go until my ear touches the ground before pushing back up. You don't have to go this far, but it's something to aim for some day.

Kiss goodbye to your pencil-neck

The bodyweight neck bridging exercises in this chapter are deceptively simple. But if you devote a big chunk of quality training time to them, you'll find that they really are the last word in neck training. They've been used by many greats of the past, and they'll last you a lifetime.

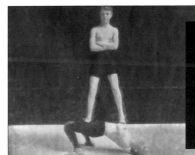

One of the truly legendary conditioning courses is Martin "Farmer" Burns' 1913 series of wrestling lessons. Burns paid heavy emphasis on bodyweight training for strength, and his favorite exercise was the neck bridge (his sons are shown in this photo).

Before we finish the chapter, I'd like to pass on six killer neck training tips I've acquired through my own years of training:

NECK TRAINING TIPS

TIP 1: WARM UP. Always warm up your neck muscles and ligaments before you train. If preliminary neck bridges are still quite difficult for you and you need a gentler warm up, try *manual resistance head raises.* Link your hands behind your head and pull slightly against the force of your muscles as you nod up and down and from side to side. Use a good range of motion. One set of twenty to thirty reps will loosen up a tight neck nicely.

Continued next page.

NECK TRAINING TIPS CONT.

TIP 2: SUPERSETS. Training the front and sides of your neck gives the muscles at the back of your neck a rest, while also keeping them warm and primed for training. Similarly, training the back of your neck keeps the front and sides of your neck ready for work. For this reason, it's a good idea to alternate these areas in your neck workout—do a set of wrestler's bridges, and follow it by front bridges, and so on.

TIP 3: SYMMETRY. For injury prevention and peak functioning, all areas of the neck should be trained equally. Strive for balance in your neck training by performing the same number of sets and reps for front bridges as you do for wrestler's bridges, and vice versa.

TIP 4: RECOVERY. The neck has a lot of ligaments, and because their blood supply is poor, ligaments take longer to recover from exercise than muscles do. For this reason, don't work your neck hard more than twice a week. Believe it or not, just once a week works for a lot of guys.

TIP 5: SCHEDULING. The neck is a small body part and once you get used to it, it doesn't require much time or energy to train. You can train neck anytime, but after your regular bridges is a good idea because the spinal muscles are already warmed up.

TIP 6: STATIC HOLDS. Don't ever try to move your neck past the point of deep fatigue—this can lead to injury. If you are advanced, a good way to safely increase the intensity of your neck bridging is to add *static holds*. Once you finish your reps, hold the start position under tension for a few seconds. For maximum endurance, build up to sixty seconds. This technique works well with both wrestler's bridges and front bridges.

Lights out!

This chapter represents the condensed knowledge of years of training and research in an attempt to discover the perfect neck training program. And wouldn't you know it, the end result is *simple* (only two types of movements), *quick* (it takes around fifteen minutes, once or twice a week), *progressive* (there are years of harder workouts in store) and entirely based on *bodyweight training*. Even while I was doing pushups, pullups and squats every day, I still didn't realize that the ultimate solution to neck training lay hidden in old school calisthenics methods. I naturally assumed it would require harnesses, machines or other gadgets. It took a wrestler—trained in an art as old as mankind—to show me the truth. I guess you live and learn.

No matter how much knowledge I've gained throughout my training career, I always keep coming back to the same basic lessons. No matter what body part you want to train—calves, wrists, neck, even the eyes and mouth!—there's a bodyweight exercise that'll get the job done better than any equipment. There will be a way to make the exercise productive, and a way to make it progressive, right up to the limits of human potential. The knowledge is out there if you look hard enough. I know, because during my long stretches inside prison I did the looking.

11: Calf Training

Ultimate Lower Legs— No Machines Necessary

Despite the importance of the calves, it's fair to say that convicts who train probably ignore their calves more than any other muscle group. I've even seen the neck worked more than the calves inside prison, due to the number of boxers in the joint. And this is nuts, because if any "minor" body part deserves a little extra R-E-S-P-E-C-T, it's those lower legs.

Strong calves are crucial for athleticism. Nobody can run fast, jump high, or move their body explosively without plenty of calf and foot power. The seat of the body's strength lies in the waist and hips, but for the body to work as a unit the force generated by these areas must be transmitted through the feet. Watch any strongman competition, and you'll notice that these guys all have humongous calves. Strong calves are functional. Anybody who has run out of gas and had to push their car uphill will have felt their calves burn and ache as they struggle onwards and upwards. Hundreds of thousands of people in America today suffer with ankle and foot problems—through acute injuries and chronic, nagging pain—because their calves and feet are too weak.

Calves are also vital to bodybuilders. In competition, all body parts are judged on a points system, relative to various standard poses; and the calves are visible in virtually all of those poses. In his autobiography *Arnold: Education of a Bodybuilder,* Arnold Schwarzenegger emphasized the importance of calves to the whole "look" of the lower body. He pointed out that if a guy has big thighs and small calves, most people would say what bad legs he had; but if an individual has great calves and slim thighs, you'd probably think how impressive their legs were. This is true, for reasons of geometric contrast; since the calves are at the end of the legs, extra size there gives the illusion of the whole leg being more massive, and more aesthetically shaped. So whether it's pure athleticism, health or aesthetic reasons you train for, extra calf training may have big benefits to offer you.

The role of
specialized calf work

Calves should get their share of training like any other body part. But they might be getting that share of training automatically. If you are working hard on your *squats,* the calves will receive their portion of work. If you are doing explosive lower body work like *sprinting, hill/stair sprints, fireman sprints* or *car pushing* your calves will be getting a lot of great muscular exercise. (See *Convict Conditioning* volume one, chapter six for instruction and information on these great exercises.) Because the calves play such a central role in lower body training, you are already training your calves when you train your thighs. In these cases you may not need to add any specific calf work to your routine.

But there are circumstances where extra calf training might be appropriate. For example, if you have been plagued by foot, ankle or shin injuries in the past, powerful, muscular calves play a big part in protecting these areas from re-injury. This is even true in the case of knee injuries—I've spoken to football players who've blown out their ACL and swear that regular, concentrated calf training helps keep their knees stable. This isn't as unlikely as it sounds—it's a little-known fact that as well as crossing the ankles, the tendons of the calf also intersect the knees. In addition, special calf work can increase your strength levels in large compound movements like pushing or jumping, and it goes without saying that if you're embarrassed by puny lower legs when you are wearing shorts, the only solution (bar wearing long pants) is to get training your calves hard. Calf training is an interesting and rewarding aspect of calisthenics that's simple to perform and quick in results—provided you do it properly.

The myth of machines

No muscle is more associated with machine training techniques than the calves. Most bodybuilders only ever use machines to train their calves. If you ask a personal trainer about calf work, you'll find that the majority of these "experts" only know two calf exercises; standing machine calf raises, and seated calf raises. In fact, there are *dozens* of effective exercises you can do for the lower legs, many of them better than these two exercises. Far from being the best form of calf training, machine work is actually inferior to more basic methods. The largest bodybuilding machine manufacturer in the world is *Nautilus*. But for many years, Arthur Jones—the inventor and innovator behind the company—refused to put a calf training machine on the market. He believed that no machine could ever match the simple heel raise off a block, holding a dumbbell in one hand. That should tell you something about how effective machine work is for the calves. Even the guy making money from all these machines didn't want to build a calf unit, because he was convinced it would be inferior.

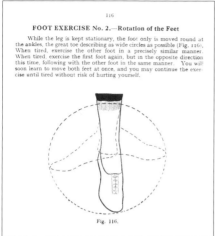

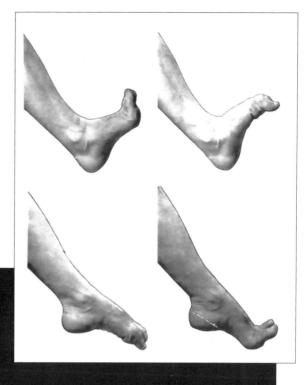

The classical systems of calisthenics all included specific exercises for the feet and lower legs. In these excerpts from J.P. Muller's 19o4 training manual you can see methods that are still considered "cutting edge" today. On the right, active flexibility techniques for the feet; above, circular

"Tougheners" for calves

Forget about machines. You don't even need free weights to build maximum calf size. All you need is your bodyweight.

Whenever I discuss calf training with bodybuilders I am inevitably met by disbelief at this statement. They can't believe that you could use bodyweight progressively to train such a small muscle. Their confusion stems from the fact that most gym-trained guys only understand one way of getting stronger—putting more weight on a bar or machine, time after time. In fact this is the most primitive way of getting stronger. It does add strength and size, but it does so at the expense of the joints and with no benefit to the important qualities of coordination and balance.

Using bodyweight techniques to become stronger is a far superior method than just adding weight to an exercise; and despite what the current crop of personal trainers mistakenly believe, you can do this for any muscle, however small. To continue getting stronger on any exercise, all you need to understand is what my own calisthenics teacher Joe Hartigen called the "tougheners" of that exercise.

All of the convict trainees stretching back centuries understood what was meant by the idea of "tougheners". A *toughener* is an element within the make-up of any given exercise that makes it harder. By manipulating the tougheners, you can make an exercise progressively more demanding, often over years of grueling training. These days, exercise scientists and Olympic coaches would use the term "intensity variables" instead of "tougheners", but they mean the same thing. Old Joe wouldn't be caught dead chewing on a phrase like "intensity variables".

After a short while into your own calisthenics training, you'll start to understand how the exercises work and be able to identify these tougheners in your own program. There are *three* basic tougheners for calves—three fundamentals you can play with to make the exercise harder over time. They are:

1. Range-of-motion: This is how far you move your heels during calf work.
2. Bilaterality/unilaterality: This is whether you use one leg or two.
3. Knee flexion: This is whether you bend your knees or keep them straight.

At a more advanced level, there are another *six* calf tougheners; *volume, inter-set rest, frequency, stance, speed of motion* and *post-failure intensity techniques.* I'll discuss some of these later, but for now let's look at the three basic tougheners listed above, and see where they get us.

Let's pick the most basic calf exercise to use these tougheners on; the *standing heel raise*, often called the *calf raise* these days. In simple terms, you just press your toes down, lifting your heels off the floor and raising your body a few inches. Descend and repeat. A simple enough concept. But it's only one exercise, right? Wrong. Let's see how progressive we can make it using the three tougheners.

For a start we will keep things fundamental and assume just *two* ranges of motion for the calf raise; you can either lift your heels up from the floor, or you can stand on your toes on a step (or any raised surface) and lift your heels up. Using a step means that the range of motion is about double what it is when you use the floor, because the heels can descend much further, all the way to their maximum flexion determined by the suppleness of the individual (compare images 15 and 16). There are lots more potential ranges between these two extremes, but let's stick with two to make things easy. So already we have two calf exercises:

> 1.   Calf raises off the floor
> 2.   Calf raises off a step

Now we consider our second toughener—bilaterality/unilaterality. In other words, on either of these exercises you can use both legs—which is obviously easier—or just one leg, which is harder. Since both the above exercises can be done with one or two legs, we now find that we actually have *four* exercises:

1. Double leg calf raises off the floor
2. Single leg calf raises off the floor
3. Double leg calf raises off a step
4. Single leg calf raises off a step

Now comes the matter of knee flexion. It's a fundamental principle of kinesiology that if you want to increase the work output of a muscle which crosses two joints, you should stretch out one of the joints while working the muscle at the other joint. The major muscle of the calf—the *gastrocnemius*—crosses two joints, the ankle and the knee. The upshot of this technical yadda is that if you really want to make your calves work hard, you need to do your calf raises with your legs totally locked at the knee. If you don't believe me, try it; stand on a step with your knees bent a little and try doing calf raises (see image 17). Fairly easy. Now lock your legs, ramrod stiff—suddenly things get significantly harder (see image 18). So using this little-known bit of sneaky anatomical knowledge, we have two more variables—bent knees and straight legs. Since the four exercises we have just listed can all be done either with bent knees or locked legs, we have doubled our exercises. Now we have eight:

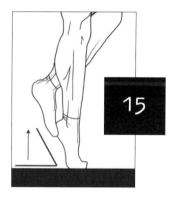

1. Double leg calf raises off the floor (bent legs)
2. Double leg calf raises off the floor (straight legs)
3. Single leg calf raises off the floor (bent leg)
4. Single leg calf raises off the floor (straight leg)
5. Double leg calf raises off a step (bent legs)
6. Double leg calf raises off a step (straight legs)
7. Single leg calf raises off a step (bent leg)
8. Single leg calf raises off a step (straight leg)

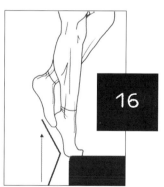

Calves are a good example of how a creative knowledge of a few different training nuances can really expand your exercise repertoire. Unfortunately in the modern clamor of "more weight on the bar" so many of these small nuances seem to have become lost. It's a real shame because they are *essential* to a master of old school calisthenics; using a little knowledge of the tougheners, we have gone from one exercise—calf raises—to *eight* different exercises. These exercises all present different levels of effort, so perhaps more importantly we have now created eight stages of difficulty for our bodyweight-only calf program.

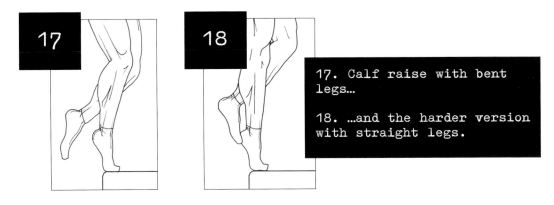

17. Calf raise with bent legs...

18. ...and the harder version with straight legs.

A sample calf series

Let's say you want to use the above eight exercises to improve your calves. Provided you take your time and really make the most out of each exercise, milking it for every bit of development it can offer you, this workout can keep you going for years. Here's a potential timetable of progression using the exercises:

STAGE 1. Double leg calf raises off the floor (bent legs)

Start off easy. Grab hold of something, or simply place your palms against the wall for support. The feet should be about shoulder width apart. Keeping your knees slightly bent, raise your heels off the floor, lifting your entire bodyweight as you do so. Pause for a full second in the top position, before slowly allowing your heels to descend again. Don't rush and pump out reps—take your time. This is a good exercise to use to get to know your calf muscles. Start with a couple of sets of twenty. This should give you a bit of a burn in the muscles; a great place to start. Gently stretch out your calves between sets for about a minute. Add a set every week until you get to four sets of twenty. Then begin adding reps. At the very most, add five reps per set every week, but don't worry about adding less if you need to go slower. Keep a written record of your reps and build up to four sets of one-hundred. If you add five reps per set each week, you will reach this goal in sixteen weeks.

BEGINNER STANDARD:	2 x 20
PROGRESSION STANDARD:	4 x 100

STAGE 2. Double leg calf raises off the floor (straight legs)

By now it's time to make the exercise a little harder on the calves. Begin the exercise again, but lock your knees completely straight. You will find that this shifts the emphasis from your ankles (the *soleus*) to the bulk of the calf higher up (the *gastrocnemius*). Drop back down to four sets of forty reps, and build up to four sets of ninety reps. Take your time in doing this. If you go fast and add five reps per set per week, you'll meet this goal in ten weeks. Continue taking a minute or so to stretch out your calves between sets.

BEGINNER STANDARD: 4 x 40

PROGRESSION STANDARD: 4 x 90

STAGE 3. Single leg calf raises off the floor (bent leg)

By now your calf muscles will be more toned than ever. The tendons will be healthy and your ankles nice and strong. Time to shift to unilateral work. Lift one leg off the floor, gently linking your non-working foot behind the ankle of the working leg to keep it out of the movement. Bend the knees by a few degrees and hold onto something for support. Now perform your strict heel raises, dropping back down to two sets of thirty reps to accommodate the fact that the weight on the muscles has nearly doubled. Alternate legs. Add a set every week for two weeks (until you are doing four sets per leg) and then lowly build up your reps again at your own pace, until you reach four sets of eighty. If you add five reps per set per week, this will take you ten weeks.

BEGINNER STANDARD: 2 x 30

PROGRESSION STANDARD: 4 x 80

STAGE 4. Single leg calf raises off the floor (straight leg)

Now repeat the procedure with straight legs, totally locked at the knee. You'll find that with a little bend in the knee, you can cheat slightly as you become tired by pushing through your legs on the difficult, painful final reps. When you start and finish with locked legs, this is impossible—you must use pure calf power. Stretching between sets, drop back down to four sets of thirty and build back up. By building up five reps per set per week, you'll reach your goal of four sets of seventy reps in eight weeks. If you need to go slower—if your form starts to get messy—only add a rep or two each week.

BEGINNER STANDARD: 4 x 30

PROGRESSION STANDARD: 4 x 70

STAGE 5. Double leg calf raises off a step (bent legs)

By now—if you have been doing your exercises under full muscular control—your calf muscles will be much fitter and possess real stamina. It's time to increase the range of motion. Hop up onto a step. If a step isn't available you can use a cinderblock or thick piece of wood—anything high enough to allow your heels to hang down. In prison I often used law manuals. If you are going to wear shoes, wear some flimsy sneakers—thick boots will take pressure off the feet and this is not what you want; you *want* this exercise to develop the soles of your feet, toes and arches as well. (A chain is only as strong as its weakest link—so make *everything* strong!)

Famous bodybuilder and the first Mr Olympia Larry Scott used to do his calf raises barefoot, and if you can too if you find this comfortable. It really depends on the platform you are using. Again, hold onto something (like a guide rail) for support. Shuffle back so that only the balls of your feet are on the step. For this exercise, your feet should be closer together—nearly touching—to put even more pressure on the calf muscles. Bend the knees slightly, and keep them more or less bent throughout the exercise. Now, slowly descend until your heels are as low down as they will go, and pause in that position. Smoothly drive the heels up as high as they will go, until you are on tiptoes. Pause for another second, contracting the calves hard. Repeat this for twenty reps.

Now that your calves are in good shape from their training, it's a good time to step up your stretching. Instead of hopping off the step and grabbing your swollen lower legs when you complete a set, keep your heels in the lowest position, pushing them down as far as they will go. At first, this stretch will seem like torture, but persist—it will improve "supple strength" and enhance your ability to tolerate pain and perform high reps. Stretch this way for sixty seconds (or twenty breaths) and *immediately* begin your second set. Shoot for two sets of thirty reps. Add a set per week for two weeks, then begin building up your reps until you can manage four sets of sixty reps. Stretch hard after each set. If you add two reps per set each week—and this will be more than plenty at this stage—you will reach your goal in fifteen weeks.

BEGINNER STANDARD:	2 x 30
PROGRESSION STANDARD:	4 x 60

STAGE 6. Double leg calf raises off a step (straight legs)

Repeat the above exercise, but with your legs entirely locked during the calf raises *as well as* during the stretching after the sets. This will really burn up those calves. The new position may mean that you gradually begin working your way fractionally backwards during the exercise. That's fine. If this ever happens during calf work just reposition yourself so that you are stable and continue. Drop to four sets of thirty and build up to four sets of fifty. Adding a couple of reps to every set each week will get you where you want to go in ten weeks. This exercise—with strict form, high reps and all the stretching—should be considered intermediate level. If you need to drop to one rep per week, even one rep every two weeks, do so. The name of the game is getting better in little chunks. As long as you can do this for an extended period, you'll get damn good. Far from screwing up improvement, slowing up often just lengthens the time you are able to make progress.

BEGINNER STANDARD:	4 x 30
PROGRESSION STANDARD:	4 x 50

STAGE 7. Single leg calf raises off a step (bent leg)

Time to get those calves *really* strong. Link your non-working foot behind your working ankle, bend at the knee and perform an extremely strict calf raise. Go at least two seconds up, one second at the top, two seconds down, one second at the bottom. This will build genuine strength. Start with two sets of fifteen, stretching after the sets by pushing your heel down as far as it will go for a minute (or twenty breaths). The added proportional weight will drive your heel down even further than in the bilateral version and the stretch combined with the strict calf raises will make for a very severe workout. Alternate your legs by doing one set then stretching, immediately doing a set with the other leg, then stretching. If you can, continue with this rep range, adding another set every four weeks. This will give your calves the chance they need to really grow and get stronger, as well as allowing the Achilles tendon and ankles to properly adapt to the rigors of the unilateral work. After two months, you'll be doing four strict sets of fifteen and—provided you have worked patiently through the exercises I have laid out—it should be relatively easy. Add no more than two reps per set weekly until you reach the target of four sets of forty-five. At minimum, this will take fifteen weeks.

BEGINNER STANDARD:	2 x 15
PROGRESSION STANDARD:	4 x 45

STAGE 8. *Single leg calf raises off a step (straight leg)*

The same exercise as given above, but with a perfectly straight working leg. You know the drill by now. The single leg calf raise off a step—with perfect form, a straight leg, a maximum stretch at the bottom and a tight contraction at the top—is one of the hardest calf exercises known. A lot of people think it's easy, but when you watch them they bend their knees and bounce, using momentum to help them from their very first rep. The key is to pause at the bottom. Don't bounce. And move smoothly; don't go faster during one portion of the rep than another. Maintain an even cadence throughout. These sound like little things, but they turn a so-so exercise into a real monster. Start with four sets of thirty (if you can) and build up by adding no more than *one rep per week* until you are doing four sets of fifty reps per leg. This will take you twenty weeks, provided you can maintain the pace. If not, go slower.

BEGINNER STANDARD:	4 x 30
PROGRESSION STANDARD:	4 x 50

Warm ups and rest

Calves need time to rest like any other muscle group and for strength they should be worked only once or twice a week. As usual, pay attention to your body and attend to its needs while you train. The ankles are usually a very robust joint, kept warm by carrying the body around all day, so you might never feel the need for a warm up. But if you do, just start the session with a high rep set of an easy exercise two or three steps back in the series from where you've reached. Whenever I do calf work I do it immediately after squats, and I find that my calves are already nice and heated by then.

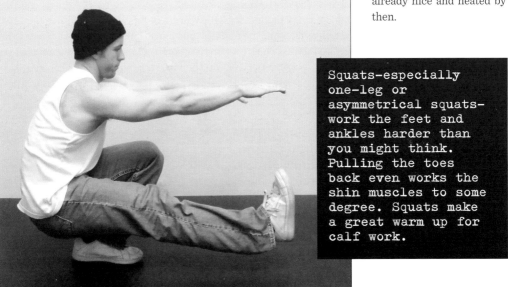

Squats—especially one-leg or asymmetrical squats—work the feet and ankles harder than you might think. Pulling the toes back even works the shin muscles to some degree. Squats make a great warm up for calf work.

Too many progressions..?

When I show guys on the outside how to train calves with bodyweight, many of 'em ask: *Why do I need a lotta slightly different calf exercises? Why don't I just jump to the hardest one?*

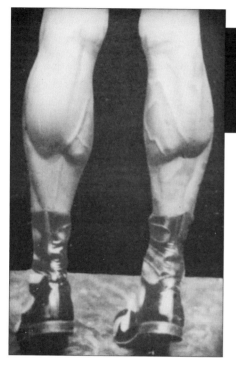

Huge weights aren't necessary to build perfect calves. These lower legs belong to Indian muscle control expert, Chanchal Prosad (c. 1930).

This is the wrong attitude. It's a big mistake to rush to the hardest exercises you can handle. Your goal is not to finish with an exercise as fast as you can—just the opposite. Your goal should be to stay with an exercise *for as long as you can possibly get conditioning gains from it.* This is the prison attitude. If you are going to be training your calves (or your pecs, or delts) alone in your cell for three years, why would you want to skip to the hardest exercise there is? There's nowhere to go from there.

This is not just a bodyweight-style training approach, either. Virtually all champion bodybuilders train this way. They don't train with limit weights from workout to workout. They train hard, but they use a "working weight" lighter than their max, and find ways to make that weight seem heavier. They milk each weight increase for all it's worth. You should do the same.

A prison athlete is not a gymnast or dancer. You don't get judged on the difficulty of your movements—just your results. In old school calisthenics, difficult movements aren't the goal. They are just *tools* to help you achieve your goals (strength and muscle). You are using these calf exercises to develop solid muscle and tendon, to put strength in the bank. This takes time. Please don't rush ahead of your body's own ability to adapt. Remember: you are using these exercises to *build* strength—not to *demonstrate* it.

Commitment to power

Maximizing a lagging body part—especially a minor muscle like the calves, famously slow to respond—really isn't complex or sophisticated. But it will require application, willpower and above all *commitment*. If you follow the above routine as I suggest, it will take more than two years to complete. For some people it will be closer to three years. This is how real muscle and conditioning is gained; slowly, patiently, intelligently. But if you follow the program as I advise, proceeding slowly, you will gain tons of strength almost without realizing it. You will thoroughly transform your lower legs. By the time you reach the end you will have packed inches of dense meat onto your calves, and they will possess more athletic ability (endurance, tendon strength, tension-flexibility) than you would have ever believed possible. Try challenging somebody who thinks they have great calf power—maybe a bodybuilder or even a runner or a military man—to doing four sets of fifty strict unilateral calf raises off a step. It'll be fun watching them collapse to the floor before they even get halfway, clutching their flaming, cramped-up calf muscles.

Never forget that long-term commitment to calisthenics training is actually far easier to maintain than interest in other forms of training. This is because cell routines are as hassle-free as training gets. The sessions detailed above will only take minutes to complete, and they'll require no special equipment. You can train your calves anywhere, anytime.

Advanced calf tips

Most trainees will find that by the time they have built up to four sets of fifty in the strict straight leg calf raise, their calves will be about as thick and powerful as they'd ever want. But the road goes ever on. If you get to an advanced stage of calf training and you feel the need to add something that'll take your lower leg fitness to the next level, explore some of these ideas, cribbed from my own little black book of calf training secrets:

- ### *INTENSITY TECHNIQUES:*

When you have trained your calves with full-range reps to failure, try "burns"—keep on doing half-range reps from the midpoint up to the top. When you reach exhaustion on these, continue just bobbing up and down a couple of inches until your calves are completely paralyzed. Then get off the stairs, place your feet together and hop up and down twenty or thirty times. When you're done with that, perform knees-high running on the spot for a full minute...if you can. If this doesn't give you the best calf workout of your life, you are probably a Terminator or something.

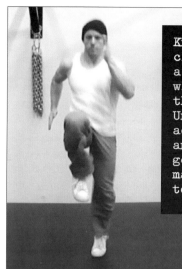

Knees-high running on the spot is a classic cell exercise. It's often used as a stamina workout, but it can be combined with calf strength techniques to push those feet and lower legs to new limits. Unlike machine training, this kind of addition builds speed, fast-twitch power, and total-body athleticism. Use it as a gentle warm up or a brutal finisher. For maximum calf development, stay on your toes!

become very strong, and using over a thousand pounds on a standing machine is common for bodybuilders. Unfortunately this weight passes through the shoulders, spine and hips, screwing up the back and ruining the body's natural alignment. Instead of thinking in terms of *strength* for shocking the calves, focus on *higher reps*. Once in a while shoot for very high reps in a set—a hundred, two hundred, or even more. Really test yourself, but be prepared for soreness the next day.

• NONSTOP SETS:

The calves respond well to high reps, but increasing beyond four sets of fifty is excessive for most purposes. If you want to work on stamina, try this instead; quit alternating your single leg calf sets. Build up to the point where you can plough through all four sets *on one leg*—with a good hard stretch after each set to break things up. This will give you calves of iron.

• INTEGRATION TRAINING:

The calf raise series I gave you isolates the calf muscles. Condition your calves to move as a unit with the entire body by exploring disciplines like *hill sprints, car pushing*, etc.

• EXPLOSIVE WORK:

Once you have built your calf strength, learn to use that strength explosively. The best exercise for this is jumping.

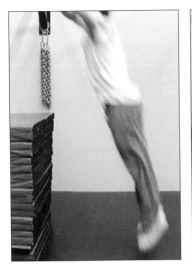
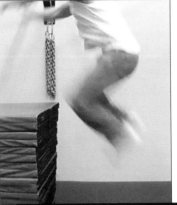
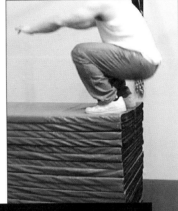

"Plyometric" training-plain old jumping!-is great for adding useful power to the feet and ankles. It's also another excellent way to work the calves in coordination with the rest of the body's muscles.

- *CIRCULAR MOBILITY:*

Keep the tiny muscles of the ankles supple and strong. Often nagging ankle pain can be removed completely by a few sets of *ankle rotations* performed on alternating days. Just sit down, raise your feet and draw circles with your toes as wide as you can for ten reps in either direction. This exercise serves as a brilliant cool down to remove tension from the legs after an intense calf workout. Try it.

- *RECIPROCAL DEVELOPMENT:*

It's difficult building incredibly powerful muscles on one side of a limb if the muscles on the other side of the limb are weak and feeble. The body seems to sense the disparity and slow down your development. If you really want to maximize your calves, work on their antagonistic muscles—the *anterior tibialis* at the front of the shin. Pull your toes and insteps up as high as you can, until the shin starts to burn. Extend the toes fully outwards again, and repeat for high reps. Keeping these muscles healthy and strong will go a long way to reducing injuries like shin splints. One guy I knew at San Quentin used to train his shins by hanging upside-down from the pullup station with his feet hooked over the bar holding him. Try this for a couple of minutes if you think you have strong shins!

If you are really interested in pushing your calves to their absolute limit, these techniques are a must. Use them sparingly and focus on your progressive bodyweight work first and foremost and you'll get the calves you want—not just muscular and strong but swift, agile, supple and healthy—with more endurance than you ever believed possible.

Lights out!

It's ironic that no body part is more associated with machines than the calves, because calves are probably the simplest muscle group to effectively train using bodyweight. This makes perfect sense if you think about it; during any given day the average Joe might not stress out his pecs, back or biceps, but with every step he takes the individual calf muscles are moving the entire weight of his body. In a sense, you are training your calves just by walking around. Have you ever noticed how fat guys inevitably have really thick, stocky calves? Some of that is chub, but probably not as much as you might think—the body tends to pile lard on around its own centre of gravity, and doesn't like putting it on the extremities like the calves. A lot of the mass is muscle, earned purely by carrying around a heavy body for thousands of reps each day.

Calves are not intimidating or macho, and they're not a muscle group that'll directly help you in a fight. For these reasons, many convicts neglect specific calf training. It's true that if you are doing lots of hard leg work, you might not even require extra calf training. But if you do, forget the status quo theory of huge weights on machines. Focus instead on bodyweight training methods, apply picture perfect form, progressive exercise, high reps, explosive work and plenty of discipline. Before you know it, your calves will resemble massive diamonds in their shape and hardness!

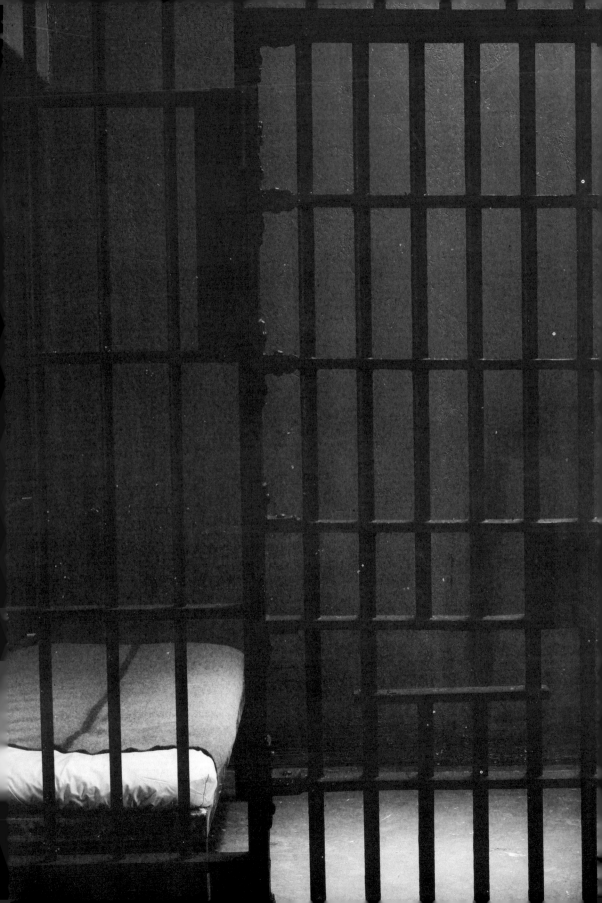

— PART II —

BULLETPROOF JOINTS

One of the most crucial aspects of strength development and bodybuilding is *joint training*. If your joints are weak, there's no way you can be strong-at least, not for long, and not without a whole heap of pain. It takes years to build real, drug-free muscle, and your body can only do it if you build your joints *up* along the way. It's a tragedy that most wannabe big dudes misuse weights and machines that wear their joints *down*!

In this section, I'll teach you how to build super-powerful joints using calisthenics, how to develop mobility without becoming lax and weak, and how to tune-up a rusted and seized physique. No equipment, no supplements, just techniques I picked up behind the bars.

12: TENSION-FLEXIBILITY

THE LOST ART
OF
JOINT TRAINING

I f the old time prison bodyweight masters had one lesson in common about how to build ferociously strong joints, it would be this: always, always train to generate what Joe Hartigen called "supple strength" in the "sinews". The old timers all would've recognized the concept of *supple strength*, but because it might mean different things today, I'm going to update the term and call it *tension-flexibility*. If there's one key or "secret" to strong tendons and soft tissues, you can find it right here.

What is tension-flexibility?

Tension-flexibility is the capacity of a muscle to remain tensed and strong even though it is stretched, or elongated.

Tendons have *evolved* to be tensed and powerful when on the stretch. It's what makes them *springy* and allows animals (or us) to jump, hop, sprint or perform explosive movements. In nature, if stretched muscles were flaccid and relaxed, most forms of strength and power would be impossible.

This view of "flexibility" is one that modern bodyweight strength athletes and gymnasts will know all about, although it's very much at odds with the *general* concept of flexibility found in the everyday fitness world. When most coaches talk about flexibility, they automatically associate it with *relaxation*. This is largely because passive training methods involve deliberate relaxation techniques. It's taken for granted that a muscle being stretched *needs* to be relaxed. But does it?

For sure, for voluntary movement to be possible, the muscles on one side of a joint must contract harder than the opposite side. But it doesn't follow that the muscles on the other side cannot contract *at all*. They can tense quite hard, in fact—as long as they're *not* tensing *harder* than the muscles on the opposite side, movement will still occur.

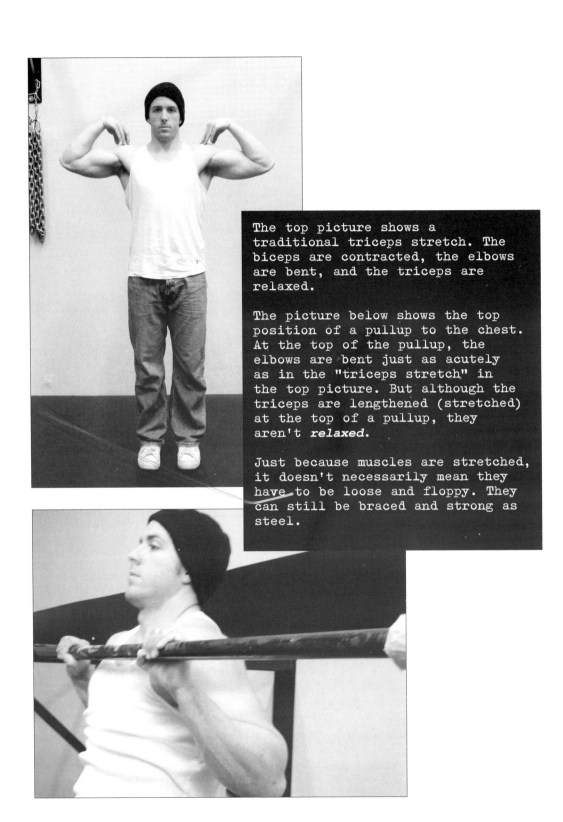

The top picture shows a traditional triceps stretch. The biceps are contracted, the elbows are bent, and the triceps are relaxed.

The picture below shows the top position of a pullup to the chest. At the top of the pullup, the elbows are bent just as acutely as in the "triceps stretch" in the top picture. But although the triceps are lengthened (stretched) at the top of a pullup, they aren't *relaxed*.

Just because muscles are stretched, it doesn't necessarily mean they have to be loose and floppy. They can still be braced and strong as steel.

We can think of lots of examples where a muscle needs to be stretched *and* powerfully contracted simultaneously. Here's one example. If you wanted to stretch out your quadriceps, and the tendons of the knee, what would you do? Most athletes would probably grab their ankles and pull their heels into their butts, like this:

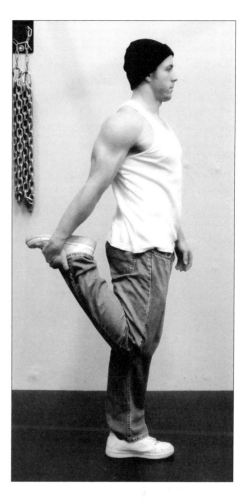

For sure, this movement is a good example of *relaxation-flexibility*. The muscles of the quadriceps are being relaxed, and the knee joint is being stretched out. But what if I asked the same athlete to pop down and do a one-leg squat?

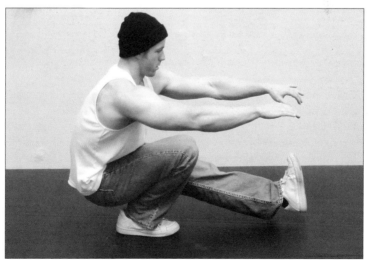

The one-leg squat is generally seen as a great *strength* exercise. It sure as hell isn't seen as a *stretching* exercise. But you can see from this picture that Max's knee is fully bent. In fact, it's bent *even more* than when he was deliberately stretching his knee by pulling on his ankle. But despite the fact that the quad and knee tendons are stretched to the limit, they are still generating a lot of tension in this position. In fact, it's obvious that they must generate a large amount of tension in the fully bent position—if they couldn't, Max wouldn't be able to begin moving and stand up straight again. Pressing variations like the *uneven pushup* are upper body analogs to the squat. In the uneven pushup, the elbows are bent to the max, but the triceps still have to generate high levels of strength and tension to press the athlete up.

It's not just the quad that's stretched in this bottom squat position, either. Scan the photo again and catch a look at Max's right hip. This joint is also being stretched. The glute is stretched so far that his thigh is compressed up against his trunk! But that glute is tensed like a rock to maintain this position, and it's about to become the motor that pushes his bodyweight up. The ankle is also highly flexed. So you can see from this simple example that a stretched muscle can also be a very powerful muscle.

Let me give you another quick example. Look at these two pictures:

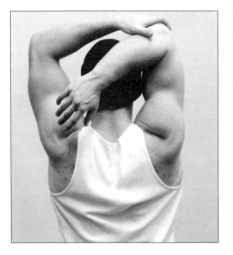 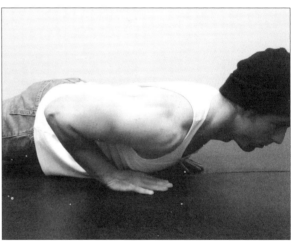

In both images, the athlete is stretching out the triceps muscle of the upper arm. The shot on the left is a good example of the kind of *relaxed-flexibility* found in passive stretching. Max is relaxing his arm muscles and pulling his forearm so that the elbow is bent as much as possible to stretch out his right triceps. In the shot on the right, Max isn't *trying* to stretch at all—he's just doing a close pushup. But you can see that, for the pushup, Max's elbow is bent to at least the same degree—in fact his bicep is pressing hard on his forearm. Are his triceps *relaxed*? No way! They are tight and tensed as hell. Even the wrists are bent and stretched, but taut as steel. If Max relaxed his muscles now he'd collapse!

Strong joints and calisthenics

The take-home message? Tension and flexibility aren't enemies. They go hand-in-hand when it comes to producing strong tendons and powerful joints. Whatever training floats your boat, make sure you gradually build supple strength, or your joints will get proportionately weaker over time—even as your muscles get stronger. This is a dangerous combination.

Many athletes are surprised that strength training in the gym seems to give them aches, pains and injuries, while calisthenics strength training keeps their joints strong, fresh and pain free. There are several reasons for this, but one of the main reasons is that bodyweight exercises develop high levels of tension-flexibility. The basic exercises involve a full range of motion—full squats, close pushups, pullups, etc. Because the extended muscles and tendons are under load in these movements, they are an ideal way to build "supple strength". Just as important, because *Convict Conditioning* is divided into gradual, manageable stages (the ten steps) it allows you to build tendon strength slowly. It helps you walk before you can run.

Compare this with a more modern approach, like bodybuilding. Far from taking steps to develop their supple strength, most of these guys do the exact opposite. Instead of building tension-flexibility in their joints by loading their tendons on the stretch, they often *avoid* full range movements. Instead of full squats, they load up the leg press with huge weights for partial reps. And they all wonder why they have knee problems after just a few months! They shun "supple strength" and favor machines which pump up their muscles using peak contractions, stimulating the muscle bellies but doing nothing for the tendons and joints.

You'll never see a big-ass bodybuilder perform a one-leg squat or a full one-arm pushup. Their joints would rip in half. These guys pile on muscle as quickly as they can, but fail to realize that the joints and tendons adapt more slowly than the muscles. Instead of smooth, gradual development, everything grows and adapts at the wrong speed. On top of this mess, many bodybuilders have bought into passive flexibility ideas. They train these huge muscles to be loose and limp under force. As a result, when they trip, slip or have to lift something awkward, bad things often happen. Big, impressive muscles *do not* equal strong, healthy joints.

The most popular in-gym moves build muscle, but not joint strength!

Compare some popular in-gym movements with their prison bodyweight counterparts, and you'll get a good idea of why calisthenics movements naturally build tension-flexibility better.

In the gym, most lifters use dumbbell curls to work the biceps. But at the bottom position, where the arm hangs down, the biceps are hardly under tension at all.

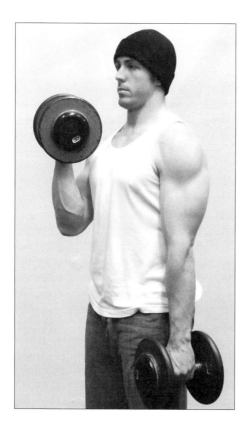

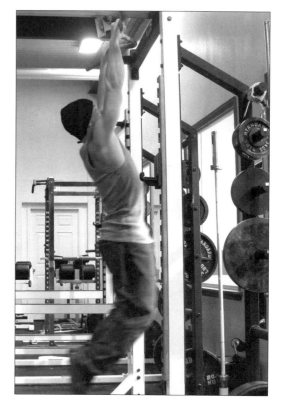

Compare this to a properly executed pullup—the arms are kept "soft" meaning that the elbows are slightly, almost imperceptibly, kinked. Not only does this prevent hyperextension, it keeps the elongated biceps under full tension when they are lengthened.

Machines are used more and more in gyms, because they deliver "peak contractions" at the top of a movement. They rarely develop supple strength. Here, an athlete works his anterior shoulder girdle with front cable raises. This will contract (and build) the *muscles* due to the contraction at the top, but what about the *joints?* Where's the tension at the bottom?

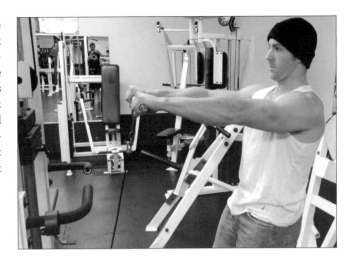

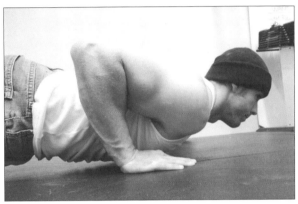

Contrast this with a *lever pushup*—the front delts are forced to retain tension strongly at the bottom, while they are on the stretch. Both the muscles and the joints are developed simultaneously.

I could produce enough examples to fill a whole book, but you get the message. Tension-flexibility is a dead concept for modern trainers.

Do you relax when you stretch? Think again.

The idea of "supple strength"—of having muscles and tendons which are *strong* while stretched—is totally at odds with most modern training methods. Contemporary methods focus on the *opposite* approach—they teach athletes to *relax* their muscles while stretching. This is the key to most "passive stretching" methods which pass for flexibility training today.

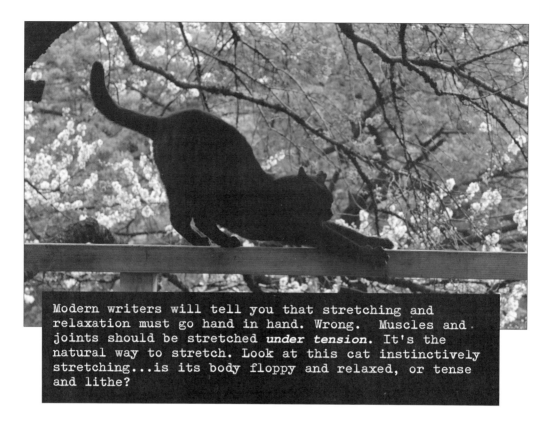

Modern writers will tell you that stretching and relaxation must go hand in hand. Wrong. Muscles and joints should be stretched **under tension**. It's the natural way to stretch. Look at this cat instinctively stretching...is its body floppy and relaxed, or tense and lithe?

Why do modern coaches and trainers teach their athletes to relax during stretching exercises? The reason is obvious. Relaxing while stretching increases the range-of-motion (ROM) of the stretch. It makes it appear that you are more flexible than you really are. But do you really need this "extra" flexibility that relaxation-stretching can give you? For sure, close pushups, deep squats and full pullups contract and extend the muscles over a healthy range-of-motion, but they will never turn you into a contortionist. The question is, do you need this extra artificial range?

Extra ROM from relaxed stretching techniques sounds kinda cool, I admit. But it's actually a double-edged sword. Relaxing into a flexibility exercise only helps you stretch further because it desensitizes the receptors in your soft tissue—called *muscle spindles*. Normally the muscle spindles work hard to stop your muscles from overstretching, but gradual relaxed stretching "tricks" them into thinking nothing's wrong. (Like when you put a frog in a pot of cool water and slowly heat it up to boiling—the frog's nervous system won't notice if you do it gradually. The principle is similar.) This desensitization process allows the muscles to stretch further than normal; but it takes time—usually at least several minutes. This loosening up period might help you increase your max ROM, but here's the nut-punch: *you need to perform that loosening up stage again if you want to access the increased ROM in the future.* You might see a lot of karate guys pull off impressive kicks in the dojo, but outside on the street, there's no way they can perform those same moves. So there's something fishy about all that extra ROM.

The old timers I trained with in jail all shared the same view, maybe for different reasons though. Joe Hartigen, my mentor in SQ, always emphasized that—far from giving you strong joints—relaxed stretching exercises gave you lax, weak joints. I heard similar views from many advanced, knowledgeable bodyweight strength guys stuck behind bars: if you want bulletproof joints, stick with your supple strength training—full range calisthenics movements with bridging and leg raises thrown in. Modern "cutting edge" articles over the last few years talk about stretching like it's the goddam Holy Grail of injury prevention, but a lot of the old timers believed the exact opposite: relaxed stretching made you more prone to injury!

Ironically, science is only now catching up with those old prison dinosaurs. In an effort to improve the performance of their warriors, the US Army recently conducted an extensive study on the relationship between relaxation-flexibility and injury prevention.* Guess what? Soldiers with the highest levels of flexibility were *more* prone to injuries than soldiers with average levels of flexibility!

Brace yourself: Myotatic reflexes save the day

Why do athletes with high levels of relaxation-flexibility get injured more than "tenser" athletes? The answer is that passive stretching methods are based on *relaxation under force*. They train your muscles to *relax* under pressure. This is totally contrary to what your body wants to do.

Let me ask you a question: why do joints get injured in the first place? Virtually all joint injuries are caused when ligaments, tendons and soft tissues *are stretched too far*. These materials can be stretched up to a point, but beyond that point, they rip and split. The results can be devastating.

Knee ligaments split, bursae are torn, shoulder capsules are ripped open, wrists and elbows dislocate and pop out of place. These horrors are all the result of joint tissues being overstretched.

Luckily, Mother Nature is real clever. Your body intuitively understands this risk of overstretching the joints, and has put safety-measures in place to prevent it happening. These natural safety measures are called *myotatic reflexes*. These reflexes are very ancient, primitive, and totally involuntary. Whenever a muscle is exposed to sudden, shocking forces, it contracts. This is a direct result of the myotatic reflex. The classic "knee-jerk" reflex is an example of this phenomenon. If you strike the tendon of the kneecap, even lightly, the quad muscles will contract to protect the joint.

*Physical Training and Exercise-Related Injuries Surveillance, Research and Injury Prevention Military in Populations. (US Army Center for Health Promotion and Preventive Medicine)

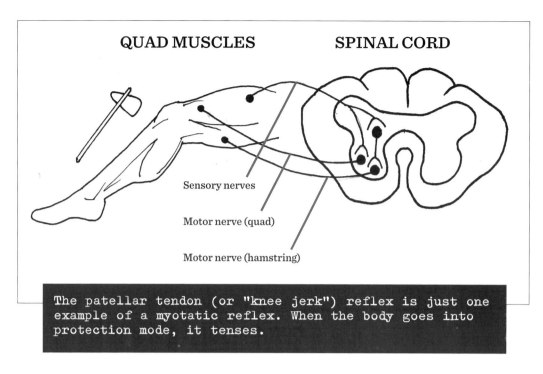

QUAD MUSCLES　　　**SPINAL CORD**

Sensory nerves

Motor nerve (quad)

Motor nerve (hamstring)

The patellar tendon (or "knee jerk") reflex is just one example of a myotatic reflex. When the body goes into protection mode, it tenses.

To put it simply, when your body gets a shock, it *tenses*. It braces itself, automatically. Do you remember the last time you were walking down the stairs and missed a step? As soon as your body felt the extra jolt of force when you hit the next step, your lower body will have undergone a series of myotatic reflexes—your leg will have tensed. It might be embarrassing to look like a spaz suddenly jerking to attention like that, but trust me, your body does it for a good reason. Tensed muscles absorb shock safely. If you relax when you take a tumble, all that extra force has only one place to go—through the joints. Without muscle and tendon to protect them, joints are fairly easy to injure. Even mild pressure in the wrong direction can easily dislocate a shoulder. If the knee is twisted in the wrong direction by just a few degrees, the ACL can be torn—forever. I could go on and on.

Relaxation and injury

One of the reasons that passive stretching is so dangerous is that it gradually de-activates your body's vital myotatic reflexes. It replaces tension with *relaxation*. Great if you are in a hot tub—not so great if you are using your body to actually do something challenging.

A relaxed body is incredibly easy to injure. This is as true for the trunk as for the arms and legs. A single punch can end a fight, if a boxer's not ready for it—and by "ready" I mean "tensed". Just ask a karate fighter. For centuries, those dudes have been performing tension exercises. When they get struck, they *need* their muscles and tendons to be taut and strong to act as armor for their internal organs. Their training supports their myotatic reflexes, and makes them more indestruct-

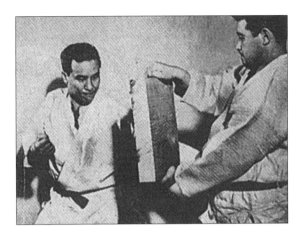

ible in combat. Gymnasts brace for a landing, as do parachutists. Even Olympic divers retain body-tension when they hit the water. In any discipline where big forces are suddenly introduced to the body and the chance of injury is high, athletes are taught how to support their myotatic reflexes by maintaining the right kind of muscular tension.

Don't believe that flower power bulls*** that a relaxed body is impossible to damage. We've all heard the old wives' tale that drunks rarely get hurt when they fall over, because their bodies are relaxed. It's just that; an old wives' tale. Talk to medics who work in the Emergency Room over any given weekend. The vast majority of injuries they are forced to deal with are alcohol related. Falling onto concrete braced is bad enough, but falling relaxed like a drunk is a sure way to really hurt yourself. It might even kill you—many drunken falls result in severe head injuries because the cervical spine is too relaxed to contract and prevent the head from striking asphalt. Excess alcohol can interfere with the nervous system and make your myotatic reflexes sluggish, but this ain't a good thing. Getting wasted might be fun, but it certainly doesn't protect you from injury. Just the opposite.

Tension-flexibility: a caveat

Exercises which generate high levels of tension-flexibility (like *one-leg squats*) strengthen the joints like nothing else. But you can't launch into them overnight. Your tendons and soft tissues can and will adapt to these exercises, but you need to give the body the correct preparations—which is the reason why progressive calisthenics begins with gentle steps which allow the tendons to strengthen at their own speed. Rushing into hard "supple strength" exercises, such as *close pushups* might give the *illusion* of ability, but athletes who slowly build up to these exercises will have stronger and healthier joints in the long run. Tension-flexibility exercises can be tough. (Which is why many bodybuilders purposefully avoid them.)

Another important point to make is that your muscles need to be elongated under load during tension-flexibility training. But "elongated" does not mean "hyper-extended". Moving your limbs in their normal range is perfect. You don't need (or want) to become a contortionist to gain maximum supple strength.

One last word of advice. When training your muscles to be strong while stretched, stick only to those exercises which mimic your natural biomechanics. Steer clear of anything forced or painful. Heavy pressing or pulldowns with a bar behind your neck might stretch your muscles under load, but they also put your rotator cuffs in a vulnerable position. The same is true for most fixed barbell presses and many machine exercises. Avoid.

BRACED FOR STRENGTH

The old time strongmen understood that hard contractions were the key to powerful joints. You didn't find them doing any faggy aromatherapy or freeform dancing to "loosen up". Instead of *relaxing* their joints, these dudes did the exact opposite: the real powerhouses utilized "support lifts", where the body was locked in one position and weight loaded on or lifted over a tiny distance. When I say "weight" I mean *real* weight! When Louis Cyr wanted to train his joints, he "back pressed" 4337 lbs. Warren Lincoln Travis held 3985 lbs in the harness lift. Strongfort kept aloft 3.5 tons in the "human bridge" support hold. The great John Grimek routinely supported over a thousand pounds overhead.

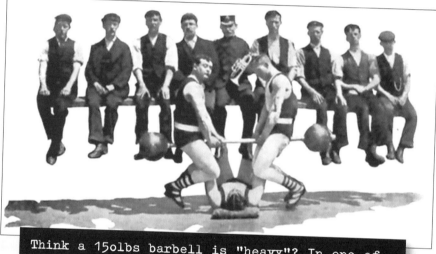

Think a 15olbs barbell is "heavy"? In one of his incredible feats, Saxon supported that barbell-plus eleven men!

These support lifts forced the muscles to flex as tightly as possible around the joints, making for a super-strong protective sleeve. I wouldn't advise anyone to actually copy feats like this, because the risks involved are too high; but this kind of work undeniably produced ultra-strong tendons and joints. The forces used were so heavy, they even went through the bones themselves, stimulating and thickening the ligaments that hold the joints together!

Lights out!

If you want high levels of supple strength, you don't need to use fancy machines, bizarre exercises or expensive "supplements". The best thing you can do is skip the modern stuff and stick to good old-fashioned calisthenics, using bodyweight. Be progressive—begin training the movements in a full-range of motion, but with very little resistance (*jackknife squats, wall pushups* and *vertical pulls* are great examples). Build up slowly until you are moving the bulk of your bodyweight (*full squats, full pushups* and *full pullups*), then push things further by going on to only one limb (*one-leg squats, one-arm pushups* and *one-arm pullups*). This is the approach I learnt in prison, and it not only gives you incredibly powerful joints, it also helps you get that power *safely*, because you give your tendons and soft tissues time to adapt to the demands of tension-flexibility. Following this kind of "supple strength" routine should be the cornerstone of your training if you want strong, healthy joints.

13: STRETCHING—THE PRISON TAKE

FLEXIBILITY,
MOBILITY,
CONTROL

It seems like, on the outside, everyone everywhere is all about getting flexible. They are bending themselves into weird mathematical shapes, learning the splits, yadda yadda yadda. A gym just ain't a gym without stretching mats. Stretching is an integral part of each and every workout. (It even gets its own special sessions.) Many athletes are spending more time stretching than working out! Flexibility is seen as a core component of fitness, these days. If you don't favor stretching, you're a dinosaur, a barbarian.

You don't see this behind bars.

Inside jails, athletes focus on *strength* first and foremost. Where flexibility exists, it exists hand-in-hand with strength. You see it in bridges, high leg raises, in calisthenics exercises performed with a full range of motion. Flexibility for its own sake? You might see guys doing light stretching in between sets to loosen up muscles over-pumped with blood and waste. You might see guys stretching and flexing a little to help them prepare for a specific muscular exercise. And you will probably see cons gently stretching out muscles tightened up by scar tissue and injury. Beyond that? Nothing. Nada. Prison athletes don't see the point of stretching—and they certainly don't practice stretching for its own sake.

Guess which approach I buy into?

Flexibility should be a by-product of calisthenics

Prison athletes don't focus on stretching, because they understand that flexibility without strength is useless. Good mobility should come as a by-product of correct strength training. The calisthenics masters I trained with had no interest in "flexibility". They were primarily interested in proper "extension" (i.e., *range-of-motion*) of strength techniques. This is what naturally gave them "supple strength". They often spoke of "tendon training" or joint work, but never *flexibility*. Being a contortionist for the sake of it? They weren't interested in that. Why would they be? This worship of flexibility is a modern idea.

Old time bodyweight athletes didn't stay up nights worrying about their flexibility. They thought only in terms of *strength*. Strength is *control*—whether control of your body, control of a weight, or what-ever. (Shoving, pushing or heaving something may represent *power* or *speed*, but not *strength*.) Having the strength to control your body is *essential*. Having levels of flexibility which exceed that control is *not* essential—it's *counter-productive*. What's the point of possessing muscles which can be stretched beyond the point your strength can control? That just leaves you liable to injury.

Strength + flexibility = mobility

People often confuse *flexibility* with *mobility*. This is a mistake. Mobility is *the ability to move your-self.* Mobility, therefore, is based on strength first, and flexibility second. Examples of mobility—running, leaping, dodging—are dependent upon muscle power primarily. Tight muscles are undesirable, sure. But the flexibility athletes really require is automatically generated by *muscular movement,* rather than passive stretching exercises. Truly mobile, agile animals all possess supple strength; tension-flexibility, rather than relaxation-flexibility. Think *panther,* baby!

This idea of mobility as primarily *strength-based* is as true in everyday life as it is in athletics. Standing on one leg and lifting up the other leg to put a sock on requires a certain level of strength (control) to raise your foot up to your hands. It doesn't matter how *passively* flexible you are—how high you can raise your foot up when someone else is pushing it. This is not mobility. If you can't raise your foot by yourself, that theoretical flexibility is wasted. Useless.

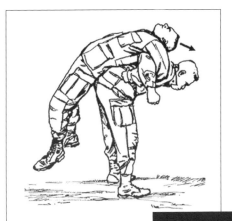
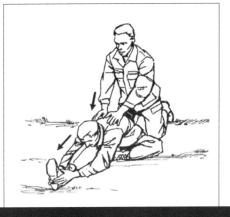

If a buddy bends your spine for you, does that count as true mobility? Compare these two passive stretches with bridges and L-holds (ch. 14).

Convict Conditioning and flexibility

This is where most prison athletes are coming from. The old bodyweight guys weren't savages who were too dumb to appreciate the cutting-edge benefits of stretching. They just saw the true relationship between flexibility and strength more clearly than most modern athletes. They knew damn well that having high levels of flexibility without the strength to control it is like having a raging inferno without a strong steel furnace to constrain and direct it. It might look impressive, but in reality it's useless and dangerous. The strength has to come first.

This old school attitude is reflected in *Convict Conditioning*. I want you to build *strength* and *mobility*. Flexibility? Only as it goes hand-in-hand with strength. I teach all my students to train their muscles with a deep range of motion. Even where I promote half or partial movements, these are always combined in a workout with full range techniques. Full pushups, full squats, full pullups. Always.

Look at specific joint training techniques I promote—like the *twists*, *bridges* and *L-holds* of the *Trifecta* (see chapter fourteen). To the untrained eye, they might *look* like flexibility exercises. But in fact, when performed correctly, they require more *strength* than flexibility. The *muscles* should be leading the movement—where the movement fails, it's because the leading muscles cannot contract hard enough. "Flexibility" is just along for the ride. You *will* iron out tight muscles using my methods, and you will certainly maximize your mobility, because mobility is strength-led. But you won't become lax or over-loose like many injury-prone modern athletes. You can't. Your strength and flexibility will be in perfect balance.

Passive vs active stretching

When I train my students, I focus on strength, first and foremost. If I see someone wasting their time performing silly stretching exercises instead of training their muscles hard, I usually slap the bastards. As a result of this, some of the people who know me have come away with the message; "Coach Wade doesn't believe in flexibility". That ain't right. I *do* believe in the importance of flexibility. But I believe in *strength-led* flexibility—where muscular contraction controls the range of motion. (This is often called *active* stretching.)

Passive flexibility is a different matter. There are various types of passive stretching, but I define passive stretching as:

Elongating relaxed muscles and soft tissues using an exterior force.

Examples of an exterior force might include:

- **External weight** (as in a stretch deadlift)
- **Momentum** ("bouncing" a stretch)
- **Leverage** (as in trapping your foot and bending forwards)
- **Pushing with another body part** (for example, bending your wrist back with your opposite hand).
- **Machinery** (like those dumbass splits machines you see in kung fu magazines)

I don't count *gravity* as an exterior force. The body's own weight under gravity is something we evolved to stretch against. Every time you do a deep squat or pushup you are stretching the muscles under gravity. More importantly, you never *relax* during these exercises. Your muscles are in control. In my definition, *passive stretching* occurs when your muscles are *relaxed* and are stretched by something *external*. It could be because a partner is stretching you (see the image on page 165), or it could be because an object—like a barre—is stretching you (see photo opposite).

I don't believe in *passive*, relaxed stretching, for reasons I gave in the last chapter. But active stretching is a good idea if you want to improve your mobility. I usually advise a pretty minimalist approach to *active* stretches—just a few powerful strength-led stretches for the entire body (the three *Trifecta* holds of chapters 14-17 are active flexibility techniques). But there are a wide range of active stretches to choose from. For a more complete discussion of the science and discipline of active stretching, check out Pavel Tsatsouline's excellent *Super Joints*. It's the ultimate manual on the topic.

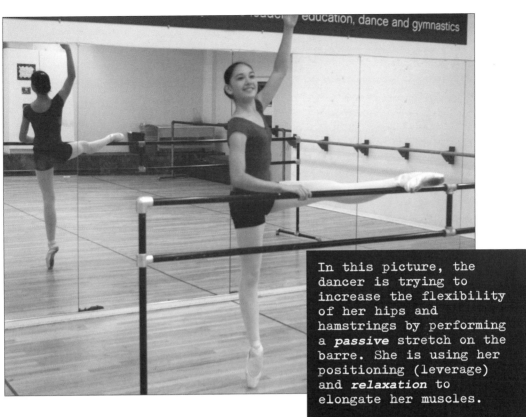

In this picture, the dancer is trying to increase the flexibility of her hips and hamstrings by performing a *passive* stretch on the barre. She is using her positioning (leverage) and *relaxation* to elongate her muscles.

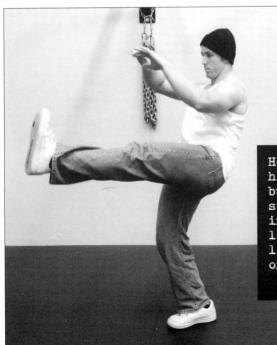

Here, Max is also stretching his hips and hamstrings, but he's doing it by *active* stretching-applying *tension* instead of relaxation. (Your leg has to extend straight out like this at the bottom of a one-leg squat.)

The correct role of passive stretching

Don't throw the baby out with the bath water, though. Just because I don't promote passive stretching as a *workout*, it still has its uses. Passive, relaxed training has value in three ways:

1. As a rehabilitative method, to stretch out tight scar tissue and promote blood flow—when active stretching would cause re-injury;

2. As a low-intensity therapy following high-intensity bodyweight training, to assist the circulation and help remove wastes from pumped-up muscles;

3. In special circumstances, to free up overly stiff movement patterns to allow athletes to perform calisthenic techniques (for example, learning to get into position for the *front bridge*).

Beyond these three? No passive stretching is required. The hours most athletes free up to do passive stretches are *wasted*.

If you want flexibility, what should you do?

That's easy—try *active stretching*.

Active stretching and bulletproof joints

If you want bulletproof joints, you need to focus on calisthenics. If you do add some stretching, it should be *active* stretching. Passive stretching is useless for protecting the joints—in fact, it makes the joints *more* vulnerable to injury, not less (see page 158-159).

What's so hot about active stretching? Here's some basic reasons for y'all:

- Active flexibility goes hand-in-hand with tension flexibility

If you've read chapter twelve through (if not, why not?!) you'll know why I'm big on tension-flexibility, or "supple strength"—the ability of your body to generate force safely, even when your muscles and joints are stretched. It's the best way to strengthen your muscles. Fortunately, active flexibility training is an excellent way to safely improve tension-flexibility.

Passive stretching trains you to *relax* your muscles as you stretch them; relaxation is a key part of the method. During active flexibility techniques, some of your muscles are already firing to the max just to move your joints—far from causing overall relaxation this results in a radiation of tension around the limb, trunk, or whatever you are working. Once you are aware of tension-flexibility, you can easily include it during active stretching. Once you are in the stretch, don't relax. Brace yourself—tense everything hard!

Joint Circling

If you want to refresh tight or tired muscles, you don't need to resort to passive stretching. Try *joint circling* instead. Joint circling is not really "stretching", but an opening and closing of the joints to promote circulation of fresh synovial fluid. This is a low intensity, low skill way of "oiling" your joints (see page 177). Joint circling actively revives the joints and increases blood flow without damaging the muscles at a cellular level, unlike hard stretching. This means you can do it several times daily if you feel the need.

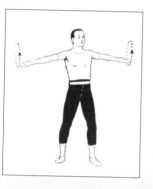 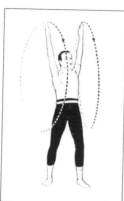

JOINT CIRCLING DRILLS:

• Neck	• Mid-spine
• Shoulders	• Hips
• Arms	• Knees
• Elbows	• Ankles
• Wrists	

Arm circles are a prime example of joint circling. Just make circles with your arms—bigger circles each time. (Try two sets of 2o reps, in both directions, as a great warm up for creaking shoulders.) Joint circling is simple and should feel good. Find a way to make the joint a pivot to circle your arms, wrists, knees—anything that feels a bit stiff or sore.

- Active flexibility teaches your body to work as a unit

Passive flexibility methods focus on the body in a very partial, isolationist way. If you are stretching your hamstrings, for example, you are stretching your hamstrings. The opposite muscles—the quadriceps—are not being stretched. They aren't doing anything, really. Ideally, they should be *relaxed*. Tension is avoided like the plague in passive flexibility training. As a result, whenever you perform a passive flexibility exercise, only one side of the body (or limb, or joint) is getting the workout.

In a way, this approach is a parallel of the bodybuilding fallacy of isolating the muscles during training. Both methods treat the body as if it were simply a collection of parts. Unfortunately it's not—it's a complex system. Everything works together. In the real world, it's never true that one side of the body stretches while the other side relaxes. In real-life movements, one side of body has to contract hard to make the other side stretch out! Active stretching methods mimic real life. The area that stretches only stretches to the degree that the opposing muscle group can contract.

When a training method works in harmony with the body and helps you improve your contractile ability and your flexibility *at the same time,* you know that's a method you should look at.

- *Active stretching is safer than passive stretching*

This simple fact also makes active stretching far safer than passive stretching, for healthy people. It's easy to get injured performing passive stretches, because an exterior force is moving the body. But during active stretching, *the body moves itself.* The nervous system acts as a natural "safety valve" preventing overstretching. Trust Mother Nature!

- *Active flexibility training increases strength*

So many guys out there are working their butts off lifting weights or performing complicated bodybuilding routines, it's easy to forget that active flexibility training is the most natural, basic strength booster. For sure, very simple active flexibility exercises won't give you nineteen-inch arms and thirty-inch quads, but they can give you something healthier; the power to control your muscles and generate very high intensity contractions. Most people just aren't used to contracting their muscles as hard as possible. Ask a couch potato to slowly raise his locked leg to the side, and he'd probably only be able to lift his leg a couple feet off

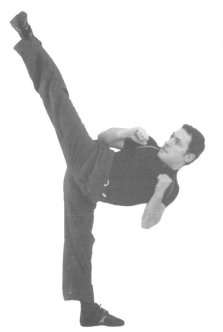

the ground. Imagine the special hip strength it takes to raise one locked leg out to the side like Van Damme...now apply that kind of contractile strength to every single muscle in the body, and you get the idea.

"Q. How strong do the hips need to be to raise the leg this high—in slow motion?

A. Pretty freakin' strong, son."

Without high intensity contractions, true strength is impossible. Active flexibility exercises are like a tune-up for the nervous system; because they force you to tighten your muscles as far as possible, they amplify the neural patterns which are responsible for intense muscular contraction. Even if you did no other training, a program of active flexibility exercises would boost your strength in the healthiest way possible. But if you *add* active flexibility work to a regular strength training routine (especially a body-weight strength routine) both programs will work in synergy, enhancing each other and augmenting your results significantly.

- Active flexibility training increases your "functional" ROM

Many people use passive flexibility exercises because they think it's the best way to increase the range of motion of their muscles and tendons. This is simply untrue. It is true that by learning to relax and stretch passively—using an external force like a partner, a weight or a leverage position—you can push your muscles further in any direction than by active flexibility techniques. Many athletes quickly latch on to this fact. But what they don't realize is that this extra range of motion is *completely useless.* The only time you can actually *access* that range of motion again is when you are progressively warmed up (to deactivate the muscle spindles) and when your body is subject to external forces.

Think about this for a second. When you passively stretch, you are training to generate an ability you can't control. It can only be "turned on" by external factors, like violent momentum or an exterior force. Essentially, you are training to lose control of your muscles!

Active flexibility is totally different. Whereas passive flexibility practices will increase the *maximum* ROM of your warm muscles, active flexibility maximizes the *functional* ROM of your muscles. Because active flexibility involves moving the body under complete muscular control, I call the resulting increase in range of motion a "functional" increase. Unlike the ROM developed through passive stretching, it's something you can really use. ROM which is not matched by strength is pointless. In fact, it's *fake*. What's the point of being able to *force* your body into the splits, if your muscles are only powerful enough to lift your leg to thigh height?

By using active methods you can and will increase the ROM of all the joints in your body. But you will do this safely, in a balanced way, and at your body's own speed. Nothing is forced; nothing is fake.

Lights out!

Let's plane this down to a simple, take-home message for the future bodyweight legends of tomorrow, okay?

• There are two types of stretching; strength-led, which you control (*active stretching*) and stretching using an exterior force (*passive stretching*). Passive stretching usually involves learning to relax your muscles to help stretch further than normal.

• Just as bodyweight experts prefer to train using their own bodies instead of external weights, so most prison athletes prefer to use their own strength and avoid being stretched by an exterior force. When they stretch at all, it is strength-led stretching, and even then, they think of it as *joint training*, not *stretching*.

• Passive stretching has some benefits, but these mostly lie in stretching out injured bodies, which can't yet take the stresses of active stretching. Passive stretching is a *therapeutic* method—not an *athletic* method.

The "secrets" to healthy joints with a functional range of motion are simple, but they've been forgotten on the outside. When you train, focus on bodyweight movements, and build to a full range of motion on basic exercises. When you do choose to stretch, focus on active stretching—the muscle-led stuff—and forget passive stretching as long as possible.

What if you are already engaged in a productive bodyweight routine, and want to take your joint training even further? What if you want truly *bulletproof* joints? During my decades of prison training, I've picked up a handful of advanced tricks which—when combined with a "supple strength" routine—will maximize your joint health in only minutes a day. Sometime in the late eighties, I alchemized these tactics into a simple routine. I call this beauty the *Trifecta,* and it gives radical results! It will take a body from stiff and immobile to lithe, young and agile—in only minutes a day.

We'll look at it in the next chapter.

14: The Trifecta

Your "Secret Weapon" for Mobilizing Stiff, Battle-Scarred Physiques -For Life

hen I left SQ in '88 I was thirty-one years old. At around that time, I began hanging out with some friends of some friends, back in Richmond. One of my new buddies was a big-ass tattooed Irish freak called Carter.

Carter was as large as a house and strong as hell. He was pretty much a free weights animal. He rarely used machines in the gym; not because he didn't like 'em, but because they couldn't hold enough weight to test him. Sometimes he'd get his training partners to jump on the leg extension stack to add another 250 pounds for negs, crazy stuff like that. He didn't compete, but had some damn respectable powerlifts under his (rapidly expanding) belt. He could bench 350 and change, and didn't need a shirt (or much of a warm up) to do it. He had deadlifted six plates a side, though he told me that was a thing of the past, since his back had "gone" in '85. Fairly decent curls with eighty pound dumbbells were no problem, and he would press kegs, steel drums and logs with his buddies for fun. He was a big, powerful monster, but friendly in a gruff way—kind of like a bear.

But despite all his power, Carter had some problems. He was on the wrong side of forty, and his body no longer moved the way it used to. He complained to us that he often had to sleep with his arms over his head, because his shoulders hurt so much. When he woke up, he had to gobble some painkillers he left on the nightstand just to get out of bed. Even once he was up and moving he walked stiffly, like an old guy. If he sat down or had to get on the floor, he needed to put his hands on his knees just to get back up...this, despite the fact the dude could probably back squat a Harley for sets of ten. "I don't so much have a body as a collection of injuries," was one of his sayings.

Although Carter and I had very different ideas about training, we sometimes shot the s*** about different topics like muscle-building, high-rep training, stuff like that. But one night over a few beers, we eventually started talking about injuries, and Carter damn near broke down telling me about all his aches and pains. He knew I was in good shape from coming out of my San Quentin term, and he asked me for some advice.

"If your body was as f***ed as mine, what would you do, Paul?"

"Simple," I told him. "I'd quit the heavy weights. Right now. I'd start up with a program of simple calisthenics. Full body s***. When you start feeling better, throw in some rope climbing then maybe some handstand work. You'll keep your strength, lose that gut and be feeling like a new man in no time."

Carter looked down and shook his head.

"No way man," he said. "I'm a born lifter. Gonna be lifting iron till the day I die." This brother was addicted to the weights. He went on; "Can't you just give me some kind of secret prison routine to loosen me up or s***?"

I took another glug of beer (I drank, back in the day), wiped the suds from my mouth, leant back and thought about it.

Unleashing the "Trifecta"

A couple days later I came back to Carter, and gave him a workout with only three exercises in it. These techniques weren't even movements—they were *holds*. Once he learned to perform these holds, he did them at least every other day. Within ten weeks, Carter had eliminated 90% of his joint pain, and was optimistic that he'd lose the remaining 10%, too. He'd not only regained all his mobility, but he claimed he was more lithe and agile then when he was a teenage basketball player at Lincoln High...despite all his extra bodyweight. Carter loved the routine I gave him so much he started calling it the "Trifecta"—*the perfect three*. I lost touch with Carter a while after that, as our lives went in different directions. I heard from the man again about five or six years later; he was back deadlifting. He was still doing the Trifecta religiously.

Does this all sound too good to be true? Well, don't take my f-ing word for it, pal. Just try it yourself, for five weeks. Then you'll see. But before I show you the actual program, let me try to convince you a bit about how and why it works.

Joint training–
3 tricks of the trade

Whenever someone asks me for the key to strong joints, I always talk about progressive calisthenics first. I discuss calisthenics movements because they gradually develop the right kind of "supple strength"—or *tension-flexibility*—in the tendons which I talked about in the last couple of chapters. But some people— like Carter—just have no interest in a diet of pushups, pullups and one-leg squats. They need to feel the steel. So instead I thought about alternative ideas I had learned about joint training beyond the principles involved in supple strength. I asked myself: *is there anything athletes can use—in addition to their strength training program—to improve joint function and health?*

I instantly came up with three ideas; three of the most powerful tactics in joint training there are—period.

They are:

1)   Focus on the functional triad;
2)   "Oil" your joints;
3)   Use active stretching.

I combined these three ideas into a simple, fairly easy to learn routine. This routine—hastily scribbled out on the back of a napkin—became the program now known as the Trifecta. Let's look at these three points, one-by-one.

1)   FOCUS ON THE FUNCTIONAL TRIAD.

Back in the day (50s/60s onwards), weight-training writers sometimes used to talk about the "beach muscles"—the muscles visible on the front of the body. I'm talking about the shoulders, the pecs, the biceps, the abs and the quads. These muscles are sometimes considered the "physique" muscles. If you want to look good for chicks while you're on the beach, these are the muscles that gotta stand out. At the same time, it was recognized that the *real* strength muscles—the muscles which lift the weight in a huge deadlift, clean or pull—lay at the *back* of the body. I'm talking now about the hamstrings, the glutes, the calves, the spinal erectors and traps. These muscles feature in all the great lifts and are incredibly strong. For a lot of guys training before the seventies, it was understood that a dichotomy existed. There were "beach muscles" at the front of the body, and "work muscles" at the back.

Modern bodybuilders generally forgot this concept, but coaches and strength writers kept it alive. They updated it a bit, though—and added some snazzy pseudo-scientific language to make it all sound ever-so-smart. They called the "beach muscles" the *anterior chain*, and the "work muscles" the *posterior chain*.

This basic idea still holds true. But many lifters forget what bodyweight strength athletes could never forget—the body is three-dimensional. As well as the anterior chain (front) and posterior chain (back), the body also has a *lateral chain*, comprising the muscles of the *side* of the body. I'm talking about the tensor muscles at the side of the legs and hips, the obliques of the waist, the serratus and intercostals of the ribcage, plus the famous "lats" running under the armpits.

These three chains form what can be called the *Functional Triad*:

THE FUNCTIONAL TRIAD

ANTERIOR CHAIN
- Pectoral (chest) muscles
- Frontal deltoids
- Biceps
- Abdominal muscles
- Front hips
- Quadriceps (front thighs)
- Tibialis (shin) muscles

POSTERIOR CHAIN
- Upper back muscles
- Rear deltoids
- Triceps
- Spinal muscles
- Glutes
- Hamstrings
- Calf muscles

LATERAL CHAIN
- Latissimus dorsi (lats)
- Serratus
- Intercostal muscles
- Obliques
- Hip abductors
- Tensors (side thigh)

Some thinkers talk about more than three muscular chains—some stretch it out to six! But for me, this is over-thinking it. There are only three fundamental chains. Train those right, and you got all your bases covered.

Understanding the Functional Triad is essential if you are going to train your joints. Most mobility work is totally unbalanced. Bodybuilders have stiff, over-trained *anterior* chains; heavy "ground up" lifters have over-trained *posterior* chains; most martial artists build flexibility in their *posterior* chains and *lateral* chains, but not their *anterior* chains; and so on. This is all unbalanced training. It builds dysfunctional asymmetry into the body and invites injury.

There is only one "cure"—a functional joint training program which restores harmony and balances the body by training *all three* of these chains equally.

2) "OIL" YOUR JOINTS.

The most muscular, powerful athletes in the world train intensely and *infrequently*. They work their muscles and tendons hard, then give them time to rest, recover and grow stronger. This is the perfect recipe for mass and strength—even "supple strength".

Unfortunately, although this kind of work thickens and strengthens the muscles and tendons *around* your joints, it doesn't necessarily do as much for the ligaments, cartilage, and soft tissue *inside* your joints.

There is virtually no blood flow inside your joints. Whereas your muscles and tendons get their nutrition from the *blood*, cartilage is fed by a thick solution called *synovial fluid*. This fluid is rich in oxygen and proteins and contains everything the joints need to thrive and grow stronger. Synovial fluid also acts like a lubricant, like the motor oil in your car. It removes waste, feeds the insides of your joints, cushions them and protects them from damage. It's great stuff. But whereas the blood is pumped round the body by the heart, synovial fluid is only generated and circulated by movement—it's the *opening* of the joints that freshens this fluid and send healthy supplies to cartilage.

That's why strength training alone will not optimize your joint health. Training hard too often will wear down the joints, and training less frequently starves the joints of synovial fluid. There's only one solution. For optimal joint health, you should perform your strength training with enough rest time to recover; and on non-training days, you should perform mobility exercises to nourish and "oil" your joints.

The best way to "oil" your joints is by using calisthenic "holds". Maneuver yourself into a stretch, and then hold at the top. If there's a "secret" to why yoga helps so many people become pain free, it's this method. A good example of such a hold would be a back bridge—push yourself to a peak stretch, then hold at the top. This type of stretch opens the cartilage (in this case, the discs of the spine) to the maximum degree, allowing an optimal amount of fresh synovial fluid to circulate.

In *Convict Conditioning*, I focused on *moving* calisthenics, rather than "holds". Moving calisthenics fatigue the muscles quickly, and builds muscle, strength and endurance. Because the muscles aren't moving a load, *holds* don't exhaust the body as much. This is ideal when it comes to joint training—it allows you to train joints much more frequently and still recover. I advise people to use mobility work on non-strength training days, but that's just a rule of thumb. Once you are conditioned, you can perform holds every day; some people perform holds several times a day, to refresh their joints and shake out the cobwebs. This daily work would be impossible with hardcore *moving* bodyweight techniques. You'd burn out in no time.

SYNOVIAL JOINT

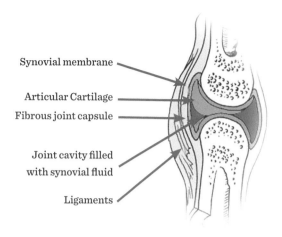

Synovial membrane

Articular Cartilage

Fibrous joint capsule

Joint cavity filled
with synovial fluid

Ligaments

Synovial fluid is the "water of life" for the joints. It is responsible for:

• Shock absorption
• Lubrication
• Nutrition
• Waste management

Healthy supplies are *essential* if you want superhuman joints.

Performing daily stretch-hold techniques won't just feed and water your joints. It also increases *mobility* in the quickest possible time. Brutal, hard-ass strength training increases strength, but it can be hard on the body at a cellular level. Over time, it results in adhesions and scar tissue, in the muscles and joints. These will kill your flexibility stone dead—it's the major reason why most veteran lifters are stiff as boards. Daily work with stretch-holds will cure this problem. Calisthenic holds ease out tightness naturally, removing adhesions, waste and toxic build-up. Many athletes force their stretches with bouncing techniques or the use of external weights or machines. This might give short-term results, but in the long-term it causes microtrauma to your muscles, just like weight-training. Avoid these methods, and stick to calisthenic-based holds performed smoothly and under your own power. If you use weights or momentum to stretch, overstretching is inevitable. If you use the power of your own muscles, your nervous system acts as a natural safety-valve.

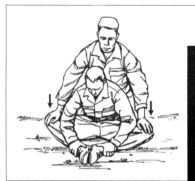

"Buddy" stretches are a popular
example of a passive stretch. But
if somebody else is controlling your
range-of-motion, how much is too much?
With active stretches, your body's
own neuromuscular systems control the
range-of-motion. You get a perfect
stretch for your level of ability each
time, every time.

In the last couple pages, I've given you some major secrets for life-long healthy joints. They are secrets most athletes overlook. They are:

- Stick to movements that *refresh* your body rather than tire you out;
- train *frequently* to feed the internal anatomy of your joints, and;
- work on *calisthenic-holds* instead of aggressive stretching routines.

This sounds simple and basic, but the most powerful ideas often are. I know what you're thinking—*but Paulie, what "calisthenic-holds" should I be using?*

Glad you asked...

3) APPLY ACTIVE STRETCHING TECHNIQUES.

If you've already read chapters twelve and thirteen, you'll know I'm not a big fan of training to get your muscles and joints lax and loose. This is how most people today train, but it's not how prison athletes do it. Real bodyweight powerhouses—the ones with truly bulletproof joints—don't train to become flaccid and relaxed. They train for *tension.*

Muscles which are *flexible yet tense* are the key to strong joints which can safely absorb force. Which would you rather have for your car's shocks? Spongy rubber or hard steel springs? The strong steel would flex and absorb forces far better than the rubber, which would rip or tear before it absorbed anything.

Apply this principle to your Functional Triad training! Forget pussified relaxation-type techniques. Loose, relaxed *passive* stretching is out for now. I want you to train your joints by using antagonistic muscle-power rather than relaxation. This method is *active stretching* (as described in the last chapter) and it encourages supple strength, mobility and agility all at once.

Active stretching is simple: *you stretch out one half of the body by contracting the opposite half.* Let's apply this to the Functional Triad:

- If you want to stretch your anterior chain, you do it by contracting your posterior chain—as in a *bridge hold*.

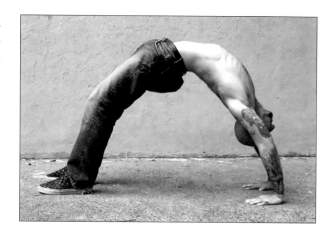

- If you want to stretch your posterior chain, you do it by contracting your anterior chain—as in an *L-hold* (also known as the *L-sit*).

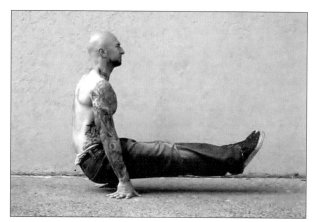

- If you want to stretch your lateral chain, you do it by contracting your lateral chain on the opposite side—as in a *twist hold*.

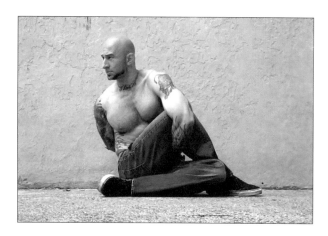

FUNCTIONAL TRIAD ANATOMY CHART

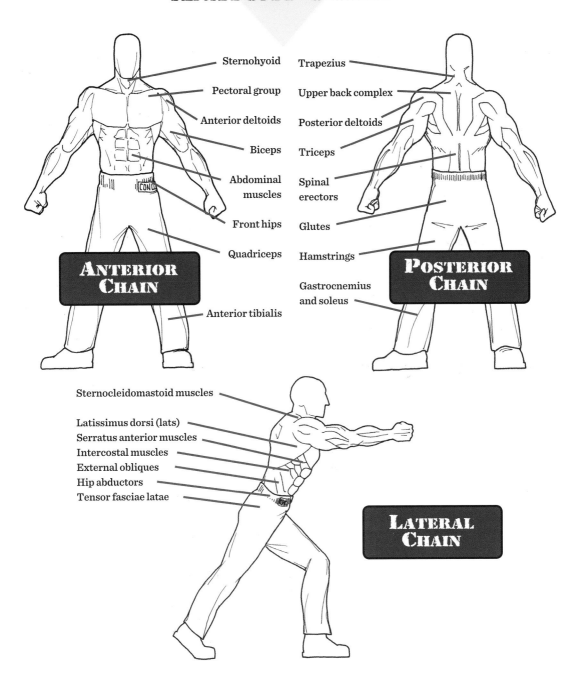

ANTERIOR CHAIN

- Sternohyoid
- Pectoral group
- Anterior deltoids
- Biceps
- Abdominal muscles
- Front hips
- Quadriceps
- Anterior tibialis

POSTERIOR CHAIN

- Trapezius
- Upper back complex
- Posterior deltoids
- Triceps
- Spinal erectors
- Glutes
- Hamstrings
- Gastrocnemius and soleus

LATERAL CHAIN

- Sternocleidomastoid muscles
- Latissimus dorsi (lats)
- Serratus anterior muscles
- Intercostal muscles
- External obliques
- Hip abductors
- Tensor fasciae latae

TRIFECTA
CHAINS TRAINED

BRIDGE HOLD

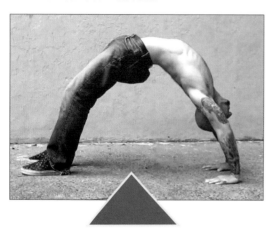

Strongly contracts the:
• POSTERIOR CHAIN

Actively stretches the:
• ANTERIOR CHAIN

L-HOLD

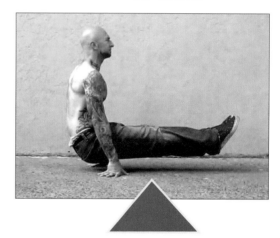

Strongly contracts the:
• ANTERIOR CHAIN

Actively stretches the:
• POSTERIOR CHAIN

TWIST HOLD

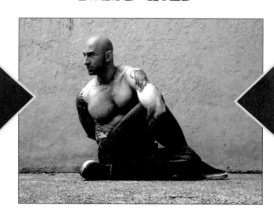

Strongly
contracts the:
• LATERAL
CHAIN

(plus rotator cuff)
On one side of
the body

Actively
stretches the:
• LATERAL
CHAIN

(plus rotator cuff)
On the other side of
the body

These three movements form the basis of the "Trifecta". They are like *gold*. When used together, they represent much more than a great joint training program; they really are a genuine "quick fix" for making a beaten up old body lithe, cat-like and mobile again. Even if you did nothing else—no weights, no cal, nothing—your entire body would stay young, agile, flexible and pain free just from the sensible application of these three techniques.

Don't worry if the techniques, as I've shown them, are too tough for you to do right now. You can build up to them if you need to. Everyone—no matter how out of shape—can start benefitting from the Trifecta, right now. In the next chapter I'll show you easier versions.

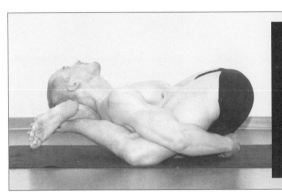

Some yoga masters become amazingly flexible—but that's not the goal here. The Trifecta movements are designed to "normalize" stiff connective tissue, and gently guide your joints to their ideal ROM. They aren't meant to be advanced yoga!

The power of the Trifecta

Students of mine who have used this Trifecta have found that it works like magic. But there's nothing paranormal about it. It's just a refinement of every effective, powerful joint training idea I've picked up over the years. These three exercises build *function, strength* and *mobility* at the same time. This is a scary combination!

Any gymnast will tell you that this kind of training will make you stronger. This is because you have to contract your muscles *hard* to perform the Trifecta holds. If you aren't used to bridges, try them to see what I mean. The issue isn't so much the *weight* being lifted, but the high levels of *muscular contraction* required to perform the hold. Most people just aren't used to contracting their muscles very hard. Like I said in the last chapter, active flexibility exercises are like a tune-up for the nervous system; because they force you to tighten your muscles as far as possible, they amplify the neural patterns which are responsible for intense muscular contraction. At the same time, the muscles on the opposite side of your body are stretched, not in an exaggerated way, but to the limits of their functional ROM. This is true of all active stretching work, but these three exercises work *entire chains* of muscles, so are much more efficient than using active stretching in isolation. The *whole system* benefits.

Because these are pretty "big" movements involving most or all of the body, your muscles have to fire strongly to keep you stabilized. This is a great way to develop the *tension-flexibility* I raved about in chapter twelve. When you do an L-hold, your lower back stretches, but it doesn't *relax*. It's strong as iron, because the waist is a girdle and your stomach muscles are pulling hard on your vertebrae. Your back muscles *need* to fire strongly to keep your spine stable and safe. Likewise, bridging stretches your anterior chain, but the quads and waist have to stay taut to retain the position. Twists are an amazing torso exercise—do them right and all your muscles get a contractile workout. The Trifecta provides total-body "supple strength".

The Trifecta also enhances musculo-skeletal "function". The major reason for poor function, crummy alignment and injury in the human body is *lack of symmetry*. Some parts of the anatomy can contract well, others can't; one side has a good range of motion, the other side is stiff, and so on. These three movements eliminate that kind of dysfunction. For L-holds, one side of the body *contracts*, the other side *stretches;* the same is true for bridges and twists. This means that the ability of your antagonist muscles to stretch always matches the ability of your agonist muscles to contract. It's a yin-yang thing. Everything is in harmony. Everything is balanced. When you practice all three holds in one session, you are working your body in 3-D, and this effect is enhanced.

The rejuvenating benefits of the Trifecta go beyond simple function, strength and mobility, and into the realm of practical therapy. Because these three techniques are "holds" instead of movements, they don't build up waste products or fatigue the muscles as much as regular calisthenics. This means you can practice them every other day, every day, or sometimes even several times a day, if you are in shape. This is a perfect way to "oil" the cartilage, feed your joints and begin healing old injuries.

I could give you a lot more reasons why these three are so awesome, or why they are so powerful when applied together in a program. But the bottom line is, you have to *work with them* to really understand. You'll *feel* the results in your own body soon enough.

Programming the Trifecta

There are lots of different ways to program the Trifecta movements. You can perform one hold a day, rotating over three days, two holds a day, and so on. I've found that working all three holds over a single session can be very effective. This works all three major muscular chains and tones and enhances function in the entire system. Feels pretty damn good, too.

SAMPLE TRIFECTA WORKOUT

1. BRIDGE HOLD:

1 x 10 second hold
2 x 5 second holds

By now your spine is fully warmed up and loose for the stretch that follows:

2. L-HOLD:

4 x 5 seconds

Your spine and hips are now pumped with blood and your joints are free. A perfect time to twist:

3. FULL TWIST:

1 x 20 seconds (per side)

And that's your mobility work—a done deal.

This approach isn't written in stone. The Trifecta stands a lot of tweaking; for example you could "superset" the holds, performing 5 seconds of a bridge, five seconds of an L-hold, five seconds of a twist, then repeat until you reach your desired time. There are lots of options. In the spirit of being your own coach, you should experiment and see what works for you. Here are some guidelines to help:

PROGRESSION:

Most athletes will need to build up to L-holds, bridge holds and full twists. No problem. I've included progressions for each exercise in the next few chapters. Start easy and find the technique that's just right for your level of development. Find movements you can do *perfectly*. Don't struggle—remember, this is joint mobility work, not strength training!

INTENSITY:

The holds should energize you—not drain you. Hold the position until you feel stimulated, not exhausted. If you push too hard, you'll get sore and you won't be able to perform the Trifecta frequently—which defeats the object. Pick easier versions rather than the hardest you can do; save the difficult stuff for your strength workouts. Never go to "failure".

TIMING:

How long you hold the positions is up to you. It depends on your strength, conditioning and mobility. Less than two seconds is pointless, because the exercise ceases to be much of a "hold". Experiment and find something that feels refreshing, even stimulating, without being tiring. A good rule of thumb is at least twenty seconds per session. This can be split into chunks. For example:

- 5 x 4 second holds

- 4 x 5 second holds

- 1 x 10 second hold
  + 2 x 5 seconds holds

- 2 x 10 second holds

...and so on.

Just remember to build up to this and use "easy" holds at first. You are supposed to be "oiling" your joints, feeding them—not wearing them down.

FREQUENCY:

If your joints are in good shape, you can get away with performing the Trifecta twice a week along with strength training. For long-term joint training, I'd advise training three to four days per week, on non-strength training days. If you really want to iron out kinks, improve poor mobility or heal old injuries daily training is an option—but keep the holds easy to moderate rather than hard. Programming multiple daily workouts becomes a drag. You can do multiple daily sessions, but keep them spontaneous rather than planned.

SPONTANEOUS SESSIONS:

If you are feeling stiff, don't be afraid to improvise an impromptu hold workout! If your back is tight, pop down and do a few L-holds. If your shoulders are dead, try some twists, and so on. You'll feel a whole lot better afterwards. Multiple daily sessions can be a lifesaver if you are forced into being sedentary for a while—maybe stuck at a desk, or watching too much TV.

INTEGRATED WORKOUTS:

If you don't want to commit a huge amount of time to the Trifecta, but want to increase your mobility anyway, you can integrate these moves into your workouts. They work great as a pre-workout warm up. More advanced guys can use them as post-workout therapy.

SEQUENCING:

If one of your chains is either sore or a little tight, perform the hold that *contracts* it before the hold that *stretches* it. For example, bridges contract your back—L-holds stretch your back. If your back is a little stiff, performing bridges before L-holds will heat up your spinal muscles, loosen your back and make the L-holds feel easier.

GOING BEYOND:

I don't believe in extreme flexibility. There's no proof that becoming a circus freak contortionist increases strength, helps the joints or improves athleticism. But there's plenty of proof that higher levels of flexibility gives you lax muscles and makes you more prone to injury. Once you've built to the bridge hold, the L-hold and the full twist hold, you have reached optimum *functional* ROM. More extreme versions of these exercises exist, but you just don't need them. Joint mobility training is not like powerlifting—more is not better.

Lights out!

With the tips I've just given you, you should be about ready to begin training the Trifecta. You just need to find the right three holds for your current ability level. The next three chapters have every step you'll need to gain (or regain) pain free, adaptive joints with perfect mobility.

...what are you waiting for? Try 'em out now!

15: The Bridge Hold Progressions

The Ultimate Prehab/Rehab Technique

Whenever athletes ask me about building strong joints and tendons, I usually wind up telling them to how to develop supple strength. There are lots of great bodyweight exercises which build tension-flexibility in the elbows, knees, wrists, etc. But I always follow up that advice by clearly saying: *start with the spine first.*

The spine represents the deep centerline of the body-structure. It's analogous to the universal joint in a car, or the main load-bearing girders in a building. If this centerline is out of kilter—even slightly—the rest of the body is automatically out of symmetry. This includes the hips, shoulders and limbs—even the fingers and toes. This is not just a hippy-fied matter of "health" and "well-being". Trust me, it relates directly to raw power, brutal strength and hardcore joint invulnerability. Your entire musculo-skeletal system is built around the spine. If your spine is not strong and aligned, the rest of your joints will not be strong and pain free for long. It's just not possible.

Let's face it, when most people talk about weak joints or "aches and pains", bad backs come smack bang at the top of the complaints list. According to recent studies, 80% of Americans have some kind of back problem; and that's not just the elderly or infirm, either. It's most people. And the number one cause of all this pain and poor function? It's *weakness in the deep muscles of the spine.* When these muscles are frail, the vertebrae which make up the spine cannot stack properly. They get pulled into uncomfortable positions under load (even just gravity). This leads to bad posture. Eventually the discs become "fixed" in these weaker positions, and this leads to lop-sided locomotion and even more disproportional weakness. The end result is pain, rupture and poor movement. Athleticism is an impossibility. There's a reason why pain therapies like the Alexander Technique, the Feldenkrais Method and Pilates emphasize posture and a strengthening of the spine. Deep strengthening exercise is the *only* way to relieve back pain and restore function. If you go to your doctor with pain, he'll throw some pain pills at you. They won't do jack s*** except poison your body and mask the symptoms temporarily.

Luckily, there is a permanent cure for the deep-muscle weakness that causes back pain. It's the ancient *back bridging* family of techniques. I devoted a whole chapter to these active flexibility movements in *Convict Conditioning*.

> The deep muscles of the spine are a hundred times more important for health and strength than the pecs or biceps. Modern athletes neglect these muscles, but athletes of previous generations took pride in their "back power".

Isometric vs dynamic bridging

In *Convict Conditioning* I focused on *dynamic bridges*—bridges where you move up and down, no different from a pushup or a squat. This dynamic style is fairly common in jails, because it's the best way to build muscle, endurance and joint strength all in one. If you are purely interested in bridging to align your spine, strengthen your joints and refresh your discs, you don't need to bust your ass repping out on dynamic bridges. You can do *isometric* (or *static*) *bridging* instead—where you just push up into position and hold at the top. Doing this benefits the joints, but doesn't tire out the body as much—which means you can do it more often. Easier, more frequent bridge holds will increase mobility faster and "oil" the joints as I discussed in the last chapter.

Evolving your bridging

With a little dedication even the most inflexible, screwed-up-tight bastards will be able to achieve a fairly respectable bridge hold. It shouldn't take too long. But you should start things slowly. Over the next few pages I'll outline four simple progressions to lead you to the perfect bridge. Those of you familiar with *Convict Conditioning* will recognize the logic behind these progressions.

By now you should understand that performing bridge holds for *joint health* is different from performing dynamic bridges for muscular strength and endurance. Remember:

* Aim at performing your bridge hold for 20 seconds per session (this can be broken up into multiple sets).
* Aim for *perfection* of movement—not *difficulty* of movement.
* Don't push your muscles, get sore or go to "failure".
* Joint "oiling" sessions should be energizing, not exhausting.
* Train frequently to stay mobile, but don't break your muscles down.

'Nuff said. On to the progressions.

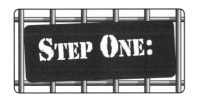

STEP ONE:

SHORT BRIDGE HOLD

PERFORMANCE

Lie on your back, with your feet flat on the floor and around 6-8 inches from your butt. This is the start position. Press down through the feet, lifting the hips and back clear of the ground until only the shoulders and feet are supporting the bodyweight. At this point, your thighs and trunk should form a straight line. This is the hold position (see photo) Keep this position for the desired time, breathing as smoothly as possible. Return to the start position by slowly reversing the motion.

EXERCISE X-RAY

The *short bridge hold* is an ideal way to begin "oiling" the hips and spinal vertebrae. Because the knees are bent, the anterior chain is gently stretched without too much strain being placed on the back. Beginning functional mobility training with short bridge holds will tone and condition the alignment muscles running up the spine and build some basic flexibility into tight stomach muscles. The knees (which are *synovial joints*) also get some gentle therapy from this hold. The perfect way to begin joint work.

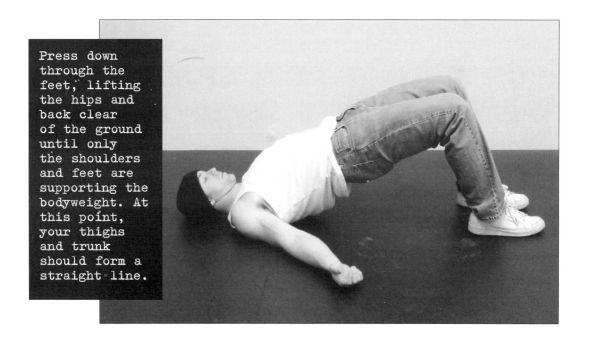

Press down through the feet, lifting the hips and back clear of the ground until only the shoulders and feet are supporting the bodyweight. At this point, your thighs and trunk should form a straight line.

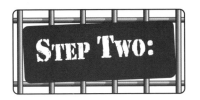

STRAIGHT BRIDGE HOLD

PERFORMANCE

Sit up straight on the ground with your legs stretched out in front of you, feet shoulder width apart. Place your palms on the floor on either side of your hips. Press down through the hands, as you simultaneously push your hips upwards until your legs and torso form a straight line. Draw the chin up and look at the ceiling. This is the hold position (see photo). Keep this position for the desired time, breathing as smoothly as possible. Return to the start position by slowly reversing the motion.

EXERCISE X-RAY

With the *straight bridge hold*, the upper and lower limbs are made to work as struts. This begins working the deep muscles behind the shoulders, while gently stretching out the muscles at the front of the shoulders and chest. Straightening out the legs activates the leg biceps more and generates tension-flexibility in the tendons behind the knees. The straight-leg position also mobilizes the midsection better, loosening up the hip flexors, which can be notoriously stiff in strength athletes.

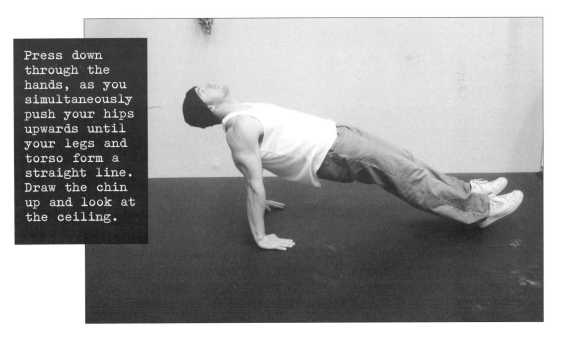

Press down through the hands, as you simultaneously push your hips upwards until your legs and torso form a straight line. Draw the chin up and look at the ceiling.

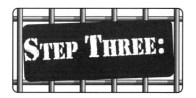

STEP THREE: ANGLED BRIDGE HOLD

PERFORMANCE

Angled bridges require an object which is about the height of a prison bunk. Lie back on the edge of the bunk or bed with your hips clear, and your feet flat on the ground and shoulder width apart. Place your hands either side of your head, with your fingers pointing towards your feet. Press down through the hands, pushing the hips up, arching back until your head and body are entirely clear of the bunk. Look at the wall behind you. This is the hold position (see photo). Keep this position for the desired time, breathing as smoothly as possible. Return to the bunk by slowly reversing the motion.

EXERCISE X-RAY

The *angled bridge hold* continues from where the *straight bridge hold* left off. It still contracts the posterior chain while stretching the anterior chain but with this version of the bridge the joints of the upper body really begin to gain some benefit as well. The "hands alongside head" position opens up the ribcage, gently frees up tight rotator cuffs and begins building supple strength in the wrists and elbows, which are stretched under a light load.

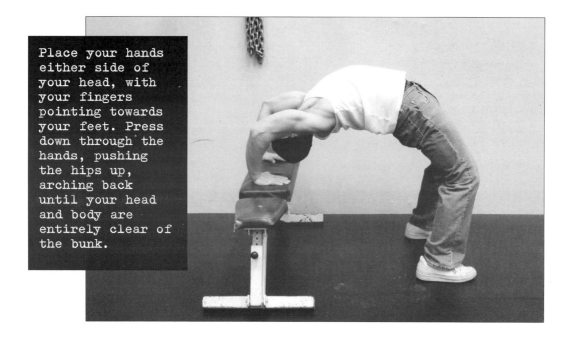

Place your hands either side of your head, with your fingers pointing towards your feet. Press down through the hands, pushing the hips up, arching back until your head and body are entirely clear of the bunk.

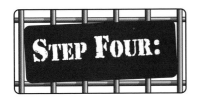

STEP FOUR:

HEAD BRIDGE HOLD

PERFORMANCE

Lie on your back, with your feet shoulder width apart, flat on the floor and around 6-8 inches from your butt. Place the hands alongside the head, with the elbows pointing up, the palms flat on the floor with your fingers pointing towards your toes. Push the hips as high as you can, lifting the body from the floor. Keep your head in contact with the ground as you go, pivoting it back until the crown of your head is touching the floor. Remember to push up using your arms—the neck is just along for the ride. This is the hold position (see photo). Breathing smoothly during the hold. Lower yourself gently.

EXERCISE X-RAY

The *head bridge hold* is kind of different from moving *half bridges* as detailed in *Convict Conditioning*. For this version I want you to use your head like a lever, similar to a *wrestler's bridge* (see chapter 10), but much less intense. Because your head stays in contact with the ground, this hold is less pronounced than the *full bridge hold*, and places less strain on the rotator cuffs. Head bridge holds make for a perfect transitional exercise.

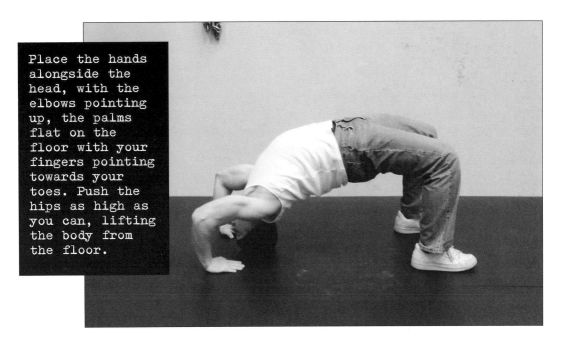

Place the hands alongside the head, with the elbows pointing up, the palms flat on the floor with your fingers pointing towards your toes. Push the hips as high as you can, lifting the body from the floor.

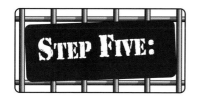

STEP FIVE:

BRIDGE HOLD

PERFORMANCE

Lie on your back, with your feet shoulder width apart, flat on the floor and around 6-8 inches from your butt. Place the hands alongside the head, with the elbows pointing up, the palms flat on the floor with your fingers pointing towards your toes. Push up through the hips, lifting the body from the floor. Allow the head to tilt backwards between the arms, so that you can look at the wall behind you. Continue pushing through your arms and legs until your arch is as high as possible, then "set" yourself by bracing your body. This is the hold position (see photos). Keep this position for the desired time, breathing as smoothly as possible. Get down by slowly reversing the motion.

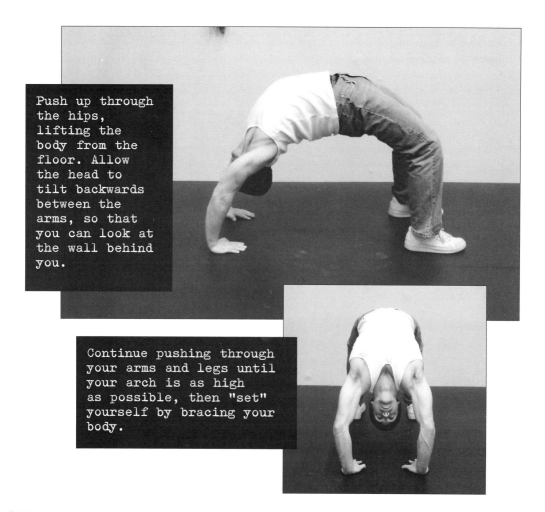

Push up through the hips, lifting the body from the floor. Allow the head to tilt backwards between the arms, so that you can look at the wall behind you.

Continue pushing through your arms and legs until your arch is as high as possible, then "set" yourself by bracing your body.

BULLETPROOF JOINTS: THE EFFECTS!

The bridge hold conveys enough benefits to fill a book! Here are just a few:

• Bridging strengthens the posterior chain. Unlike most barbell exercises, it also works the deep layer of spinal muscles. When strong, these muscles are like armor for the entire back, keeping the vertebrae correctly aligned, healing old back injuries and reducing the chance of new ones.

• Bridging also acts as powerful active stretching for the entire anterior chain; freeing up stiff hip flexors, as well as undoing "knots" in the stomach, thighs and knees.

• Many martial artists (training for high kicks) only bend forwards when stretching. This makes the back of their body flexible, while the front is tight as hell. Back bridging rebalances the body, stretching the front and offsetting any uneven flexibility.

• The backwards-rotational shoulder position will strengthen the small rotator cuff muscles within the shoulder in a way that linear weight lifting *cannot ever* accomplish.

• The muscles and connective tissue inside the shoulder girdle has a poor blood supply; this is why the area is prone to "nagging" injuries that never heal. Frequent practice of the bridge hold injects these areas with fresh blood, and increases circulation throughout the day, enhancing healing time.

• The stretched-under-load position of the arms develops excellent levels of tension-flexibility in the elbows and wrists. This "supple strength" carries over into strength training and daily activities, reducing the chances of elbow and forearm problems like tennis elbow, golfer's elbow, carpal tunnel, etc.

• Many bodybuilders suffer from slumped shoulders, caused often by excessive bench pressing. Bridge holds pull the pectoral muscles back, curing postural problems, expanding the ribcage and increasing lung capacity.

Going beyond?

A lot of athletes will be wondering where they are supposed to go after mastering the bridge. The answer is: Nowhere. You can find more difficult back-bending exercises—hell you can keep going till your heels touch your skull—but that won't improve joint health. If anything, it'll make you *too* loose, and ripe for an injury.

That said, I very rarely see people perform a *perfect* bridge. In a truly ideal bridge, the arms and legs are straight; and this requires muscular power and connective tissue flexibility which few people (except yoga experts or pro dancers) possess. So don't push yourself to move past the bridge hold. The bridge represents an ideal backwards range-of-motion for the spine. If you get to the stage where a perfect bridge hold becomes truly effortless, congratulations. In terms of spinal functionality, that's not a "plateau"—it's the peak of the mountain.

Lights out!

The bridge hold will bulletproof your spine, and tune up alignment muscles other training methods just can't touch. But you don't need to rush to the full bridge hold. Go slow, go easy, practice often to keep your joints fed and oiled and be kind to your body.

Training the spine for health and function is different from hardcore strength training. Harder types of dynamic bridging—like the *stand-to-stand bridge*—don't require more flexibility than the bridge hold, but they do work the muscles of the spine and trunk a lot harder. If you want to work your back for strength, set aside one or two sessions per week to practice dynamic bridging as laid out in the first book. Keep the Trifecta for a joint-focused tune-up, not as hardcore strength work!

16: The L-Hold Progressions

Cure Bad Hips and Low Back— Inside-Out

J ust like the spine which runs behind, the waist/hip girdle is another key area where modern athletes are likely to run into trouble. Everyone today is obsessed by *external* appearance—the visible thickness of the "six pack" (*rectus abdominis*) muscles. But what about the deeper, internal alignment muscles, such as the *psoas*, the *hip flexors*, the *iliacus*, the *transversus*? These key muscles are far more important to strength and function than the external gut muscles, but they are usually ignored—even deliberately. Pick up an "ab training special" off the newsstands, and the chances are that the writer will be telling you "secrets" for keeping the hip flexors out of your ab movements. This is madness! The external muscles are grown at the expense of the deeper, alignment muscles. And people today wonder why the modern population (and ex-athletes in particular) are plagued by hip problems: tendonitis, sciatica, osteoarthritis, and so on. How can you expect to have a strong lower body when the muscles which align your trunk and hips are out of whack? It'll affect every move you make!

Old time physical culturists understood this importance of the deep abdomen. In their quest for huge strength and external muscle, modern Western thinkers have largely forgotten it, but in the East they still understand. Look at a kung fu master—he breathes and moves from his *center*. Bruce Lee was well versed in this way of thinking; unlike American "muscle-men" of his era, he didn't believe that strength came from having big arms. He knew that power and function comes from the *waist*, which is why he trained his alignment muscles (hips, midsection, spine) first. The same principles hold true in Japanese martial arts. Anyone who has studied aikido or classical jujutsu will be familiar with the terms *tanden* or *hara*—a vital concept relating to the *deep center* of the body.

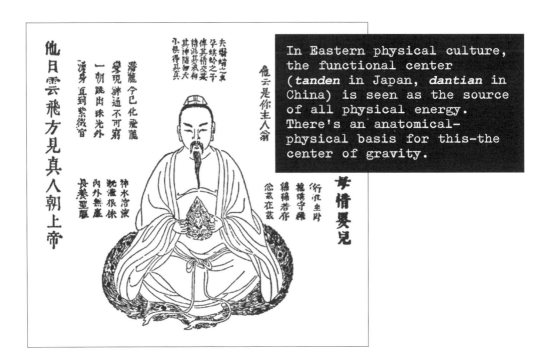

In Eastern physical culture, the functional center (*tanden* in Japan, *dantian* in China) is seen as the source of all physical energy. There's an anatomical-physical basis for this—the center of gravity.

Entire fighting systems are based around this concept in Japan. A lot of bulls*** has been built up around it over the years, but the original concept was not as mystical as you might think—Japanese fighters understood that strength moves outwards from the center of the body. That's why they placed the soul at the naval, and that's why a Samurai wishing to destroy himself stabs his gut. In Japan, this act is called *hara-kiri*—or "cutting the hara".

Martial artists worth their salt understand that developing the deeper muscles of the abdomen is about more than building a great six-pack. You need to train the muscles and tendons which stabilize the trunk and legs. Crunches, isolation exercises and machine work are *out*—powerful active flexibility techniques which require holding the legs up and out are *in*. I don't care how "sexy" your belly looks. If you can't hang from an overhead bar and hold your locked legs out perfectly horizontally, the deeper muscles of your stomach and hips are weak. You need to do something about it.

Hanging leg raises vs L-holds

Hanging leg raises are an ideal way to strengthen the deep muscles of the hips and gut, but they are too demanding to perform frequently—and as I explained in chapter fourteen, the synovial joints need regular "oiling" so tiring exercises are out. For the maximum bang for your buck, keep hanging leg raises in your training routine for strength and stamina, and add in some *L-holds* more frequently as part of a Trifecta program.

L-holds are an excellent little trick to throw into any "bulletproof joints" routine. Not only does focusing on the top position of the leg raise maximize contraction of the deep muscles, it also stretches out the spine and develops "supple strength" in the lower back. Because the waist muscles anchor onto the spine, the lower back has to work hard to stabilize itself during powerful anterior chain contractions—which makes L-holds an excellent, safe way of smoothly building tension-flexibility in the back, making it stronger and much more injury-proofed. You can do L-holds while hanging, but doing them off the floor is more convenient for frequent practice because it requires no equipment.

Evolving your leg raise holds

Remember—the Trifecta is meant to be a *subjective* program, to improve subjective qualities such as the way your joints feel and respond. It's not geared towards producing *objective* results, like strength feats. When you begin using leg raise holds, pick an exercise that feels right for you—don't view it as just a stepping stone to the next exercise. When you just can't *feel* the hold you are on working any more, try a harder variation.

A twenty second hold workout (broken up into several "sets") is more than enough to stretch you out and oil the joints. If you are set upon racing through the progressions, adding more time/more sets will help. But why focus on tricks? If it's real hardcore gut strength you want, just put more energy into your hanging leg raises!

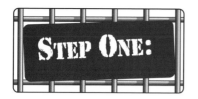
BENT LEG HOLD

PERFORMANCE

For this hold, you'll need to find a sturdy chair with some arms. (If you are in a gym, you can use parallel bars.) Grip the chair with straight (or slightly kinked) arms. Brace your upper body, and lift your knees up. At the top, your thighs should be at least parallel to the ground (see photo). Over time, as this hold gets easy, try to lift your knees higher for a better active stretch. Eventually you'll be able to pull your knees close to your chest (a *tuck hold*). Keep your feet and legs together and try to breathe normally during the hold.

EXERCISE X-RAY

Most athletes have been trained to work their "abs" with their lower backs on the floor—as for crunches. They have been told that this takes the hips and lower back out of ab movements. Since these muscles were designed to work in unison, this method only results in physical imbalance. The *bent leg hold* functions as an excellent corrective exercise, as it not only strengthens your alignment muscles, it also begins generating tension-flexibility in the lumbar muscles, which are stretched while firing to stabilize the trunk.

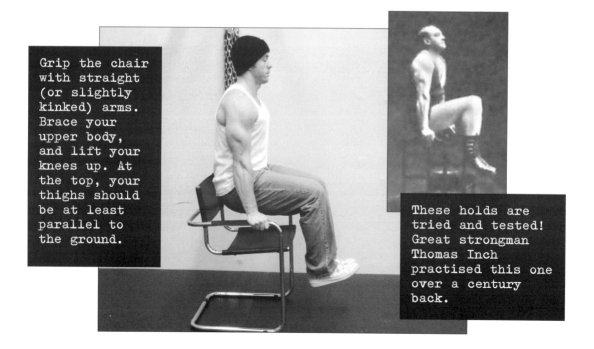

Grip the chair with straight (or slightly kinked) arms. Brace your upper body, and lift your knees up. At the top, your thighs should be at least parallel to the ground.

These holds are tried and tested! Great strongman Thomas Inch practised this one over a century back.

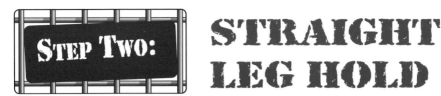

STEP TWO: STRAIGHT LEG HOLD

PERFORMANCE

For this hold, you'll need the same chair or base you used for the previous technique. Grip the chair with straight (or slightly kinked) arms. Brace your upper body, and lift your knees up. At the top, your thighs should be at least parallel to the ground (this is a *bent leg hold*). From here, straighten your legs until they are locked out straight. This may mean your feet dip down so that your legs are diagonal (see photo). That's fine—just make sure those legs are locked out. Keep your feet and legs together and breathe normally.

EXERCISE X-RAY

Once your back and midsection have adapted to the demands of bent leg holds, it's time to take things further by straightening your legs. This is the purpose of the *straight leg hold*. Because the muscles of the posterior chain are interconnected, the stretching of the hamstrings caused by the locked out legs also increases the stretch in the lower back and waist. This increases tension-flexibility in these areas, strengthens the muscles of the hips, and prepares the athlete for the harder holds that come next.

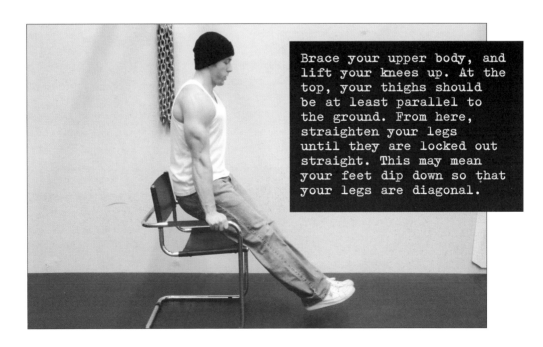

Brace your upper body, and lift your knees up. At the top, your thighs should be at least parallel to the ground. From here, straighten your legs until they are locked out straight. This may mean your feet dip down so that your legs are diagonal.

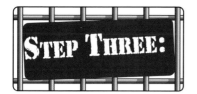
N-HOLD

PERFORMANCE

There are various names for this technique, but in jail I usually heard it called an *N-hold*. (In the *L-hold* your body forms an "L" shape; in this hold it makes like a backwards "N"). Get down on the floor, with your hands by your hips. Your legs should be together, and well bent. Straighten your arms, brace your whole body and push down until your butt and feet leave the floor—only your flat hands should be in contact with the ground (see photo). If this is too difficult at first, make it easier by placing a couple of books under each palm. When this is easy, try the fists, then the palms again.

EXERCISE X-RAY

The N-hold doesn't look a million miles different from the *bent leg hold*, but trust me—working off the floor represents a whole new level of ability. To keep your feet and butt off the ground, your trunk has to work hard to pull the hips above the level of the palms. This is harder than it sounds, but the payoff is worth it: the harder muscular contractions build increasingly impressive supple strength in the spine, which has to stay tight to keep up.

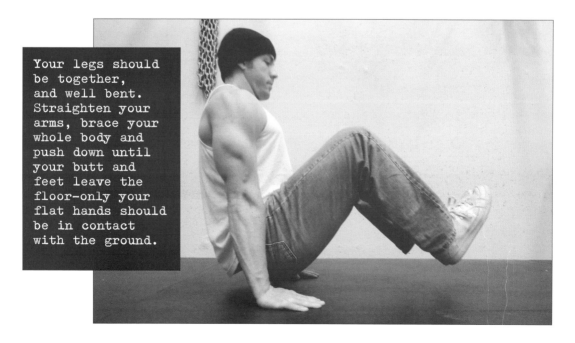

Your legs should be together, and well bent. Straighten your arms, brace your whole body and push down until your butt and feet leave the floor-only your flat hands should be in contact with the ground.

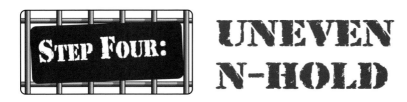

STEP FOUR:

UNEVEN
N-HOLD

PERFORMANCE

Get down on the floor and perform an *N-hold* (see previous page). Once in the hold, straighten out one leg as far as you can—ultimately, you want to be able to lock your leg right out, while the other leg stays bent. At no point should your lower body touch the floor (see photo). Draw your leg back in, then repeat on the opposite side for the same amount of time. As you get stronger and more comfortable in this one-leg out position, slowly start extending your bent leg out as well; it's this kind of transitional experimentation which will lead you to a full *L-hold*.

EXERCISE X-RAY

The *uneven N-hold* is a very gradual, natural way to move on from the N-hold. Straightening out one leg increases the leverage and the strength demands on the hip flexors, whilst simultaneously stretching the hamstrings and lower back. If you have committed some time reaping the benefits of the *straight leg hold* this variation should not pose much of a problem. The supple strength will be there.

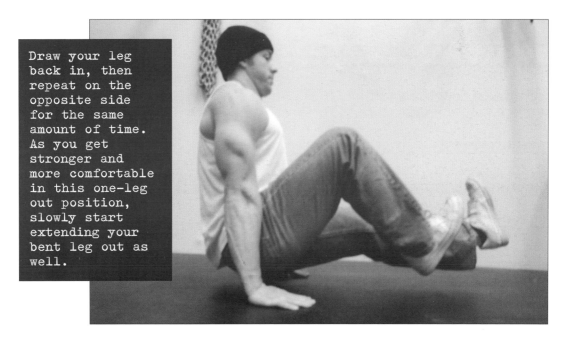

Draw your leg back in, then repeat on the opposite side for the same amount of time. As you get stronger and more comfortable in this one-leg out position, slowly start extending your bent leg out as well.

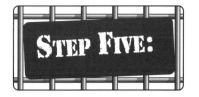

L-HOLD

PERFORMANCE

Get down on the floor, with your hands by your hips. Your legs should be together and locked out straight, with the toes pointing upwards. Straighten your arms, brace your whole body and push down until your butt and legs leave the floor—only your flat hands should be in contact with the ground. Your legs should be at least parallel with the ground (see photo). As with all the floor holds, you can make things easier at first by pushing from books, or from the knuckles (see inset). If the *L-hold* becomes too easy, increase the stretch by slowly raising the locked legs (called a *V-hold*). Breathe normally during the hold, and keep the gut in tight (this is true for all leg raise holds).

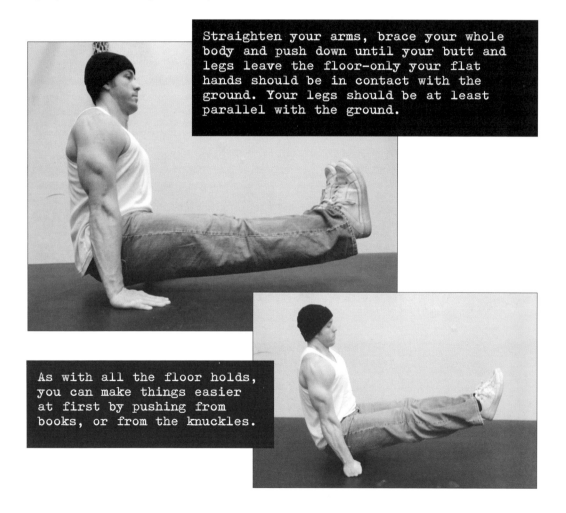

Straighten your arms, brace your whole body and push down until your butt and legs leave the floor-only your flat hands should be in contact with the ground. Your legs should be at least parallel with the ground.

As with all the floor holds, you can make things easier at first by pushing from books, or from the knuckles.

BULLETPROOF JOINTS: THE EFFECTS!

The L-hold is an excellent movement for promoting mobility and integrity in stiff "trouble spots" including the hips and low back:

- Most athletes stretch their posterior chain by bending forwards, or using gravity to stretch *passively*. The L-hold stretches the posterior chain *actively*, using tight muscular contraction. As a result, the L-hold builds functional range-of-motion: flexibility that can be *controlled*.

- The functional range generated by L-holds leads to more realistic, healthier, safer and stronger movement patterns.

- The lower back must retain tension during the stretch, to stabilize the hips. This builds tension-flexibility, or "supple strength".

- Increased levels of supple strength in the low back make it much more impervious to acute injuries caused by lifting. What athlete wouldn't want a bulletproof back?

- The L-hold tones the deep tissues of the hips, strengthening the muscles close to the bone and reducing the possibility of chronic hip pain and injury.

- The L-hold is the perfect way to open the vertebrae in the lumbar spine, allowing synovial fluid to circulate to feed and oil these joints.

- Breathe smoothly and keep the belly tucked in tight for all leg raise movements. This strengthens the *transversus* muscles, reduces the potential to develop hernia and is a cure for sagging guts.

- Using the L-hold as part of a *Trifecta* program increases blood flow and nutrient injection in the lower back area, healing inflamed tissue, old injuries and even damaged discs.

- Holding the position frequently will free up adhesions and stiffness in the hips, make the legs feel light, and free up rigid or prematurely fused vertebrae in the lower spine.

Going beyond?

As I already suggested, if you feel the L-hold is just too easy—it's not stretching or contracting your chains enough—then just up the ante by raising your feet, while keeping the legs locked. This is the *V-hold*.

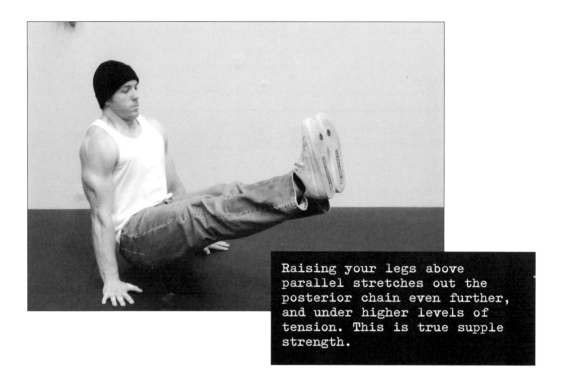

Raising your legs above parallel stretches out the posterior chain even further, and under higher levels of tension. This is true supple strength.

The L-hold and the V-hold aren't really different exercises; it's more accurate to say that the V-hold is an extension of the L-hold. Ultimately, they are extensions of the same fundamental technique, whatever you want to call it.

Once you can perform the V-hold, you have reached a point very few human beings get to—and you really don't need to push your system any further to get the joint-training benefits you're looking for. Sure you can find *harder* leg raise/abdominal movements, but remember, that's not the point. Strength is great, but the Trifecta is about regularly feeding, oiling and healing battered bodies, while gently extending and loosening up premature rigor mortis. Learning specialist gymnastics or circus tricks is cool if that's what you're into, but will it help you with these particular goals? Nope.

The movements contained in this chapter are all you'll ever need as part of a bulletproof joints program.

Lights out!

Here's some simple math for ya:

Low back pain + weak hips = the "curse" of modern athletes

Sad but true. Often, these problems are seen as just being part of life; aging; overuse; or a design flaw in the human body. They are none of these things.

Modern abdominal training—those endless reps of crunches on the gym floor—are often associated with back pain and spinal discomfort. Why? Should working your abs give you back pain?

No. *Isolating* your abs will give you back pain. Many active people who experiment with Pilates for their "core" are forced to perform leg raise movements sitting down, *but with their backs off the floor.* Guess what pro athletes like Tiger Woods, Pat Cash and Curt Shilling "discovered" when they performed those movements? Their chronic back pain went away. As soon as they dropped super-popular ab isolation movements and began working their abs and back together with leg raise holds, their joints started getting stronger, more functional, and a damn sight healthier.

Don't panic. You don't need to screw around with over-complex new systems like Pilates to get the same results. Forget all the other posing and just take the active element you need—L-holds, baby.

17: Twist Progressions

Unleash Your Functional Triad

I f you want powerful, strong joints, there's no point just training your arms and legs. Functional movement is based on *physical alignment* and it radiates outwards from the trunk—in particular the spine, hip girdle and shoulder girdle. It's totally pointless having strong muscles anywhere on your body if these three key areas are weak.

This is something modern bodybuilders just don't understand. They train for muscular arms or thick, brawny legs, but they can't appreciate why they still suffer from chronic and acute injuries. This is because they are focusing on their *external muscles*—the showy stuff—but they have allowed the deeper, *alignment muscles* of their bodies to become weak and stiff. This is nuts. The alignment muscles are what keep the entire musculo-skeletal system where it should be for optimal health and function. It's like the foundations of a building. Growing huge external muscles on top of weak deep muscles is like building a skyscraper on top of a crummy, shallow foundation. Trouble is bound to happen!

Erase deep shoulder pain and weakness

In this part of the book, we've already discussed a weak spine (fixed by *bridge holds*) and a weak hip girdle (fixed by *L-holds*). But the shoulder girdle is another prime example of "deep" alignment muscles which most gym trainers ignore. Most lifters pack slabs of meat onto their pecs, lats and delts, around the shoulders, but the *internal* muscles—the rotator cuffs, for example—don't get any training at all. Without active flexibility work to help them, they will get irritated constantly—until they eventually give up the ghost and freeze altogether. Speak to any long-term weight-trainer, and he'll probably tell you how he's suffered some terrible, "freak" shoulder injury. In fact, these "accidents" are nothing of the kind. If an athlete combines high levels of pressing strength with stiff, weak rotator cuffs, injury is inevitable. Unfortunately, most athletes don't know much about active flexibility at all; and they certainly don't know how to perform correct active flexibility work for the shoulder girdle. In their ignorance, these guys treat the deep rotator cuff like it was any other muscle—and try to work it with teeny baby dumbbells or low-power elastic cables. Endless reps with fixed weights won't strengthen your rotator cuffs—in fact it will probably just make your shoulders more irritated over time.

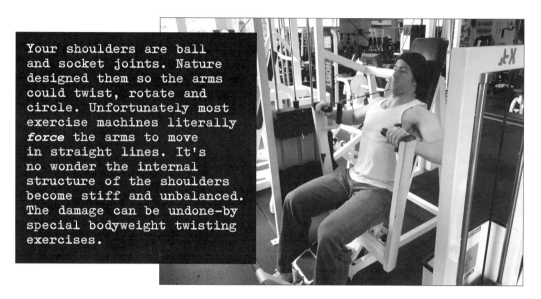

Your shoulders are ball and socket joints. Nature designed them so the arms could twist, rotate and circle. Unfortunately most exercise machines literally *force* the arms to move in straight lines. It's no wonder the internal structure of the shoulders become stiff and unbalanced. The damage can be undone—by special bodyweight twisting exercises.

The finest way to train your rotator cuff is with bodyweight—active flexibility twisting exercises which gently stretch out and free up your rotator cuffs, and give them the kind of special "supple strength" I discussed in chapter twelve. Trust me, if you learn how to twist correctly, you can kiss your shoulder problems goodbye. I'll show you how in the next couple of chapters.

The Big Seven?

I'm gonna tell you something now. When I set down the "Big Six" of *Convict Conditioning*—pushups, squats, pullups, leg raises, bridges and HSPUs—I came damn close to adding twists to that list. That's how much I believe in the power of twisting. Done right, twisting is great for the back, and boosts the hell out of trunk and torso flexibility—something few athletes think about much (most of them follow the lead of martial artists, and only stretch out their legs). Twists have an almost magical ability to iron out shoulder pain, plus the fact that they work the lateral chain—something I didn't specifically include much of in the Big Six.

In the end, I didn't add them. They aren't really a strength exercise, and they seemed kinda out of step with the other six, which are much more old school. But none of this has changed the high esteem I have for twisting.

Let's twist again

If you are doing *Convict Conditioning*-based workouts, you are already getting *some* of the benefits of *bridge holds* (from dynamic bridging) and *L-holds* (from leg raises). If you don't want or feel the need to perform a separate joint health/mobility program like the Trifecta, no problem. But if you take nothing else from this book, *at least add a program of twists*.

Twice a week is enough; three times is better. You can add them to your bodyweight workouts or pick a different day—but do them. The effects twists have on the body are awesome. They align the spine, free up stiff backs, heal and strengthen the rotator cuffs, and tone and stretch the sides of the body. They even stretch out the elbows and forearms in a healthy way.

So—are you ready to add twisting to your program, now and forever? Excellent, my man. You won't regret it. Over the next few pages I'll show you how.

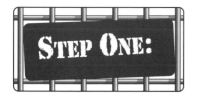

STRAIGHT LEG TWIST HOLD

PERFORMANCE

Sit on the floor with your legs together and outstretched. Bend one leg until your foot is inside the knee of your straight leg. Keep the foot of your bent leg flat on the floor. Twist your opposite shoulder towards your bent knee, and secure the elbow on the outside of that knee. Allow the neck and head to naturally follow the turn of the torso. Place the palm of your other hand behind you, and prop yourself securely on that outstretched arm (see photo). Hold the posture for the required time, trying to breathe as normally as possible. Repeat the hold on the opposite side for the same amount of time.

EXERCISE X-RAY

This basic twist hold should be achievable for any person without a major injury or disability. The athlete learns the basic sitting position essential for all twists, but the twist here is mild due to the natural arm positions and the straight leg. Just holding this position for a period of time is an ideal way to undo knots and stiffness in the hips, back, upper back and shoulders. As an added bonus, the biceps of the straight arm gets some flexibility work. This hold is a godsend for ultra-tight lifters who want to move on to harder twists.

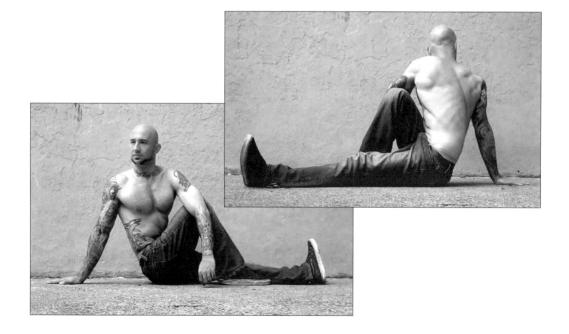

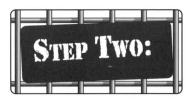

STEP TWO:

EAST TWIST HOLD

PERFORMANCE

Sit on the floor with your legs outstretched. Bend one leg and place the foot flat on the floor, to the outside of your opposite knee. Bend the other leg until your heel comes in contact with your glutes, keeping that leg on the floor. Twist your opposite shoulder towards your raised knee, and secure the elbow on the outside of that knee. Place the palm of your other hand behind you, and prop yourself securely on your outstretched arm. Allow your neck to naturally continue the twist, and look obliquely back (see photos). Hold the posture for the required period, trying to breathe as normally as possible. Repeat the hold on the opposite side for the same amount of time.

EXERCISE X-RAY

This hold is slightly harder than the last. Bending the leg and moving it inwards will stretch the muscles running up the thigh and hip (*quads, tensor* muscles, *gluteus medius,* etc.). Since all the muscles of the lateral chain are interconnected (hence the term *chain*), this increases the stretch higher up. With this stretch, the waist, upper spine and shoulders begin to feel the benefit. Remember to keep the stretch *strength-led*—don't force anything.

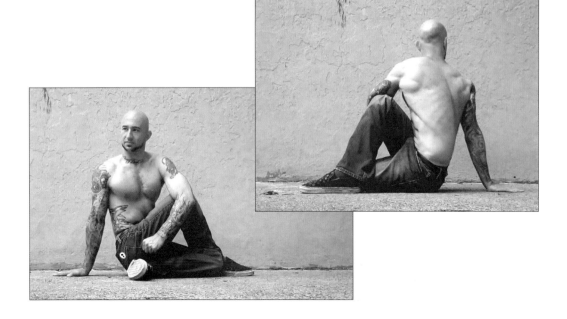

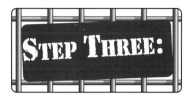

HALF TWIST HOLD

PERFORMANCE

Sit on the floor with your legs outstretched. Bend one leg and place the foot flat on the floor, to the outside of your opposite knee. Bend the other leg until your heel comes in contact with your glutes, keeping that leg on the floor. Twist your opposite shoulder towards your raised knee, and slide your hand down your outer calf, so that it runs parallel to your shin until the fingers touch your instep. Place the palm of your other hand behind you, and prop yourself securely on your outstretched arm. Rotate your neck to look behind you (see main photo). Hold the posture for the required time, trying to breathe as normally as possible. Repeat the hold on the opposite side.

EXERCISE X-RAY

I consider this a halfway point for athletes looking to master the *full twist*—if you can hold this for 1-20 seconds while breathing smoothly, you're halfway there. The arm-along-leg position requires a strong twist from a flexible spine—you're starting to make progress. The neck is also worked now. If this standard version becomes easy, you can anticipate the next step by taking your rearmost hand from the floor and looping it around your torso.

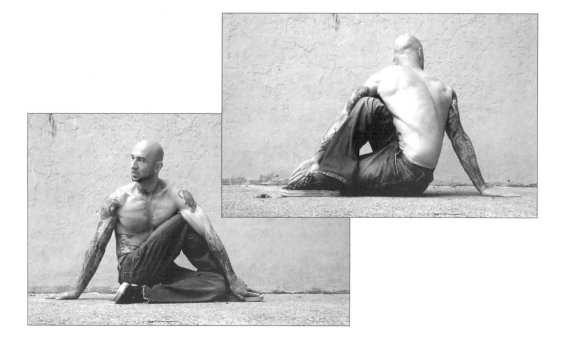

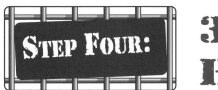
3/4 TWIST HOLD

PERFORMANCE

For this exercise you need an object—anything about a foot long (a hand towel is a perfect option). Sit on the floor with your legs outstretched. Now perform the *half twist hold* (see page 216). The hand of the arm alongside the shin should be holding the towel. Once alongside your shin, push the hand holding the towel back and under the elbow. Reach around your body with the other hand, and try to grab hold of the towel. This may take some practice at first. Once you grab the towel, rotate your neck to look behind you (see photos). Hold the posture for the required time, trying to breathe as normally as possible. Repeat the hold on the opposite side.

EXERCISE X-RAY

In terms of difficulty, this hold lies somewhere between the *half twist hold* and the *full twist hold*. Previously, the rear arm has been in contact with the floor, but now it snakes its way around the trunk. This forces the athlete to twist harder, and stretches the shoulder girdle and lateral chain further than ever. Progression is simple as pie—try to inch the fingers closer each time things feel easy. Impossible as it might seem, one day they'll touch!

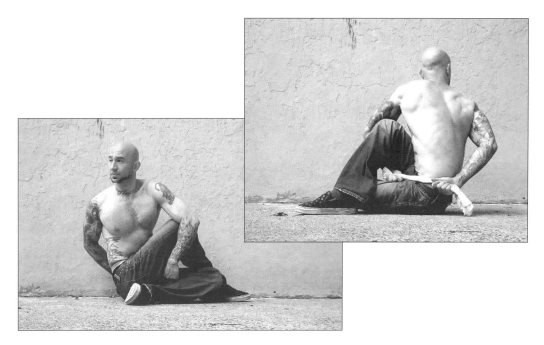

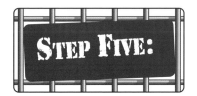

STEP FIVE:

FULL TWIST HOLD

PERFORMANCE

Sit on the floor with your legs outstretched. Bend one leg and place the foot flat on the floor, to the outside of your opposite knee. Bend the other leg until your heel comes in contact with your glutes, keeping that leg on the floor. Twist your opposite shoulder towards your raised knee, and push the hand of that shoulder holding back and under the elbow. Reach around your body with the other hand, and touch fingers. Hook the fingers, or lock them in a "monkey grip" (see top photo). Lift your chest, and rotate your neck to look behind you (see bottom photo). Hold the posture for the required time, trying to breathe as normally as possible. Repeat the hold on the opposite side.

EXERCISE X-RAY

This hold should be considered the advanced template for all twist-stretching. Anyone who attains it will be more functionally flexible than the next hundred athletes. If you feel the need, you can move past this stretch by gripping further than the fingers. Be warned that, beyond this point, every extra inch of reach is exponentially harder to attain. I got to the point where I could grasp my wrist instead of my hand, but it took a solid year of work.

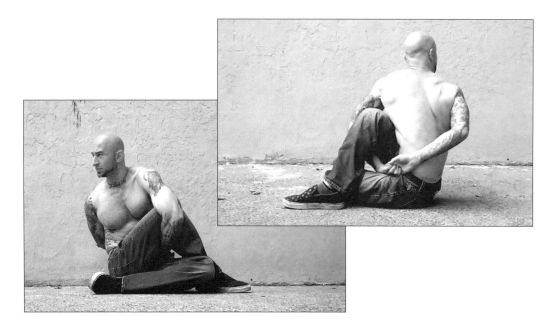

BULLETPROOF JOINTS: THE EFFECTS!

Bodyweight twists are an excellent candidate for the "ultimate" in active stretching exercises—particularly for strength athletes. Reasons why include:

- Many athletes train to move their bodies up-and-down, and front-and-back: but how many train to *rotate*? Twists take care of this "missing link" in most training programs, increasing flexibility and strength in the deep muscles responsible for rotation.

- The unique arm/shoulder socket position of harder twists stretches and tones the *rotator cuff* from the inside out, without need for weights, cables or other equipment. This deep stimulation frees up the shoulders and radically improves mobility. It increases blood flow, enhances healing, cures old injuries and eliminates nagging shoulder pain—for good.

- Over time, consistent performance of the full twist will break up calcium deposits in the shoulder, and even eliminate painful spurs.

- Twisting is the best way to safely work the *internal oblique* muscles. When combined with an exercise for the *external obliques*—such as human flag training—you have a perfect oblique program.

- Many athletes suffer from upper back pain because they hold on to excess tension in the muscles between the shoulder blades (heavy rowing and curling doesn't help). Twists actively release the shoulder blades in the most efficient way possible, dissipating tightness in the deepest layers of upper back muscle and fascia.

- Deep twisting massages the internal organs, keeps them healthy, and even aids digestion.

- When done right, twists reverse stiffness and damage done to the hips and back caused by misuse or underuse, helping to prevent hip cramps and backache. Because hip twisting is key to so many sports (think punching, kicking, batting, throwing, etc.), even a short course of twists will improve athleticism and sports performance.

Going beyond?

No doubt about it, most people have trouble twisting. This is because it's not part of their regular movement pattern. The average fit person would have serious trouble achieving the *full twist hold*, and bodybuilders—well, forget it. The full twist represents an ideal range of rotational motion, but it can be achieved, with patience and dedication.

Of course, the *ideal* range of motion for normal joints is not necessarily the *maximum* range. Maximizing your flexibility beyond the exercises I've set out won't improve your joint health or athleticism. It'll only make you more prone to injury. If you want to learn more advanced twists, you'll have to learn that stuff from a yoga master. But you don't really need it. Build up gradually to the full twist hold, and retain that mobility by practicing the twist at least two or three times a week. That's all you need for perfect lateral chain function.

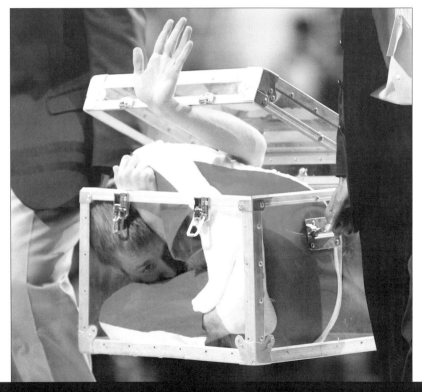

With training, the human body can be taught to twist to an amazing degree-like the contortionist above. Tricks like this are real impressive, and take years of dedication to master. They stretch the body to the point where even the ligaments-which should be like steel cables-become looser. Strength athletes looking to build bulletproof joints should avoid this like the plague.

Keep it strength-led

One more quick tip before lights out. Twists convey a lot of benefits, but these are maximized when you do things the right way. The most common mistake I see during twists is *reaching and pulling*. Athletes jerk or throw themselves around, trying to twist using momentum or by yanking with the leading hand.

Avoid this. Remember, twists are meant to be an active flexibility technique—they are *strength-led*. They are no different from bridges or L-holds. Don't twist by reaching, jerking and pulling. Twist using muscle power alone. Rotate using the contractile strength of your trunk muscles—then pause at the limit of your movement. The technique you use should be determined by the limit of your rotation—not the other way round.

What if you can't rotate and twist as much as you want? That's fine. Work at the level you are at. Don't force things. *Forcing* a stretch can only be done by losing control of what you are doing (passive stretching), and that defeats the object. The Trifecta holds—all of them—are meant to iron out movement kinks and improve functional mobility. They aren't goddam limbo contests, where you get points for bending yourself out of shape.

Lights out!

Most people never stretch the muscles of their lateral chain, and rarely perform rotational movements. Throwers are the exception; pitchers, putters, discus and javelin throwers. These sportspeople need to unlock the rotational power of their torsos, but even these athletes are often too stiff or worse—stiff and strong in an unsymmetrical way. If this is you, you can benefit from twist holds more than most.

More average bears will also get some big time results from twisting. I've always said that if you only add one type of stretch to your strength routine, it should be twist holds. They undo a huge amount of excess tightness in the torso and shoulder girdle brought on by heavy strength work, and at the same time loosen up the lower back and hips. Plus, they make an old upper body feel like a young upper body.

Seriously—try it for a month or so. You've got nothing to lose but pain and rust.

— PART III —

WISDOM FROM CELLBLOCK G

Advanced calisthenics is about more than
just pushups. I trained alone in my cell
for years—nearly two decades, in fact.
During my prison journey, I was lucky
enough to find some wonderful teachers,
but none of us had the luxuries athletes
on the outside take for granted. There
were no juice bars or health food stores.
No saunas, masseurs or chiropractors. We
had to learn about a lot of stuff through
experience; painful trial and error. If
we had injuries, we had to learn to cope
alone, for the most part. I've learned a
lot about coping alone, with everything
from the negative temptations of prison
life to the nasty stuff going on in my own
head.

This section is my attempt to pass on some
of what I've learned in those areas of an
athlete's life that stretch beyond simple
sets and reps.

18: Doing Time Right

Living the
Straight Edge

I n this book, and its predecessor *Convict Conditioning*, I've written at length about different training techniques. I've discussed proper form, ideas for routines, and even the principles of productive exercise necessary to lock onto your training targets. These components are the elements that go to make up anybody's workout program.

But I'd be misleading you if I told you that getting bigger, stronger, fitter, faster, *better* was all about your workout program. It's not. Put in perspective, your workouts form a relatively small chunk of your life. If you train for an hour every day—which is more than enough for any athlete, provided you are working hard—that equals only a little bit over *four percent* of your total time. It's really not much, is it?

That four percent is vitally important. But the way you spend the remaining ninety-five-and-change can really make the difference between so-so results and *phenomenal* results. Everything you do throughout the day—what you eat, how long you sleep, what you put into your body—these things all have an impact on how effective your training is for you. These effects might seem little in isolation, but when they are combined and multiplied over the course of weeks and years they add up to *huge* differences. I've seen many hundreds of convicts train behind bars, and I can say for sure that *lifestyle* is a major factor in the relative success or failure of all these men. It's no good training like an animal in your cell if your life outside your workouts is sloppy and self-destructive. On numerous occasions I've seen athletes with inferior potential become far greater than their genetic superiors purely because of the discipline they apply to their lives beyond the training.

A great many guys bust their ass in the gym, but think nothing at all of staying up late to go out drinking with the boys. I've written any number of grand routines for my students living on the outside, only to watch them sabotage these programs through a lack of rest and recuperation. In prison, I had to personally witness far too many natural athletes with huge potential literally destroy their latent talents through the abuse of recreational drugs.

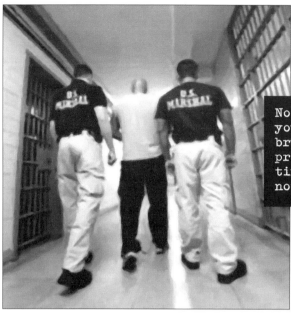

No matter how committed you are, no matter how brutal your training program is, most of your time in prison is spent not training at all.

Discipline unlocks talent

The key to straightening out these problems lies in just one quality—*discipline*. If being incarcerated in correctional facilities taught me one thing, it taught me the value of living a disciplined, regulated lifestyle. In prison, there is a time to get up, a time to work, a time to exercise, a time to eat, a time to socialize (if you're lucky) and a time to go to bed. It's almost a military-type regimen. I saw this drive a lot of new fish crazy—particularly the guys from welfare neighborhoods or the projects. These kids have more freedom than any other generation in history. They get up when they like, see who they like, smoke what they like and go to bed when they like. Many of them haven't had to face any kind of discipline their whole lives. Certainly not from their parents, most of who were "raised" pretty much the same way.

Guys like this benefit the most from the harsh, regulated lifestyle of living by the buzzer. After the initial shock, a lot of them come to value the order prison forces upon their lives. I know I did. If you can't get some kind of pattern, some form of schedule and discipline into your life, you'll never achieve any of your fitness goals. In fact, achieving *any* worthwhile objective requires a regulated life.

In this chapter I'd like to break away from the cold, bright science of working out, to explore the often chaotic and murky question of *lifestyle*—the way you spend your time when you're *not* working out. Let's continue the journey we've started and examine several of the factors that exist outside your training time that may—or may not—influence how effective your program is for you. Perhaps a grizzled ex-con can teach you a trick or two, by virtue of his own mistakes. Maybe not. We'll see.

Rest and sleep

Rest is the most important element in recovery from hard training. It's more important than nutrition, supplements, active therapies, or any other factor. When you perform hard calisthenics, you cause micro-trauma to the muscles and joints; pour toxins into your muscle cells; you strain your nervous and hormonal system to some degree. Most importantly, you deplete the sugar (called *glycogen*) in your muscle cells. Your body is perfectly capable of repairing all this damage and replenishing internal muscular energy, but it requires *time* to do so.

Determining just how much time you need to fully recover before training your muscles again is an individual matter. It depends upon your innate recovery ability, athletic experience, as well as the volume and intensity of your training methods. Some people can work a strength exercise three times per week and still make gains—most people would be better off leaving it a full week before working a particular exercise again, particularly if they are performing their exercises in a very hard, disciplined manner. The only way to really ascertain how much rest you need is by experimenting with different programs. If you are continually getting stronger in your movements—by adding high-quality repetitions, and moving to harder exercises—then you are getting enough rest. If you struggle to increase your reps, or if your performance actually *declines*, it's probably because you're not resting long enough between sessions. Ideally, you want to fine-tune your rest periods so that you train as often as possible within a context of maximum productive rest. This is a very delicate equilibrium to maintain. You can only locate it as a result of lots of hard, intelligent training. There's no other way.

Without a doubt, sleep also plays a major factor in recovery. When I was first incarcerated, I barely slept a wink for the first two weeks or so. Nightmares are incredibly common in prison, due to the high level of anxiety many convicts experience through the day. As a result, there are always guys screaming and shouting stuff in their sleep. Plus, there's usually some mad fool on your block yelling something at night to prove a point. These nocturnal noises terrified me when I was a new inmate, and night after night I would lay awake in the dark, listening to the voices and feeling my stomach turn over. I almost prayed for the next day to arrive, although when it did I was good for nothing; I was edgy, depressed, exhausted and paranoid. I certainly couldn't have got any decent training done, let alone made any progress.

A lot of inmates use little foam rubber earplugs to block out the disturbing nighttime cacophony, the disposable kind often used in loud factories. My third week in I managed to lay my hands on a pair of these, although I found that they made my ears sore and rendered a bad situation even worse. It probably took me three months before I adapted to the prison atmosphere and got a full, uninterrupted eight hours sleep.

These days I can sleep pretty much anywhere, no matter what's going on around me. In fact, once you get used to it, prison is great for sleep. There are no opportunities to stay up late, partying. The power goes off at lights out, so you can't watch TV or even read a book. You just go to bed. As a result, most inmates in America probably get more sleep than working stiffs on the outside. When I was in lockdown in Marion, we were in our cells twenty-three hours a day, and as well as a full eight hours, most guys got one or two naps in during the afternoon. This surplus of sleep, plus all the free time and energy on your hands, combines to make high security penal institutions ideal environments for effective calisthenics training.

On the outside, it can be difficult to get enough sleep, particularly if you live a wild or hectic lifestyle. The best advice I can give you is to aim at *regularity* in your sleeping patterns. Mimic what happens in prisons; give yourself a fixed time for lights out, a time which is at least nine hours before you need to get up. If you follow this pattern repeatedly, your body will eventually get used to the routine and figure out what it needs to do.

Activity levels

Don't be misled into thinking you have to be incarcerated and lying around in a jail cell all day to make gains in strength and muscle. Certainly, lots of hard physical work outside your regular training program may affect your development, but not nearly as much as people think. Canada's greatest ever Strongman Louis Cyr built most of his strength working in a lumber camp. The Mighty Atom was a dock laborer while he was making his best gains. Famous weightlifter and bodybuilder John Grimek used to work exhausting shifts in a steel foundry before going to the gym to do his training. The list goes on.

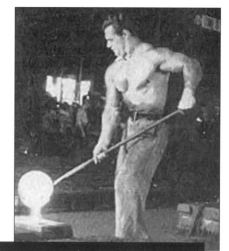

It's not true to say that all prisoners have it easy, either. This may be true in some prisons—particularly supermax institutions—but most convicts have to work while they are inside. When I was in Angola Pen, I toiled full days on the famous prison farm, and did my training in my cell after work duty. I was once buddies with an inmate from Alabama who who spent his days working on the chain gang in blistering heat, and still found the energy to do his pushups and sit-ups on the side of the road!

John Grimek built the world's strongest, most muscular body—after a full day's toil. What's your excuse?

If you have been training regularly and you suddenly begin a job where you need to perform manual labor for twelve-hour shifts, five days a week, your training will almost certainly suffer. Whenever we experience a radical alteration in our set routine, it takes a while to become accustomed to the new workload. But if you give the body the extra calories it requires to do all that work, you'll find that in a short time your energy systems will acclimatize and you'll be able to make regular gains from hard strength training again. The body has much greater powers of adaptation than people give it credit for. Just give yourself time.

Stress

Everybody talks about "stress" as this major factor in recovery. I just don't buy all this New Age crap. Seems like stress is a major part of everyday life nowadays. Everybody has "stress", and they don't hide their shame in telling you all about how stressed out they are. People attribute overeating to stress, they attribute illnesses to stress, and they take time off from work sick due to stress.

Nobody I ever met in the joint uses this kind of language. It would make you a target very rapidly. In prison you try to *hide* stress; stress is a weakness, stress makes you look vulnerable. Compared to prison, this "stressful" life on the outside never seemed that stressful to me anyways. I always thought that people who spend most of their time bitterly complaining about money worries and relationship problems should spend a few months locked up, constantly under threat of being raped in the shower rooms or offending the wrong veterano and being shanked during your lunch break. That might put the "stress" of modern life into perspective.

Maybe my outlook is a bit warped. Because of the long stretches I have spent inside prisons, my view of the outside is a bit like a time-lapse film. Things are always a little different, a little worse, when I see the streets again. I was shocked by what America had become when I last got parole. My role models were John Wayne and Charles Bronson; today the kids have role models like Paris Hilton and Britney Spears. Is it any wonder that we live in an era of complete self-obsession? The relative economic wealth of our nation combined with a decadent, corrupt media have made us into little children, neurotically wrapped up in our own thoughts and feelings and the contents of our personal little skulls.

Forget your thoughts and feelings and focus on *getting the job done*. Guerrillas fighting in warzones don't have time to get stressed—they're focusing too hard trying to stay alive. Nomads in Africa don't have time get hung up on how stressed out they feel when a drought strikes. They are far too busy trying to locate water and get it home to their kids. Fire your shrink and challenge yourself to some pushups instead. I guarantee you'll feel better.

Harden the hell up, America.

Conjugal visits/the Bone Yard (...sex!)

Okay, here's yet another section where I'm going to look pretty old-fashioned. (I'm getting used to this now.) Many state prisons have a "Bone Yard". The Bone Yard is a place set aside for (what Californian jails call) "Extended Family Visits"...that's *sex* to you and me. In federal jail, conjugal visits don't happen; and my time in federal made me think more and more about the relationship between sex and training.

Many of the old time strongmen believed that excessive sexual activity played a significant role in depleting strength and endurance. It wasn't just strength athletes who believed this; prior to the 1970s, a lot of boxing trainers used to demand that their fighters abstained from bedroom activities in the week prior to a big match. The prevailing opinion was that the sexual act drained energy reserves that could be channeled into physical achievements instead. *No sex before a fight!* the coaches ordered.

The notion that sex somehow saps the body of energy is a very ancient idea that can be found in many cultures. Taoists believe that sexual power, *jing*, becomes transformed into physical energy, *chi*. If you waste jing, you lose chi. The Hindu practice of "tantric" sex is based on the idea that sexual energy can be retained and stored to improve bodily health. If you look back far enough, you'll find similar theories all around the world.

These days, sports scientists tend to laugh at these archaic ideas. They are seen as being primitive superstitions. But I'm not so sure. I know a lot about sexual frustration from years of being locked up in prison, and I'm convinced that this frustration forces you to expend energy in other ways. For a lot of red-blooded convicts, this built-up tension only finds release through hard, physical training. When you are sexually satisfied, you become incredibly relaxed, almost dopey. The last thing you want to do is set after set of pushups. But if you're not getting any, your body becomes charged, wired, on edge—the perfect state for athletic activity.

Sex is one of the best things in life, so I'm certainly not telling you to become a monk or kick your girl-friend out of bed. But be aware of your sexual activity and how it relates to your strength levels. If you are going for personal records in your training, steer clear of sex a few nights before your big workout. You might be surprised by the results.

Skin dips

Smoking is a real bugbear of mine. The habit is common in prisons—far, far more common than it is beyond the bars these days. Convicts often have a lot of time to kill, and most guys on the inside have bigger problems than worrying about getting lung cancer in twenty years. The average con only thinks in terms of days or maybe weeks anyway. Thinking about your life in bigger chunks than that would drive you totally nuts, especially if you have a lot of time to serve.

Smoking tobacco is a major currency in the joints where it's allowed. Regular whole cigarettes—called "tailor-mades" on the inside—are as rare as gold. Cheaper, hand-rolled smokes are far more common. They are usually known as *skin dips, rollies* or *paper wafers*. Even these are jealously guarded treasure. Never come between a dude and his skin dips, that's for sure. When smokers can't put their hands on rolling papers, they can get pretty creative. I've seen guys use everything from toilet paper covers to the prison-issue Bibles to make papers. I've heard that smoking cigarettes is at least as addictive as heroin, and from what I've seen over the years I'm convinced that's true.

I guess I'm lucky, because I never got the taste for skin dips. I tried smoking as a kid—I guess all kids do—and it made me puke. I never went back to those foul cancer sticks, and I'm glad. Smoking, far from helping you through your sentence, actually makes doing time *more* difficult. When smokers *do* have tobacco, they desperately try to hold onto it for as long as possible, while paradoxically smoking their way through it compulsively. When they *don't* have tobacco they feel like crap, and all they can think about is getting more smokes. It's a lose-lose situation. Smokers on the inside are definitely more miserable than smoke-free cons.

Despite what you may have heard, you can still smoke if you are an athlete. I've met lots of prison athletes who smoke—some were pretty good at whatever kind of training they did. Joe DiMaggio used to like to suck on a cigarette, and so did Jesse Owens and even Babe Ruth. These guys were true greats, but the reality is that if they didn't smoke, they would have been even greater.

When you train hard—whether for strength, stamina, or in any real sport you can name—you suck in great gulps of air. The oxygen in this air passes through the lungs and is distributed to the muscles via the blood. Oxygen is a vital element for the generation of energy in all living species. The more energy demands are placed on an organism—as in physical training—the more oxygen is required, and humans can only get this through *breathing*.

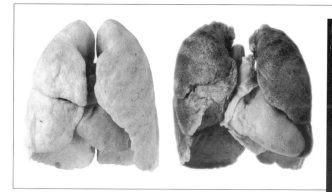

Over the years I've taken just about everything I can swallow or inject—from shrooms and hippy crack to LSD, DMT and bathtub crank. I've been an idiot, so I don't expect anyone to listen to my advice on avoiding smokes. Instead, if you puff, just look at these images of two sets of lungs. On the left, a nonsmoker. On the right, a chain smoker.

Anybody who tries calisthenics or one of the drills in this book will immediately know all about this. Fitness *absolutely* depends upon this breathing-oxygen relationship. But when you light up that cigarette, you are doing the best thing you could possibly do to screw up that relationship. Tobacco smoke contains numerous toxins that destroy the alveoli and capillaries inside the lungs which are essential to air exchange. The damage starts from the very first inhalation, but over time matters become worse as smoking causes sticky tar to build up in the respiratory system. This tar acts as an impenetrable barrier between the lung tissue and the air you draw in, which is why heavy smokers always seem to have a hard time getting enough air into their lungs when they get out of breath.

Even once you get some oxygen into your system, smoking does a great job of corrupting it. Carbon monoxide, a component of tobacco smoke, enters your system and binds up with hemoglobin, the oxygen-carrying molecule in your bloodstream. As a result, the body's army of hemoglobin molecules become depleted, and the blood becomes much less capable of carrying oxygen to the starving muscles (including your heart) which need it most. Absorbing tobacco into your body—even just by chewing the stuff—radically increases the heart rate, draining endurance. Smoking even causes or contributes to diseases like chronic bronchitis, heart disease, and emphysema as well as various forms of cancer. All of these will devastate your training. They could well kill you.

If you currently smoke and want to optimize your physical potential, try to quit or at least cut down. If you don't smoke, don't even consider starting.

Prison hooch

Drinking is kind of rare inside the joint. In this respect, it seems to be the opposite of smoking. Fewer and fewer people on the outside are taking up smoking, but where it's still allowed, a great many convicts smoke themselves silly. Alternatively, there's a pretty big drinking culture in America, but not very much of that goes on inside prisons.

The reason for this comes down entirely to *availability.* Tobacco is allowed in many institutions, alcohol is not. (Recreational drugs are also contraband, but drugs can be more easily smuggled in—in body cavities, for example—than a bottle of bourbon.) There's a really good reason for this. Nothing makes men turn into assholes quite like booze.

This is not to say that cons go without the occasional alcoholic beverage—oh no! Many booze-hounds on the inside make their own moonshine, commonly known as *prison hooch, raisin jack,* or *pruno.* Different prisoners have their own recipes for this foul rotgut. The standard procedure involves throwing some water and fruit into a trash bag—raisins, fruit cocktail, apples and grapes are popular. In the old days, prunes were a favorite choice of the discerning wino, hence the name *pruno.* This gross mixture is called the *motor.* From here, the squishy, lumpy motor is basically kept warm—in a hot water basin, or against a heated pipe—for up to a week, to brew. Sometimes extra ingredients like stale bread or ketchup are added to the mix, in the belief that the yeast and sugar these goodies contain will speed up the fermentation process. "Fermentation" is a generous way of putting it. "Making it putrid" is much more accurate. Once this gunk is done, it's strained and drunk. The stuff is very nearly as potent as methylated spirits. A whole block can get wasted on a single bag of pruno.

I've had the honor (?) of being offered pruno several times, and each time I've refused because the stuff smells like vomit. This is not an exaggeration—I've been told that drinking pruno is exactly like drinking cold puke. Even hardened old winos have to hold their noses clamped shut as they sip the stuff to try and stop themselves from throwing up.

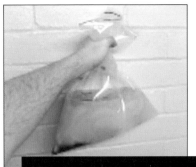

So what about booze for guys on the outside? Well, public health organizations are now telling us that moderate consumption of alcohol has some health virtues. That's as maybe, but as far as I'm concerned, there are no athletic benefits conferred by alcohol. Beer, wine and spirits only serve to make you fat and sluggish—the precise opposite of what a prison athlete wants to be. If you currently drink too much and are looking for a way to cut down, try brewing up some of your own pruno. A few gulps of that stuff will put you off liquor for years.

The vomit-inducing stew known as pruno. Avoid at all costs!

Junk, dope, horse

I have made a lot of mistakes in my life, and I'll hold my hands up and admit that the biggest mistake I ever made was experimenting with drugs when I was in my early teens. In a short space of time I moved from eating marijuana to taking amphetamines, and eventually I began abusing cocaine and heroin. If it wasn't for these evil substances, I would never have found myself in prison in the first place. I took my addictions with me inside the walls of San Quentin, and that made the early years of my stay there unbelievably hellish. As I write now, I am totally drug-free and have been that way for a little over twelve years.

The impact drugs have on prison life is unbelievable. Nobody on the outside really understands how bad the situation is—not the police, not the media, and certainly not the politicians. Drug trafficking is a massive prison industry. Illicit substances are smuggled in by correctional staff, by visitors and family members, and by mules and "keister bunnies" (guys packing drugs up their butts). Drug drops are picked up by convicts outside on work detail. In some places, drugs are simply thrown over the damn wall. As a result, hard drugs are everywhere. It's just as easy to get them on the inside as on the outside. Easier, in some institutions. I mentioned earlier that prison life has some benefits to offer athletes; things like discipline, regulation, routine, etc. This is true, but it's not all one-way. There are serious pitfalls to prison life also, and the presence of drugs is the worst pitfall of all.

The price the prisoners themselves pay for this poison is beyond belief. Drugs cement the gang dynamic, which is connected to gang war on the streets. Supply and demand combined with competition over drug turf on the inside generates a huge amount of violence. Drug debts lead to beatings and even killings. All drugs lead to is pain.

I could tell you a lot about the various illnesses and symptoms drug use can give you, but people who go on endlessly about that are really missing the point. Drugs *do* damage the body—in certain doses and combinations they can kill you quicker than a speeding truck—but it's the *mind* that's made to suffer from drug use far more than the body ever could. When you are addicted, the only thing that really matters to you is your next score. As soon as you sink to this level, all your ideas and behaviors seem to get hard-wired backwards. Crime is inevitable. I would say that for nine out of ten of the people who wind up in prison, drugs play some kind of role in their fall. The effects of drugs are insidious, and reach a lot deeper than you could ever imagine. Although I physically let go of drugs a long, long time ago, the drugs did not let go of me. Many of the contacts and circles I moved in when I was heavily involved in the lifestyle stayed with me for a long time after my system was clean, and this led to a cycle of destructive behavior that lasted for many years.

I've seen this vicious cycle in myself and many, many of my friends. It seems so obvious now, but it wasn't always that way. It never is. Nobody starts taking drugs to become a disgusting, pathetic, skinny, physically ill wreck with no future. Nobody injects heroin become they want to become a heroin addict. Nobody smokes crack the first time because they want to become a paranoid, violent sociopath. People do these things because they are exotic; because they are cool. Because they are fun. It's part of the illusion of drugs. This illusion is incredibly powerful, which is one of the reasons why it's pretty pointless telling young people to steer clear of recreational drugs. The ones who are smart enough to see beyond the false picture will keep safe. The ones who cannot see beyond the illusion will not be able to make out their problems approaching—until it's too late.

Over time, I gradually let go of the drugs. This was not easy, mostly because I have an addictive personality. I thank God that I found physical exercise, because in many ways that became my new "drug". I didn't think so at the time, but I realize now that this is what happened. Without calisthenics, I'd probably be dead right now. As it is, I've never been healthier or fitter, and my strength levels are through the roof. I hope to continue improving well into my old age.

Juicin' it: anabolic steroids

Most people—even the dumbest of jocks—understand that booze, smokes and recreational drugs will play havoc with your physical conditioning. But in the eyes of the general public, *steroids* and similar athletic drugs are a different matter entirely. Although John Doe may well have some understanding that—over the long term—steroids might be damaging to a guy's *health*, he will probably laugh at the idea that steroids can have a negative effect on your *physical performance*. After all, they are "performance enhancing" drugs, right? Most of the top sportsmen in America are probably hepped up on steroids! Just look at the huge pro bodybuilders; everybody knows that all these dudes are on massive doses of steroids. So how can steroids be *bad* for your training? If it's anything, it's cheating, right?

This is how the general public view steroids and similar drugs. The public are wrong. They only see half the story.

Anabolic steroids—compounds like *Dianabol, Winstrol*, and *Nandrolone*—mimic your body's own male hormone, *testosterone*. Testosterone, as the name suggests, is made in the testes (that's your balls, dude). It's this testosterone that kicks in when you hit puberty, and all those lean muscles suddenly spring up out of nowhere. When you take steroids, a similar phenomenon occurs, albeit in an amplified way. You go through a second adolescence—mood swings and voice changes too—all of which results in a quantum leap in your muscle mass levels.

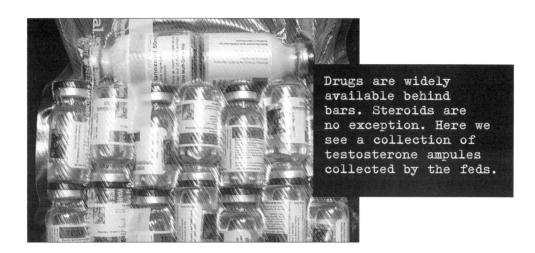

This sounds fantastic, and in a sense, it is. At least for a little while. But there's a major drawback. When you start pumping all that artificial testosterone into your system, your own cojones figure that they're not required for active service any more. They give up the ghost. Effectively, a steroid user's own internal production of testosterone grinds to a halt. (This is why steroid users inevitably have shrivelled balls. Sorry guys, but you know you do.) Eventually—like all drugs—the effects of steroids begin to diminish as the body becomes increasingly tolerant to them over time. As a result, users have to "cycle" the drugs, which is basically a nice, medical way of saying that they have to quit taking the stuff to make the drugs effective again at a later stage.

This is where the s*** really hits the fan. What do you think happens when you stop taking steroids? Do you go back to the level of muscle, strength and fitness you had before taking the drugs? Nope. These qualities depend largely on your hormone levels, testosterone in particular. When the juicers were taking external testosterone in the form of pills and injections, their own, internal testosterone factories (the balls) shut up shop. As a result, when users come off steroids they have very low levels of testosterone—much lower than the average male. As a result, muscle literally falls off the body, and is replaced by flab on a daily basis. Before very long, a steroid user will have less muscle and strength than he had before he started taking the drugs. You read that correctly—using steroids eventually makes you *smaller* and *weaker*. If you ask big users, they'll tell you that often this deterioration is visible practically every time they look in the mirror.

The physical effects of this down-cycle are horrible, but the psychological effects on tough guys are absolutely *devastating*. Imagine going from a situation where you were the biggest, most pumped up guy on the block, to suddenly looking more like Pee-wee Herman than Hulk Hogan. Aggression and self-confidence take a massive and painful beating. Of course, after a break, steroid users have the option of taking the drugs again. But the damage to the mind and body are already done, and all that the user can possibly gain now is a growing sense of *dependence* on all this artificial crap.

We all know that plenty of elite sports guys are on steroids, but this radical drop in ability doesn't bother them—they only have to stay at their peak during a relatively brief competitive season. That's where they make their big bucks. The rest of the year they can come off the drugs, and if their performance plummets, so what? Many prisoners have come round to the fact that steroids are not the way to go to build a great body year-round. When you are on the drugs, the highs are great—if you can accept the bitch-tits, hair loss and shrunken nuts—but when you have to come off them the lows are incredibly destructive, both physically and mentally. This makes you very, very vulnerable on the inside.

If you want great strength, athleticism and a maximum physique 365 days of the year, forget about steroids. Inject some *willpower* into your ass instead. I promise it'll do you good.

Lights out!

In a lot of US prisons, "straight edge" is slang for a certain kind of convict lifestyle. To get by, most inmates become drawn to gangs, drugs, and all the other destructive pursuits that inevitably follow with that. A straight edger is different. He is somebody who serves his time alone, and with discipline; kind of like a warrior monk. You keep your head down, mind your business and stay pure and focused. A straight edger doesn't put any poisons—like alcohol, drugs or nicotine—into his body. He keeps control of himself.

This philosophy is something I became increasingly attracted to when I was behind bars. Most of the really serious athletes on the inside approached their incarceration this way. I found that the more rigorously I applied this attitude, the more I got from my training. When I relaxed it, the slower the results were to show up.

You don't have to be locked away to be a straight edger. There are plenty of unhealthy distractions and illicit temptations on the outside. If you are really starting to take your training seriously, follow the advice I give in this chapter.

Go straight edge.

19: The Prison Diet

Nutrition and Fat Loss Behind Bars

There really is no universal law when it comes to feeding prisoners, beyond the broad scope of the Eighth Amendment and the specific legislation which applies to any areas where food is served. As a result, different state penitentiaries follow different internal regulations regarding the diets of their inmates. The only nationwide requirement seems to be that the inmates get three squares a day, but in my experience the content of these meals varies greatly.

A lot of bodybuilders make a really big effort to eat "clean" when they first get locked up. They'll eat the good stuff the canteen worker puts on their tray—meats, eggs, vegetables—and forgo any junk like fries, pudding, etc. Sometimes they will try to trade their junk with other prisoners, to get more of the nutritious foodstuffs. This effort rarely lasts beyond the first three weeks. Before long the craving for calories outweighs their desire for a purely healthy diet and they end up eating as much food as they can, whether it tallies with their former lifestyle or not.

I have a fast metabolism and in the early days I found it difficult to get full up in prison. The situation was made worse by the fact that during most of my years in the joint I was training every single day, sometimes for many dozens of sets of hard bodyweight exercises. I still got by though, and eventually I learned to thrive on a prison diet. Sure, most prison menus are not great, but they certainly aren't starvation diets, at least for most guys.

In a sense, prisons are no different from the streets outside—there are plenty of fat dudes incarcerated. In some places (not all) you can buy extra food at the commissary with money on your ID card. In less secure prisons, food sent in by families on the outside is big currency too. Believe it or not, some cons even cook in their cells. I've never known any institution that allows inmates to have stoves or microwaves in their cells, but in some places prisoners are allowed a tiny electric immersion heater, only big enough to boil water for a cup of instant coffee. These are called "stingers". Some convicts who have the extra food make cup soup or noodles in their stingers.

Where none of these luxuries exist, many of the lifers who are big powerlifters and bodybuilders make an effort to get placed on work duty in the kitchens. This way they have access to lots of extra goodies, provided they are careful. A lot of veteranos also bully weaker inmates and new fish for their food. This happens kinda often. Plus, there is contraband; supplements, vitamins and protein concentrates get smuggled in just like steroids and heroin.

I never resorted to any of these tricks, probably because I was too lazy. I just made the most of what I was given on my tray. A lot of guys find the three-meals-a-day system a real shock, because on the outside they could eat what they want when they like. On the outside you can get a KFC bucket in the middle of the night if you really want to, or snack on a candy bar between meals. It's not like that in prison, and it takes your body a little while to adjust to being told what to eat and when. After a few months your blood sugar levels adapt to the regular routine though. I always eat three times a day even when I get out now. It sounds weird but I've just got used to eating that way. My stomach thinks something's wrong if I don't eat like that. If you are confused about your diet, I'd advise you to try eating this way too.

Eating behind bars

Because individual prisons self-regulate their own dietary guidelines, it's impossible to show you a standard menu. Foods differ depending on season and a prison's location, also. I can give you a good idea of the kind of things prisoners eat, however. You can find two days worth of sample menus given below, and on the pages following I've included an official three week menu dispensed by the Federal Bureau of Prisons.

This kind of diet is so far from what is currently considered a "fitness" diet, that many people might believe that nobody could gain strength or muscle on a diet like this. But thousands of convicts—some of them truly formidable athletes—do just that, despite being on a diet like this for years.

SAMPLE PRISON MENUS

MENU 1

BREAKFAST:
Corn flakes with milk
Toast and jelly
One orange
Cup of coffee

LUNCH:
Spaghetti and meatballs
Cheese salad
Two doughnuts
Glass of milk

DINNER:
Meatloaf with onion gravy
Boiled rice
Green beans
Three cookies
Glass of cola

MENU 2

BREAKFAST:
Bran flakes with milk
Toast and jelly
Two apples
Cup of coffee

LUNCH:
Chicken wings
Mixed vegetables
One brownie
Glass of milk

DINNER:
Hamburger
Mashed potato
Cornbread
Jello
Glass of water

Federal Bureau of Prisons
Certified Food Menu – Week 1

Sunday	Monday	Tuesday	Wednesday	Thursday	Friday	Saturday
Fresh Apple Pkg Bran Cereal 3 Slices Bread 2 Cups Skim Milk 1 Cup Coffee 2 Pkg Jelly 2 Margarine	Fresh Orange Pkg Oatmeal 3 Slices Bread 2 Cups Skim Milk 2 Pkg Jelly 2 Margarine	Fresh Apple Pkg Grits 3 Slices Bread 2 Cups Skim Milk 2 Pkg Jelly 2 Margarine	Fresh Orange Pkg Bran Cereal 3 Slices Bread 2 Cups Skim Milk 2 Pkg Jelly 2 Margarine	Fresh Banana Pkg Oatmeal 3 Slices Bread 2 Cups Skim Milk 2 Pkg Jelly 2 Margarine	Fresh Orange Pkg Grits 3 Slices Bread 2 Cups Skim Milk 2 Pkg Jelly 2 Margarine	Fresh Orange Pkg Bran Cereal 3 Slices Bread 2 Cups Skim Milk 1 Cup Coffee 2 Pkg Jelly 2 Margarine
Fresh Apple -Spanish Omelet -Potatoes Pkg Cream Wheat 3 Slices Bread 2 Margarine 2 Cups Skim Milk 2 Pkg Jelly 2 Margarine Kosher Beverage	-Beans and Franks -Potatoes 2 Mustard 3 Slices Bread 2 Margarine Fresh Apple Kosher Beverage	1 Pkg Sardines Pkg Potato Chips 1 Vegetable Juice 3 Slices Bread 2 Salad Dressing 2 Mustard 2 Margarine Fresh Orange Kosher Beverage	-Beef Meatloaf -Brown Gravy -Mashed Potatoes -Mixed Vegetables 3 Slices Bread 2 Margarine Fresh Banana Kosher Beverage	1 Pkg Bologna Pkg Potato Chips 1 Vegetable Juice 3 Slices Bread 2 Salad Dressing 2 Mustard Fresh Orange Kosher Beverage	-Chicken Wings -Sauce -Mashed Potatoes -Sweet Peas 3 Slices Bread 2 Margarine Fresh Apple Kosher Beverage	1 Pkg Tuna Pkg Potato Chips 1 Vegetable Juice 3 Slices Bread 2 Salad Dressing 2 Mustard Fresh Apple Kosher Beverage
-Spaghetti -Meatballs -Tomato Sauce -Sweet Peas 3 Slices Bread 2 Margarine Fresh Apple Kosher Beverage	-Fish Fillet -Tomato Sauce -White Rice -Lima Beans 2 Tartar Sauce 3 Slices Bread 2 Margarine Fresh Apple Kosher Beverage	-Turkey Cutlet -Gravy -Mashed Potatoes -Mixed Vegetables 3 Slices Bread 2 Margarine Fresh Orange Kosher Beverage	-Ckn Cacciatore -Tomato Sauce -Mushrooms -Macaroni Pasta -Carrots 3 Slices Bread 2 Margarine Fresh Apple Kosher Beverage	-Veg. Chili -White Rice -Mixed Vegetable 3 Slices Bread 2 Margarine Fresh Orange Kosher Beverage	-Salisbury Steak -Brown Gravy -Mashed Potatoes -Lima Beans 3 Slices Bread 2 Margarine Fresh Apple Kosher Beverage	4oz Peanut Butter 4 Pkg Jelly Pkg Potato Chips 1 Vegetable Juice 3 Slices Bread 2 Margarine Fresh Apple Kosher Beverage

- Tray contents
- Institutions serving satellite meals or other areas with restricted access to hot water may substitute hot cereals with Pkg Bran Cereal.

Federal Bureau of Prisons
Certified Food Menu - Week 2

	Sunday	Monday	Tuesday	Wednesday	Thursday	Friday	Saturday
Breakfast	Fresh Apple Pkg Bran Cereal 3 Slices Bread 2 Cups Skim Milk 1 Cup Coffee 2 Pkg Jelly 10 gm 2 Margarine	Fresh Orange Pkg Oatmeal 3 Slices Bread 2 Cups Skim Milk 2 Pkg Jelly 2 Margarine	Fresh Apple Pkg Grits 3 Slices Bread 2 Cups Skim Milk 2 Pkg Jelly 2 Margarine	Fresh Orange Pkg Bran Cereal 3 Slices Bread 2 Cups Skim Milk 2 Pkg Jelly 10 gm 2 Margarine	Fresh Banana Pkg Oatmeal 3 Slices Bread 2 Cups Skim Milk 2 Pkg Jelly 2 Margarine	Fresh Orange Pkg Grits 3 Slices Bread 2 Cups Skim Milk 2 Pkg Jelly 2 Margarine	Fresh Orange Pkg Bran Cereal 3 Slices Bread 2 Cups Skim Milk 1 Cup Coffee 2 Pkg Jelly 10 gm 2 Margarine
Lunch	Fresh Apple -Cheese Omelet -Potatoes Pkg Cream Wheat 3 Slices Bread 2 Cups Skim Milk 2 Pkg Jelly 2 Margarine Kosher Beverage	1 Pkg Bologna Pkg Potato Chips 1 Vegetable Juice 3 Slices Bread 2 Salad Dressing 2 Mustard 2 Margarine Fresh Apple Kosher Beverage	-Chicken Patty -Chicken Gravy -Mashed Potatoes -Mixed Vegetables 3 Slices Bread 2 Margarine Fresh Orange Kosher Beverage	1 Pkg Sardines Pkg Potato Chips 1 Vegetable Juice 3 Slices Bread 2 Salad Dressing 2 Mustard 2 Margarine Fresh Banana Kosher Beverage	-Salisbury Steak -Brown Gravy -Mashed Potatoes -Lima Beans 3 Slices Bread 2 Margarine Fresh Orange Kosher Beverage	-Beans and Franks -Potatoes 2 Mustard 3 Slices Bread 2 Margarine Fresh Apple Kosher Beverage	1 Pkg Tuna Pkg Potato Chips 1 Vegetable Juice 2 Salad Dressing 2 Mustard 3 Slices Bread 2 Margarine Fresh Apple Kosher Beverage
Dinner	-Fish Fillet -Tomato Sauce -White Rice -Lima Beans 2 Tartar Sauce 3 Slices Bread 2 Margarine Fresh Apple Kosher Beverage	-Veg Stuffed Cabbage -Tomato Sauce -Parsley Potatoes -Mixed vegetables 3 Slices Bread 2 Margarine Fresh Apple Kosher Beverage	-Beef Meatloaf -Brown Gravy -Mashed Potatoes -Mixed Vegetables 3 Slices Bread 2 Margarine Fresh Orange Kosher Beverage	-Ckn Chow Mein w/ -Chicken Gravy -Green Beans -White Rice -Peas and Carrots 3 Slices Bread 2 Margarine Fresh Apple Kosher Beverage	-Veg Cutlet -Mushroom Gravy -White Rice -Lima Beans 3 Slices Bread 2 Margarine Fresh Orange Kosher Beverage	-Spaghetti -Meatballs -Tomato Sauce -Sweet Peas 3 Slices Bread 2 Margarine Fresh Apple Kosher Beverage	4oz Peanut Butter 4 Pkg Jelly Pkg Potato Chips 1 Vegetable Juice 3 Slices Bread 2 Margarine Fresh Apple Kosher Beverage

-tray contents
-Institutions serving satellite meals or other areas with restricted access to hot water may substitute hot cereals with Pkg Bran Cereal.

Federal Bureau of Prisons
Certified Food Menu – Week 3

	Sunday	Monday	Tuesday	Wednesday	Thursday	Friday	Saturday
Breakfast	Fresh Apple Pkg Bran Cereal 3 Slices Bread 2 Cups Skim Milk 1 Cup Coffee 2 Pkg Jelly 2 Margarine	Fresh Orange Pkg Oatmeal 3 Slices Bread 2 Cups Skim Milk 2 Pkg Jelly 2 Margarine	Fresh Apple Pkg Grits 3 Slices Bread 2 Cups Skim Milk 2 Pkg Jelly 2 Margarine	Fresh Orange Pkg Bran Cereal 3 Slices Bread 2 Cups Skim Milk 2 Pkg Jelly 2 Margarine	Fresh Banana Pkg Oatmeal 3 Slices Bread 2 Cups Skim Milk 2 Pkg Jelly 2 Margarine	Fresh Orange Pkg Grits 3 Slices Bread 2 Cups Skim Milk 1 Cup Coffee 2 Pkg Jelly 2 Margarine	Fresh Orange Pkg Bran Cereal 3 Slices Bread 2 Cups Skim Milk 2 Pkg Jelly 2 Margarine
Lunch	Fresh Apple -Spanish Omelet -Potatoes Pkg Cream Wheat 3 Slices Bread 2 Cups Skim Milk 2 Pkg Jelly 2 Margarine Fresh Apple Kosher Beverage	-Chicken Wings -Sauce -Mashed Potatoes -Sweet Peas 3 Slices Bread 2 Margarine Fresh Apple Kosher Beverage	1 Pkg Bologna Pkg Potato Chips 1 Vegetable Juice 3 Slices Bread 2 Salad Dressing 2 Mustard Fresh Orange Kosher Beverage	-Beans and Franks -Potatoes 2 Mustard 3 Slices Bread 2 Margarine Fresh Banana Kosher Beverage	1 Pkg Tuna Pkg Potato Chips 1 Vegetable Juice 3 Slices Bread 2 Salad Dressing 2 Mustard Fresh Orange Kosher Beverage	-Chicken Patty -Chicken Gravy -Mashed Potatoes -Mixed Vegetables 3 Slices Bread 2 Margarine Fresh Apple Kosher Beverage	1 Pkg Sardines Pkg Potato Chips 1 Vegetable Juice 3 Slices Bread 2 Salad Dressing 2 Mustard Fresh Apple Kosher Beverage
Dinner	-Fish Fillet -Tomato Sauce -White Rice -Lima Beans 2 Tartar Sauce 3 Slices Bread 2 Margarine Fresh Apple Kosher Beverage	-Salisbury Steak -Brown Gravy -Mashed Potatoes -Lima Beans 3 Slices Bread 2 Margarine Fresh Apple Kosher Beverage	-Turkey Cutlet -Gravy -Mashed Potatoes -Mixed Vegetables 3 Slices Bread 2 Margarine Fresh Apple Kosher Beverage	-Spaghetti -Meatballs -Tomato Sauce -Sweet Peas 3 Slices Bread 2 Margarine Fresh Apple Kosher Beverage	-Ckn Chow Mien w/ -Chicken Gravy -Green Beans -White Rice -Peas and Carrots 3 Slices Bread 2 Margarine Fresh Orange Kosher Beverage	-Beef Meatloaf -Brown Gravy -Mashed Potatoes -Mixed Vegetables 3 Slices Bread 2 Margarine Fresh Apple Kosher Beverage	4oz Peanut Butter 4 Pkg Jelly Pkg Potato Chips 1 Vegetable Juice 3 Slices Bread 2 Margarine Fresh Apple Kosher Beverage

-tray contents
-Institutions serving satellite meals or other areas with restricted access to hot water may substitute hot cereals with Pkg Bran Cereal.

Before you allow your dietary practices to become too complex, take a lesson from the prison diet and focus on these basic guidelines:

• Regularity is an important factor for an athlete. Try to eat at the same time each day so that your body knows when to expect nutrients.

• Ensure that you eat enough calories to sustain your training. If you are in hard training, you don't need to steer clear of "junk" like cake, jelly or candy daily, provided you eat these things in moderation.

• Don't overeat. If you have a fast metabolism a small snack (or even two) is acceptable, but otherwise three meals a day is enough to meet your needs. If you are a very large athlete, you don't require more meals a day—just proportionately more at each sitting.

• Don't undereat. Try to get a decent meal when you sit down to eat, even if you aren't hungry then and there. Skimping on one of your main meals will only make you hungry and tired later. Eventually your body will figure out when to expect food and you will automatically have a good appetite at mealtimes.

• Eat a balanced diet. By "balanced" I mean a daily consumption of meat, grains or cereals, dairy (milk, cheese, eggs, etc.) and vegetables and fruit. If you are vegetarian, focus more on dairy.

• Stay hydrated. Drink something with each meal, and take in fluids in between meals.

Try following these rules before you blow your hard-earned dollars on protein powder, nutrition bars and supplements. You may find that your training goes even better than before, and that you don't need a fancy diet after all. I'm betting you'll be pleased with the results.

Fluid intake

The most important substance a human being needs is the oxygen we derive from the air around us. Water comes second, and food a distant third. You can survive for weeks without food, days without water and only minutes without air. Although the way supplement companies push their products, you'd think it was the other way around!

Fluid intake is another area that modern thinking has overcomplicated. Your body needs fluid frequently just to stay alive. Provided that fluid is not inherently toxic (like alcohol) or emetic (like seawater), it really doesn't matter where you get it from. The bad rap coffee seems to get these days is a good example. Many people falsely believe that because coffee is a diuretic, it dehydrates you. This is not true. Drinking coffee *does* mildly stimulate the kidneys and make you urinate, but the water taken in when you imbibe the beverage more than outweighs what you lose through urination, so the drink always hydrates you.

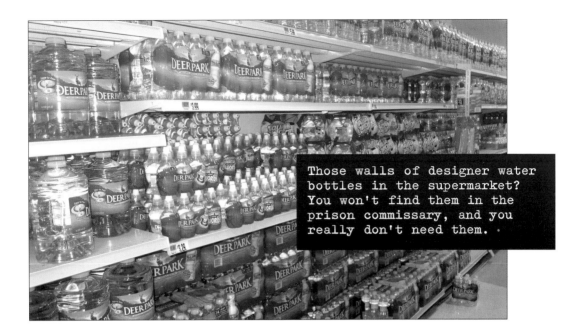

Those walls of designer water bottles in the supermarket? You won't find them in the prison commissary, and you really don't need them. ·

Good old tap water is another modern victim of marketing propaganda. When I last got out of prison, one thing I noticed was that people were carrying expensive little store-bought bottles of water around with them. There was none of this bull in any of the prisons I went to. If you wanted more water, you didn't get mineral water from the Alps, or the spring of some European health spa. You got a drink from the faucet, or you stayed thirsty.

A lot of people are worried about the impurities in modern tap water. *All* fluids contain impurities—even sterilized, bottled drinks. They always have, and they always will. But this really isn't the problem people make it out to be. The human body evolved over millions of years, and for most of that time we drank the liquids we needed from swamps, rivers and streams, puddles and the blood of our prey. Your body is pretty tough, and it has the capacity to filter out what it needs and become stronger as a result. American tap water is some of the cleanest, safest water in the world, and it costs a fraction of a cent per gallon. Make use of it.

Keep it simple, sweetheart

As you might have guessed by reading this chapter so far, I'm not a big believer in the new theories about nutrition—like the idea that an athlete needs to eat six-to-eight small meals a day, or megadose on protein. All these modern tactics do is overload the digestion and lead to weight gain in the form of fat.

Nutritional science has become so advanced that the sporting world has gotten confused and started overemphasizing minor aspects of diet such as macronutrient ratios, enzyme content andthe glycemic index. A great many fitness fanatics are genuinely *obsessed* with their vitamin and mineral intake. Some of this may be a uniquely American fixation. Back in the fifties, when Eastern Bloc athletes were routinely destroying the US competition, the Soviet coaches used to laugh at the huge volumes of vitamin pills taken by US sportsmen and women. Eastern sports scientists understood long before our guys that all the vitamins and minerals the body needs are fully provided by a normal, balanced diet. Any excess is usually excreted through the urine as waste. The running joke in Russia at the time was that the American competitors must have had the most expensive piss in the world.

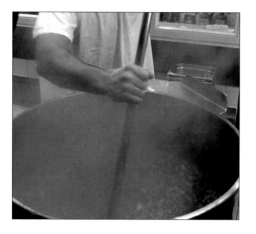

Steer clear of overcomplicating your diet with suspiciously trendy theories and modern fad ideas. People forget that the most important thing an athlete needs from food is not protein or vitamins, but *calories*—the energy to perform hard calisthenics. "Calories" has become a real dirty word these days, almost like a curse word. But that's only because we live in a society where we overeat so terribly. When I first arrived in San Quentin I was tall and lanky and had a metabolism like an atom bomb—I quickly learned to eat everything on my plate just to stop myself going hungry. Follow this example, and focus on getting three good, balanced meals every day, regular as clockwork. If you can do this, you really don't need huge doses of amino acids or special combinations of food to get big and strong. The old time inmates who perfected the training methods that became *Convict Conditioning* were lucky to have enough food to stay alive.

Protein-The Big Scam!

Protein is an excellent case in point. Most bodybuilding gurus state that you need *at least* one gram of protein per pound of lean bodyweight to gain muscle mass. A bodybuilder weighing two-hundred pounds should therefore be eating (at least) two hundred grams of protein in his diet every single day. This is way, way, way too much. You don't need a Ph.D in nutrition to realize this, just simple math.

Let's look at an example; a two-hundred pound male between the ages of nineteen and seventy requires approximately fifty-six grams of protein per day to maintain his bodyweight. This is not a number I got from a buddy, a personal trainer or the back of a comicbook—it's the official figure given as part of the *Dietary Reference Intake*, a body of recommendations utilized by many US penal institutions and derived from *The US National Academy of Sciences* and the *Institute of Medicine*. These highly respected—and *impartial*—organizations state that a two-hundred pound guy only needs fifty-six grams of protein per day. It doesn't matter whether this guy is an athlete or not, because the energy you expend comes from *calories*, not protein. If you are eating plenty of calories in the form of carbohydrates and fats, your daily energy requirements won't be "stolen" from your protein intake, so you won't require any more than the average couch potato your size. But the muscle magazines tell our guy that if he wants to be a bodybuilder or a strength athlete he needs two-hundred grams per day, not fifty-six—so where are the extra *one-hundred and forty-four* grams going?

The gurus will try to convince you that it's going straight into making muscle. Big ol' arms and pecs. Sounds cool, huh? Well, no—don't believe the hype. You'd be amazed at how many smart people have been conned by advertisers into thinking that muscle is made of protein. Actually, muscle *isn't* built totally from protein. Not even a third of muscle is made up of protein. More than seventy percent of healthy muscle is *water*. In fact, there's barely eighty grams of protein in a pound of muscle—certainly no more than a hundred grams. If the extra intake of one-hundred and forty-four grams of protein advised by modern writers was really added to water and turned into muscle, a guy consuming this much protein would gain more than *six-hundred and fifty pounds of pure muscle in a year.* To put it another way, he would have five or six times as much muscle on his body than Arnold Schwarzenegger in his prime as Mr Olympia—after only twelve months of training. Even if you somehow lost more than *three quarters* of this protein as energy or through faulty digestion or via inefficient tissue-building, our average two-hundred pound bodybuilder would still become easily the most muscular man on the planet within a year, if all this extra protein was transformed into body muscle.

Protein overload

If you still don't believe that high protein diets are unnecessary, think about a few examples from nature.

Infants require more growth material—proportionately—than even the biggest bodybuilders. In its first five months of life, a human baby doubles its size. (No bodybuilder, no matter how gifted or drugged up, could double his size in five months!) So you would assume that babies require (again, *proportionately*) high protein diets for all this growth, right? Nah. Mother's milk contains less than five percent protein.

Meditate on that for a second. When humans *really need* to grow, nature presents us with a diet *that's less than five percent protein.* That's all it takes for a baby to actualize that phenomenal growth spurt.

Compare this with cow's milk. In contrast to human milk, cow's milk contains around fifteen percent protein. Why so much more? Because whereas human babies double their weight in less than half a year, calves double their weight in just forty-five days. Cows have a lot of growing to do. Healthy human males grow to an average weight of 190 pounds, but bulls grow to twenty-five hundred pounds, and more.* The take-home message? Cow's milk has far, far more protein and growth material in it than a human being could ever need.

*For you protein fiends out there, it's worth noting that bulls—like gorillas, elephants and most other truly massive mammals—are *herbivores.* They easily sustain huge amounts of muscle mass by eating low protein diets.

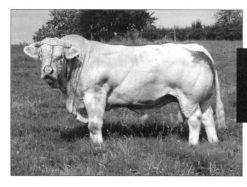

A bull does most of its growing on plain old milk. No protein powders!

So what are bodybuilders told to do with their milk? Put protein powders in it! Putting protein or whey in cow's milk is *ridiculous*. It's like adding sugar to rock candy.

What's worse is that supplement companies are constantly trying to outdo each other's numbers. A lot of protein shakes on the market now have more than fifty grams of protein per serving, when mixed up. Babies doubling their weight in a few months need a diet of less than five percent protein. But many modern bodybuilders have diets that are forty percent protein—and more! Why? All that extra protein can't be utilized by the body. But this huge intake has to be metabolized anyways, and that presents a strain on the kidneys.

Don't get me wrong. I'm not advocating *low* protein. By all means, enjoy some milk, eggs, cheese, seafood or a nice steak every single day. I *love* protein foods, and they form part of a healthy, satisfying diet. But this super-high protein craze has totally gotten out of hand. Eating muscle (protein) to gain muscle won't work. That's not science—it's *thinking by analogy*. That's the same kind of primitive thinking going through a savage's brain when he eats his opponent's heart to gain his courage!

To build solid muscle, you don't require large amounts of protein—the protein found in the average diet is more than enough to do the job.

So why do these stupid ideas get splashed across the pages of virtually every fitness magazine and website across America? Well, the answer my friend is that nine times out of ten, it's these magazines and websites that are *selling* the protein supplements somewhere along the line.

Don't believe anything you read written by anybody who's trying to sell you something. If you want to gain lean muscle and strength, you can do it easily by following the prison diet—three square meals a day.

"Small and often"...really?

Another "sacred cow" in fitness nutrition is the idea that you need to eat at least six times per day—although some writers would have you eat even more often. Hell, some writers would have a conveyor belt rolling food into your mouth 24/7—as you sat on the toilet.

The main argument for this approach to eating is that smaller, frequent meals allow for greater absorption of vital nutrients. In fact, the opposite is true. Frequent feedings keep the digestive organs constantly lined with food. This overload badly interferes with the proper absorption of nutrients when they do arrive. If you really want to improve your absorption of the food in a meal, eat moderately just three times per day and leave at least *four hours* between feedings. If you do this, when you *do* sit down to chow, your stomach will be cleared of waste and "refueled" with the necessary acids and enzymes required for the breakdown and utilization of vitamins, minerals, and nutrients. You'll get far more bang for your dietary buck.

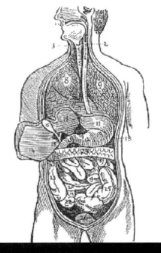

In jail, very few cons eat in the evening. They eat their last meal around five to six, then their gut slowly empties for five or six hours before lights out. This sounds like a nightmare for the average bodybuilder, who thinks that his arms and legs will drop off if he isn't filling his body every two or three hours. In fact, I'm a big believer in this way of eating. I'm convinced it acts like a safety valve to prevent obesity. It's the way people used to eat—before we became so friggin' fat as a nation. Think about it. If you constantly give your body food every few hours, when the hell does it get the chance to actually *burn fat*?

> Your intestines and other digestive organs require rest, just like any other parts of the body. Even the Ancients understood this.

In reality, being a little hungry before bedtime is no bad thing. Over such a short period, the body prefers to burn fat as fuel, rather than muscle; so you won't lose any hard-earned beef. If you get really hungry, go for a light snack, or some coffee or soda—often, what we experience as evening hunger is actually thirst. Having an empty belly before bed allows the gut and intestines to relax and recuperate, detoxifies the blood, maximizes nocturnal fat-burning and improves the quality of sleep. It also helps ensure a great appetite in the morning, which many obese people lack.

Actually allowing your belly to be *empty* before you eat might sound like a revolutionary idea, but it's what nature intended. Do you think cavemen ate 6-8 small meals a day? Nope. They burned fat while they hunted all day, made a kill and then ate it. This kept them in perfect hunting shape.

Just about every "expert" out there will totally disagree with what I'm suggesting in this chapter, but so what? You don't have to listen to me or anybody else. Just keep training. If you are consistently getting stronger on three meals a day, you *are* adding muscle. You don't need to add anything else to your diet—it'll just make you fat.

Obesity

Fat! That leads me nicely to another topic—something two out of three Americans know all about; *being overweight*. Our nation has built this problem from the ground up, largely through a combination of greed and a massive excess of food.

If you think that bodybuilders are immune to this problem, think again. Only a tiny percentage of body-builders are "ripped"—although these are inevitably the athletes you'll see on TV or in magazines. The vast majority of modern bodybuilders and strength trainers are overweight, and in many ways this is due to the overemphasis the industry places on nutrition and protein intake. I mentioned earlier that most fitness gurus recommend vastly too much protein for muscle-building purposes—as if gorging on protein will somehow make the muscles bigger. This is a stupid idea. Muscle consists mainly of water, not protein, but drinking a dozen gallons of water each day won't add tons of beef to your body. It'll just make you piss lots. If you pour unnecessary water into your stomach, it simply gets filtered through the bladder. But if you shovel excess protein into your system, that protein enters the bloodstream as amino acids which become broken down into simple sugars and fatty acids. That's right—your body turns all that super-healthy pro-tein into *sugar* and *fat*. This in turn becomes lard, packed in-between the internal organs and wobbling around on the gut.

A bodybuilder can get by with a big fat belly. He can drive down to the gym and get through his exer-cises, and even convince himself that the inches of blubber on his arms, legs and torso are "bulk". But for a master of old school calisthenics, excess body fat is a real problem. Because we use our bodyweight as resistance, every extra pound of useless fat becomes a drag, making our exercises more difficult and stop-ping us from improving. The fatter you are, the harder it will be to progress through the ten steps of the Big Six exercises. A little extra chub is one thing, but if you have a large, hanging paunch, you can forget about being great at calisthenics until you ditch that surplus weight.

Burning calories is not the solution

Many people focus excessively on exercise when they want to lose weight. This is a mistake; although activity levels play a role in increasing or decreasing fat levels, it's a relatively minor role compared to *diet*. The little bit of leisure time most people can spare for exercise isn't really enough to make an impact on their overall weight.

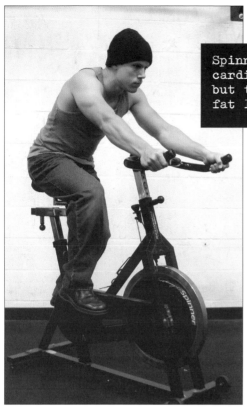

Spinning your wheels? All those cardio machines make money for gyms, but they are not the answer to the fat loss problem.

A lot of fitness promotions tell us that we can easily lose weight by upping our activity levels—perhaps by walking through our lunch break, for example. But is this really true?

Let's imagine that you are ten pounds overweight and you decide to drop this excess by adding a half-hour walk to your daily routine. How quickly can you expect to lose your extra pounds like this? Well, most people walk at approximately three miles per hour. This means that in thirty minutes you can walk about a mile and a half. Walking a mile and a half will burn around one-hundred and fifty calories. A pound of body fat contains around three thousand, five-hundred calories. Therefore, if you walked for half an hour every day single day, it would take you more than two-hundred and thirty three days to lose that ten pounds. That's over eight months, and over *one-hundred and sixteen hours solid walking.* Not a very good return on that investment, is it? To make matters worse, exercise stimulates the appetite, so people often unknowingly take in the calories they lose (and more) the same day. This is very easy to do. One-hundred and fifty calories isn't much to make up—maybe two slices of bread, a small bag of chips, or a glass of milk. For these reasons, losing ten pounds by emphasizing exercise may actually take much longer than eight months. It might take years, if it ever happens at all.

Focus on nutrition for weight loss

If you really want to lose weight, focus on *nutrition,* not exercise. By mildly reducing your calorie intake, you can easily and safely lose ten pounds in about three weeks—maybe even quicker.

If you choose to lose weight through your diet, there are several ways you can go. Calorie counting is pushed as a popular method, but in reality very few lean athletes literally count calories. What they do is establish a *baseline* by eating a regular, consistent diet they can keep track of over days, weeks and months. Once this baseline is established, the athlete can easily drop weight by gradually cutting back on the amount of food eaten as part of their standard menu.

If you want to lose that flab, apply the *prison diet* as a template and follow these simple rules:

1. **Eat three evenly-spaced meals daily.** Eating more than this prevents your body from dropping fat due to all the readily-available energy circulating in the system. One meal every four hours throughout the day is a good rule of thumb. Avoid eating in the late evening if you can.

2. **Eat at regular times.** Eating consistently at preset mealtimes stabilizes your blood sugar. When your body knows it will receive food at consistent times, you will experience fewer random cravings.

3. **Eat a balanced menu.** Try to combine the major food groups—meat, dairy, cereals, vegetables and fruit—as much as possible on a daily basis. Use the menu tables I gave earlier as a template. Drink something with each meal, too, and whenever you feel thirsty through the day. Focus on the *quantity* of your portions more than their *quality*—remember, even pure protein turns to sugar and fat when eaten to excess.

Once you have established a baseline by eating regularly this way, check the scale to ensure your weight is stable over the course of a week or two. As soon as you find that balance, losing weight will be a snap— just cut back slightly on your daily portion sizes until your weight starts to drop.

As with all things however, give your body the time it needs. Forcing weight loss will result in muscle loss too. If you are patient, there is absolutely no need for this to happen to you. Even if you are a massive one-hundred pounds overweight, you can drop all this in a single year, by losing less than two pounds per week. With discipline and regular eating, you will be at your perfect training weight in no time.

The "subconscious effect"-a "secret weapon" for fat loss

While we're on the subject of weight loss, there's one more thing I've got to mention—the unusual bonus calisthenics has on promoting fat loss. This is something I discussed, briefly, in *Convict Conditioning*. Many overweight students of bodyweight strength discover that their body fat levels reduce over time— even if they gain muscle, and even if they don't deliberately try to drop weight. This has nothing to do with burning calories. It has to do with the *subconscious effect* of bodyweight work.

*W*eight-training promotes overeating. Let's say you bench pressed two-hundred pounds for six reps last week, and this week your big goal is pressing the same amount for seven reps. The more you dwell on this goal, the more you eat—you want to make certain you are eating enough for growth, repair and fuelling, so you can meet your goal. Unfortunately, lifters inevitably overdo it. That's why most bodybuilders become chubby, at least during the offseason.

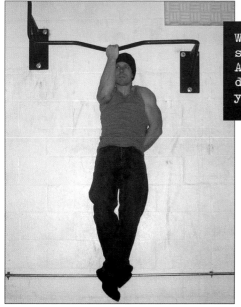

Weight loss and bodyweight strength work go hand-in-hand. Advanced pullup techniques are damn near impossible unless you are lean 'n mean.

But bodyweight work has the opposite effect on your eating habits. Let's say you did six one-arm push-ups last week, and this week your goal is seven reps. Your subconscious mind realizes that, because you are moving your body's own weight, excessive eating is the last thing you should do in order to reach your goal. The more you eat, the more weight you'll gain, and the harder those pushups will be! The same is true for squats, bridges, pullups, and all major calisthenics movements. As a result, the deeper structures of the psyche make the connection between lighter eating and success—or at least, less suffering during training. To survive, the body knows what to do. It drops the excess baggage.

Don't believe in the subconscious effect? Like I always say, I don't expect anyone to believe me. Just try it. You'll see that it works.

Lights out!

A lot of people balk at the idea of prison food. To most people, eating is associated with *freedom* and *individuality*. They hate the idea of being told what to eat and when. Modern guys and girls choke at the thought of eating a regulation menu, three times a day.

I—along with many other athletes—have found that in fact the prison-style diet can be of enormous value. Sure, on the outside people have a great deal of choice as to what they eat and when. But since nearly seventy percent of American citizens are overweight, and forty percent can't find the energy to regularly exercise, it's probably time to question just how useful "freedom" and "individuality" are as dietary standards. As a rule, fewer people get fat in prison than on the outside. It's also true that a higher proportion of men work out when they are behind bars. The prison diet must have something going for it.

The more you stick to basic, balanced, *regulated* eating habits, the closer you will be to reaching your goals. You don't need a doctorate in biochemistry to stay lean and get fuelled up for your workouts. For most guys, the more complex their attitude to diet and nutrition becomes, the more chance there is of screwing things up.

The simple rules given in this chapter have worked for me and my fellow prison athletes. They will work for you, too. They really are all you'll ever need.

20: Mendin' Up

The 8 Laws of Healing

Over the years inside prison I got hurt plenty of times. I got hurt from fights, work detail and stupid accidents, but the funny thing is I can't remember getting badly dinged up from my training, despite the fact that I often trained hard every day, seven days a week. A lot of this is down to old school calisthenics—it's an incredibly safe way to train. Go into any commercial gym and watch guys straining with heavy barbells, dumbbells and weird machines, and you'll notice they get hurt all the time. In the battle between tender flesh and unforgiving iron, the iron always wins in the end.

No matter how safely you train though, the chances are that you'll have to work through injuries at some point. The body isn't a machine. It's a strange, constantly-altering entity that can be difficult to predict and accommodate. I met a powerlifter once who could deadlift nearly eight-hundred pounds on a bar with no problem, who put his back out picking up his little girl who weighed less than fifty pounds. You can do a one-arm pullup with no pain at all, and then tweak your shoulder brushing your teeth. The body can be weird sometimes. It's the nature of human life, I guess.

During my three long stretches behind bars, I broke my nose twice, lost three teeth, strained my left bicep, got third degree burns to my right forearm, fractured (and re-cracked) several ribs, dislocated my right kneecap, tore my sacroiliac ligament, split a groin muscle and broke my ankle. I'm not complaining—a lot of guys have come away from jailtime a lot worse than I did. Prison can beat up the body bad, that's for sure.

These kinds of injuries really interfere with your training, and the problem is magnified by the fact that medical support inside prisons is rarely on a par with the kind of healthcare you get on the outside. Hacks and prison doctors are incredibly wary of inmates seeking medical help—it's usually an excuse for escape from work detail, or a chance to get access to painkilling drugs (or any drugs). Often convicts with minor injuries are just sent back to their cells to get better pretty much under their own steam. I was always obsessed with my physical conditioning routine—it was the only thing that kept me sane on the inside—and there was no way I was ever going to let something as dumb as being hurt get in the way of that. As a result, I often trained too much; but I also developed a good understanding of how to work around injuries, from the perspective of a guy who trains.

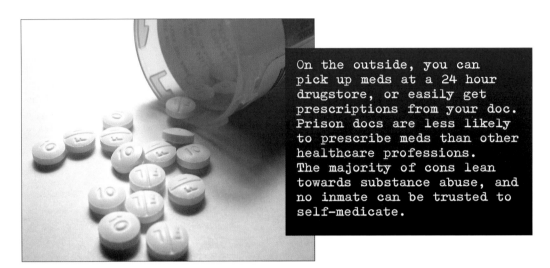

On the outside, you can pick up meds at a 24 hour drugstore, or easily get prescriptions from your doc. Prison docs are less likely to prescribe meds than other healthcare professions. The majority of cons lean towards substance abuse, and no inmate can be trusted to self-medicate.

I'm certainly not a medical expert, by any stretch of the imagination. If you're on the outside and you get hurt, seek professional attention if you can. But in my experience, doctors often don't understand the kind of help athletes need when they get dinged. The best guy to ask is usually an athlete—somebody who has been training for years, who has been hurt lots, and had to cope with injuries with very little in the way of surgery, medication, physical therapy or support. As I say, I ain't no doctor, but I pretty much fit that description.

To help you out as much as possible, I've squeezed as much of what I've learned as possible into eight general ideas, which, to me, make up the *eight laws of healing*. Older athletes will recognize a lot of what I'm saying immediately; you young punks will be able to save yourself a lot of trouble and pain by adopting these ideas early on in your careers.

Ready? Okay, lets go:

LAW 1: PROTECT YOURSELF.

The best way to handle an injury is not to get injured in the first place. This seems like a no-brainer, but it's really not. The vast majority of painful injuries are stupid little things that didn't need to happen in the first place. Teenagers are the worst offenders here—particularly the "Jackass" generation. Following puberty, kids (okay—*male* kids) are high on their own newfound sense of physical presence. They feel immortal; invincible. They delight in the rush that comes from doing dangerous things—picking fights, driving too damn quick, playing fast and loose with their health.

After a few scrapes, you begin to realize that the body definitely *isn't* invincible—you are not immortal. When you break a rib or a finger, it never feels quite "right" again. If you fully rupture a ligament, that ligament is gone forever; it never grows back. If you dislocate your shoulder, it becomes loose for the rest of your life; it dislocates much easier next time you put it under pressure. (It was a dislocated shoulder that ended Steve Reeves' bodybuilding career.) Over time, injuries begin to accumulate; even little, minor tears and tweaks, until you are continually plagued by nagging aches and pains and reduced function. Those tough guys who threw themselves around on the high school football field twenty years ago? They are still feeling it now.

You'd think that in the world of strength and fitness, people would be far more into looking after their bodies. In fact, it seems like the reverse is true. Whether to prove a point or just to satisfy their egos, guys in gyms seem prone to continually perform stupid acts that are virtually certain to cripple them somewhere along the line. They load up bone-crushing weights on dangerous exercises like the bench press and the press-behind-neck, bouncing the bar off their ribcages and spines. They hurt their joints with exercises they go back to, week-in, week-out, for years, whittling away their connective tissue and cartilage. They eat and inject all kinds of nasty s*** just to look better than the next guy, while all the time their bodies are breaking down from the inside out.

In the pen, *nobody* looks out for you. Not really. You might *think* your gang has your back, but in reality most attacks are launched by one guy on another guy in the same gang. Gang-on-gang violence is a big thing when it happens, but most of the time it doesn't. Being injured behind bars is not a macho thing like on the outside—it only makes you vulnerable, so real early on you need to cultivate a survivalist approach, an *attitude* of self-protection. This is the kind of mindset you need to have all the time if you want to make the most of your training and avoid these piled-up injuries that screw with your body and eat away at productive training time. Be perceptive. See dangers coming before they arrive. Avoid stupid, high-risk situations and treat your body nice.

This applies to the choices you make outside your training as much as it does to your conditioning career. Be careful when you train. Look at the following factors:

- Make sure your training environment is secure. Are there items strewn over the floor you could trip over? Etc.

- If you are using objects or equipment to train with, make certain that they are stable and up to the task.

- If you think a technique puts you at risk (of a fall, or hitting your head, for example), don't do it—find ways to make it safer, or drop it altogether.

- Self-protection is also about *how* you train. If an exercise hurts—I'm talking injury pain, rather than the discomfort of effort—stop. Alter the exercise so that it no longer hurts, or find an alternative.

Self-protection as a principle continues to function even *after* you get hurt (God forbid). Immediately following an injury, your first job is to identify what happened and remove yourself from any further danger. Again, this sounds obvious but it isn't. I knew a guy in my neighborhood who hurt himself doing pullups on an overhead pipe which came loose. He fell down, chipping a bone in his elbow when he slammed into the concrete. Rather than just quitting, he jumped back up in an attempt to finish his set, only to injure his elbow even further. This is a dumb macho attitude—it only makes you weaker in the long run. Be strong *and* smart.

Illnesses can interfere with your training, the same as injuries. Look after your body with good nutrition and a healthy lifestyle and steer clear of anyone you know who has colds or viruses. A bad cold can put your training back three weeks.

LAW 2: IMMEDIATE THERAPY.

When the time comes that you do get injured—and it probably will come—you need to take immediate steps to speed recovery the second you are out of harm's way.

Acute injuries to the joints are the bane of an athlete's life. Most acute soft tissue injuries arrive in the form of either *strains* or *sprains*. A *sprain* is an overstretching of a ligament encasing a joint, whereas a *strain* is the overstretching of muscle tissue. When strains and sprains occur, the wounded areas go into protective mode and begin to swell up, as the body sends excess fluid to the injured parts to act as a cushion and shock absorber. Unfortunately, sometimes the body doesn't know when to stop this swelling, and this can be a real problem because swelling interferes with the healing process.

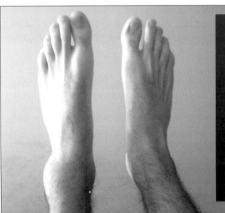

Ouch! Sprained ankles are a classic example of a sprain. You turn your foot under weight, and the ligaments are overstretched and busted up. The body responds by pumping the area with fluid. This acts great as a short-term shock absorber, but it interferes with long-term healing: it can take longer to heal a sprained ankle than a broken leg!

Once you get injured, the best thing you can do is to set about reducing swelling in order to kick-start your body's healing mechanism. The finest way to do this is to follow the acronym "P.R.I.N.C.E." which stands for:

PROTECT: This follows on from the first law. If you get injured, you must principally ensure that you prevent further injury. If you have been injured by an exercise, *stop the exercise*. If you have been injured by an object—such as a dangerous item of machinery—get away from the cause of the injury. Protect yourself immediately by identifying the problem and isolating yourself from it.

REST: The more you move an injured area around, the more it will swell up—so you must rest your injury. If you tear a muscle during an exercise, you need to stop using that muscle for the time being. If you hurt your leg in a fall, don't attempt to put weight on the leg. This is just common sense. Paradoxically, *activity* is also vital for healing in the long run (see laws 3 and 4), but right after the injury, *rest* is more essential.

ICE: When you apply ice to an injury, the cold tissues contract, preventing the excess swelling mentioned above. Ice the injured area using an ice pack, or frozen food. Make sure you have some kind of barrier between yourself and the ice pack—something like a wet towel—to prevent ice burns. A slush bath of ice cubes also works. Ice injuries for no more than fifteen to twenty minutes every two to three hours for the first two days following a strain or sprain.

NSAIDs: *NSAIDs* are Non-Steroidal Anti-Inflammatory Drugs. These are basically medicines which act to reduce swelling in an injured area by inhibiting the chemical processes which cause swelling on a cellular level. As somebody who has had limited access to these meds in jail, I can confirm that when I've used them following an injury on the outside, they work wonders. Often when injured, athletes instinctively reach for analgesics—over-the-counter painkillers like *paracetamol*. This is a mistake. If you have access to them, always appropriately use NSAIDs like *ibuprofen* or *aspirin* instead, as they will actually accelerate healing (by reducing swelling) rather than just removing the *feeling* of pain.

COMPRESSION: Compression is a fundamental and powerful way to reduce excess swelling in tissues. Wrap an injured area in a bandage, nice and snug but not tight enough to disrupt blood flow. Begin wrapping at the point furthest from your heart, and loosen a dressing if it causes pain or if the area below it becomes numb.

ELEVATION: Lifting an injured area up (above the level of your heart) drains excess fluid though the plain old power of gravity. Find some safe and secure way to place your injured limb up on something and just leave it there for a good while—at least half an hour. This is a particularly useful way to reduce swelling during the night, when you will be asleep and unable to apply ice.

Immediate therapy should be applied to joint injuries for several days—up to a week—following acute injury. As soon as the immediate pain and swelling is reducing, an athlete can move to the third law.

LAW 3: KEEP TRAINING YOUR UNINJURED AREAS.

Often athletes instinctively take a layoff after an injury. This is not only unnecessary—it actually *slows up* your body's healing process. When you injure yourself, you should get back into training your injury-free body parts as soon as you possibly can.

Let's say you break your left arm. You can still train your right arm; you can still train your midsection and legs. If you break your legs, you can still find ways to train your torso and arms. If you hurt your lower back, you can still work around the injury to train your limbs. As a general rule of thumb, if you can continue *safely* working an area, you should do so. Even if you are badly injured and can only work a single body part—maybe your grip, using dynamic tension *eagle claw* exercises—you should do it.

There are various rewards to this approach. Here's a shotgun blast of benefits:

- **Psychology.** Training boosts the self-esteem, an all-too tender quality after an unpleasant injury. It keeps you motivated and helps you to take control, doing something productive and proactive during recovery.

- **Routine.** Just laying off after an injury messes with your timetable and sense of habit. Getting back into training as soon as you can lessens the likelihood that you will drift away from the fitness lifestyle.

- **Crossover effect.** The body ultimately works as a *system*. Training one muscle group automatically transfers strength to other muscles, even if they are seemingly unrelated.

- **Fitness maintenance.** All athletic qualities are based on a bedrock of basic fitness; attributes such as *cardiovascular conditioning, neural communication, cellular health,* etc. Continued training will maintain all these qualities.

- **Hormonal balance.** Athletic training releases useful muscle-building/fat-eating hormones like *testosterone*. If you quit training due to injury, these hormonal levels plummet.

- **Circulation and blood flow.** Training the muscles improves circulation around the entire body. This in turn will speed up the healing process (see law 5).

- **Stress reduction.** Stress compounds like *norepinephrine* and *cortisol* can be destructive to the body. Continued training helps you to manage these chemicals, replacing them with painkilling endorphins.

Some people might argue that only working one side of the body—your right arm, if your left is incapacitated, for example—creates strength imbalances. This may be partially true, but there is also some crossover effect, as stated above, and as a result an untrained area will retain a higher level of strength than it otherwise would. Plus, "muscle memory" will allow you to even out your strength symmetry very soon after you get back into bilateral training.

Sometimes you might be unsure of how to train around injuries in this fashion, but where there's a will there's a way. You just gotta get creative. When pro wrestler Ric "The Equalizer" Drasin accidentally amputated three fingers in a table-saw accident, he was in the gym the very next day, lifting dumbbells using his palms rather than his fingers. A physical therapist once told me about a paraplegic guy he worked with who used to train his trunk muscles by rocking backwards and forwards while his good arm clung onto a pole. Remember, you don't need to set records while you're training around an injury—you just need to get focused and *do what you can* while being careful not to further injure your preexisting wounds.

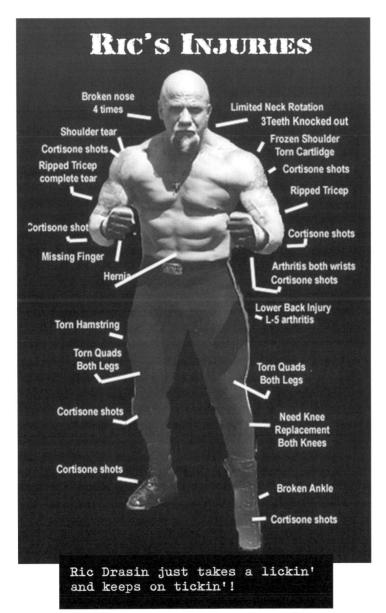

RIC'S INJURIES

Broken nose
4 times

Limited Neck Rotation
3 Teeth Knocked out

Shoulder tear

Frozen Shoulder
Torn Cartlidge

Cortisone shots

Cortisone shots

Ripped Tricep
complete tear

Ripped Tricep

Cortisone shot

Cortisone shots

Missing Finger

Hernia

Arthritis both wrists
Cortisone shots

Lower Back Injury
L-5 arthritis

Torn Hamstring

Torn Quads
Both Legs

Torn Quads
Both Legs

Cortisone shots

Need Knee
Replacement
Both Knees

Cortisone shots

Broken Ankle

Cortisone shots

Ric Drasin just takes a lickin'
and keeps on tickin'!

And there's a silver lining to be found here. Often, athletes find that they can radically improve neglected muscle groups when they injure their more highly-developed areas, because the system (both mental and physical) has more energy to invest in them. An arm injury is the perfect opportunity to improve leg strength, for example. Try it and see.

LAW 4: WORK INJURIES OUT.

As explained under law 2, the initial bodily response to injury is swelling and inflammation. This swelling must be reduced if you wish to kick-start the healing process. Once the swelling has gone down and the injured soft tissue has begun repairing itself, you should think about training that area again. How long this initial period of rest takes depends upon the severity of the injury—it could take anywhere from a week to a month, or even longer.

This is where a lot of beginners go wrong. Once they hurt themselves—maybe a knee, a shoulder, a wrist—they back away from training that area, to let it heal. Unfortunately, they discover that—six months, a year, even two years later—the acute injury has turned into a nagging, chronic pain. It never really went away. As a result, if they simply stop training an area until it feels 100% again, they will never get better.

> Passive stretching can improve circulation and is good therapy if your body is not yet up to the demands of active stretching or calisthenics.

This happens because a great deal of connective tissue has restricted blood flow, certainly compared to the main muscles. Training not only enhances blood flow, it also sets tissues into a synergistic process of growth and adaptation which is associated with incredibly powerful cellular healing agents. The old timers understood this. They used to advise athletes that injuries had to be "worked out" of joints. This idea, of literally *working* an injury away seems strange to most people, who are used to resting to try and get rid of an injury. But it works.

There is a caveat, however. "Working out" an injury requires discretion and body wisdom. It's not a license to launch back into your hardest exercises while you are still hurting. That would only lead to further damage. First of all, you have to wait until swelling has drained from the injured joint or area, ensuring that the healing process has begun. Next, you need to find a movement which involves the damaged joint or muscle, which you can perform *without pain*. Many therapists—educated from a weight-training perspective—advise the use of light dumbbells to find a movement groove that pumps up a muscle without pain. Being from a calisthenics background, I generally advocate the use of total-body exercises as soon as possible. Bodyweight-type exercises not only train the muscles, they also develop balance, coordination, core strength and functional motion, so you should always favor them over weights work while you are healing. Exercises like pushups and pullups are generally too heavy for rehab purposes, so opt for easier exercises. The movement series in the *Convict Conditioning* system of calisthenics all begin with a set of three "rehabilitation sequence" exercises, so if you are looking to work your muscles with gentle bodyweight techniques, refer to *Convict Conditioning* volume one. These milder exercises become progressively harder and are perfect for rehabilitation and physical therapy to help you get back to peak shape—and beyond.

Once you have found a movement you can perform without irritating your injury, focus on increasing your reps. Higher reps will augment blood flow far better than heavier, lower rep work, and this is exactly what you need to speed recovery. Just the simple act of repeatedly contracting healing muscles stretches scar tissue and lessens the likelihood of it spreading. Begin with a shorter, "pumping" range of motion as you are healing, and slowly build to fuller movements over time.

LAW 5: THE POWER OF HEAT.

Once you are able to work a joint again, your recovery will speed up due to the excess blood that training pumps into a wounded area. You can amplify this effect when you are not training, by the use of *thermal therapy*.

The application of heat to injuries is an incredibly old healing technique. There is evidence that the ancient Egyptians used heat to cure injuries, and the practice of applying heated compresses and poultices goes back long before the early Greeks and Romans wrote about it. Modern-day inmates lean on thermal therapy a great deal, largely because prison medics are so cagey about dishing out painkillers and anti-inflammatory drugs. Whenever I had an injury—or even just an achy joint—I'd heat up some water in my little stinger kettle and pour it into a small rubber heat pack. I found that resting the heat pack on a sore area for twenty minutes relaxed the tight tissues and really helped speed up my healing. It eases pain, too.

When you apply heat to an injured area, the local capillaries naturally expand and enlarge, and this in turn allows more blood into the area. Oxygen and nutrient-rich blood is possibly the most vital factor necessary for healing, and as a result the heat speeds recovery. All that extra blood also loosens up tissues and gently blocks pain sensations from getting back to the brain. Often, relief can come after only a few minutes. Heat therapy is a real wonder.

Get yourself a heat pack to deal with your chronic or acute injuries. I use a fluid-filled water bottle, but several varieties are available on the market, including microwavable gel and bean filled bags. You can even get electrically heated pads. Heat your pack up until it is very warm—bearable, but not burning or painful—and apply it to the point of the injury for twenty minutes on the hour. A good alternative to thermal therapy is *sitz therapy*, which involves alternating hot and cold temperature on an area (using hot and cold water, packs, etc.). The cold intervals ensure that the body can't adapt to the heat during a therapy session, and the circulation is really supercharged as a result. Try it with a faucet or showerhead, if you can get the temperature right. Be aware that the cold temperatures can temporarily numb your skin, so be careful not to scald yourself when you apply the heat afterwards.

Because the use of heat increases blood volume in an area, you should *never* apply heat therapy to an injury that is still swollen or inflamed—heat will only add to the swelling, which is the opposite of what you want. Only apply heat to an injury *after* the swelling has dissipated, preferably after you are able to work the injured area gently again (see law 4). Muscles and connective tissue can also become inflamed after heavy training, so don't heat up a tender area immediately after exercise either. In these two special circumstances, ice is the best choice.

LAW 6: BUILD BACK SLOWLY.

Let's assume it's been a while since you got hurt, and you have had some success in working the affected area again (law 4). At some point, you'll want to start heading towards your previous best performances. Note that "heading" doesn't mean "sprinting". The body is great at healing injuries, but it requires time. Give it the time it needs. When progressing back to peak shape, it's wiser to err on the side of going too slowly than going too fast, because if you go too fast and re-injure yourself you'll wind up taking more time in the long run. Where recovery is concerned, slow and steady wins the race.

Once you can use a good range of motion on your exercises with no pain, you can begin adding resistance by moving onto the harder exercises in the *Convict Conditioning* system—but do so slowly, and with tender lovin' care. Don't jump forwards several steps at a time. Work through each and every step. You can do this faster than it took the first time, but definitely go stage by stage, using your intuition and internal senses to guide you. It's impossible to give guidelines, because how fast you get back to your best depends on your healing speed and the severity of your injury, but even if you have a very light injury, *never* leap back to your previous bests. Take it stage by stage. Build up a good head of steam and you'll be smashing old barriers before you know it.

LAW 7: HAVE FAITH.

Often athletes take great pride in their physical abilities, sometimes centering their entire sense of self-esteem on what they can do with their bodies. When their abilities become curtailed—however temporarily—by an injury, this hits them hard. They can become depressed, despondent, and even suicidal in some cases. I well remember the case of Japanese marathon runner and Olympic medalist Kokichi Tsuburaya, who committed suicide prior to the Mexico City Olympics because his training was hampered by a bad back.

Injuries cause mental stress, which can lead to negativity. If we think we will never recover, we will lose the motivation to conduct proper rehab, and as a result healing slows down to a crawl. This results in stress, which leads to negativity and the cycle repeats itself—it's a self-fulfilling prophecy. If you really believe you'll never get better, you probably won't.

Luckily, the reverse is also true. Believe in yourself, and your chances of recovery *skyrocket.* Don't dwell on the negatives of your injury, no matter how bad you think it is. Most of the time, injuries loom much larger in our minds than they really are. The human body is a miracle, and people have been known to recover 100% from even horrific injuries. The sports world is full of athletes who became great again after injuries which should have ended their careers. The annals of medical history are bursting with cases of accident victims who got up and walked despite being told they never would. Have absolute faith in your own future—and you *will* heal faster.

Focus on the improvements you make on a daily basis, and above all, be *positive*. A positive attitude releases *serotonin,* a neurotransmitter that aids relaxation while boosting energy levels; perfect recovery fuel. Positivity stimulates the immune system and releases *beta-endorphins* which provide pain relief. Recent research even indicates that a good mood can increase circulating *human growth hormone*—one of the most powerful anabolic healing agents in the body.

There is a very real *biology of faith.* Tap into it!

LAW 8: HEALING IS A LEARNING PROCESS.

This law is related the previous one, and has a lot to do with staying positive through an injury. We inevitably see getting hurt as a completely bad experience, but this really isn't true. It's part of the yin and yang of life that no experience is ever *totally* negative.

If you perceive injury as exclusively bad, you are missing a trick. I've been working out for decades now, and pretty much the only time I ever really learn something new about my body is when I get hurt. Being injured forces an athlete to examine how parts of his or her body work, and encourages us to learn new forms of moving, novel methods of training. If you are paying attention, these little gems of insight will stay with you after you are fully recovered, and can be prize investments in your quest for greater and greater levels of athleticism.

Plus, there's definitely a *deeper* message to being injured. Being injured forces us big, ugly, headstrong dudes to stop for a second and gaze down over the battlefield. It gives us a chance to look inside and remember why we started working out, why we need it. Being hurt gives us a potent reminder of how fragile and precious the body really is. In older cultures, healing was seen as a divine thing, holy even. Maybe this is why.

Don't get me wrong. I'm certainly not saying you need to run around injuring yourself to obtain these profound little life lessons. Always follow law 1 and protect yourself as much as possible; injuries find a body enough without being lent a helping hand. But over the years I've learned that being injured—like being incarcerated—needn't be the end of the world. There's always a profit to be made of a bad time, if you look hard enough.

THE 8 LAWS OF HEALING

LAW 1: PROTECT YOURSELF.
Avoid injury in the first place by cultivating a convict's attitude of self-protection and awareness. Take care of your body, avoid risk-taking, and be safe when you work out.

LAW 2: IMMEDIATE THERAPY.
The moment you sustain any soft tissue injury, focus on the **P.R.I.N.C.E.** protocol:

> **P**ROTECT – Ensure that you won't injure yourself any further
> **R**EST – Cease using the injured area for the time being
> **I**CE – Apply appropriate ice therapy to the area to reduce inflammation
> **N**SAIDs – Anti-inflammatory medication will help the situation
> **C**OMPRESSION – A snug bandage will prevent fluid buildup
> **E**LEVATION – Raising an injured area above the heart will drain swelling

LAW 3: KEEP TRAINING YOUR UNINJURED AREAS.
As soon as it's safe to get back in the gym to work your *uninjured* body parts, you should do so. It will speed recovery, encourage discipline and maintain fitness.

LAW 4: WORK INJURIES OUT.
When left without exercise, sore or injured joints often become "stale" due to lack of blood flow. As soon as you can do it without pain, start training injured areas again, using gentle techniques and working up to high repetitions. This will quicken healing.

LAW 5: THE POWER OF HEAT.
Prison athletes commonly employ the power of heat as a substitute for medication. Once the swelling around an injured area is fully drained, apply thermal therapy via heat packs.

LAW 6: BUILD BACK SLOWLY.
When the pain subsides, ease back into your regular workouts gradually. Pace yourself.

LAW 7: HAVE FAITH.
When hurt, avoid despondency. Being *positive* about recovery helps you heal faster.

LAW 8: HEALING IS A LEARNING PROCESS.
Use injuries as a chance to gain perspective and learn something new about your body.

Injury-a prison experience

During my teens and very early twenties, I didn't think very much of dealing with injury. It was all just something footballers and old people did. But when I turned twenty-five something happened to me that changed my mind.

The incident in question was the famous 1982 riot in San Quentin. It involved more than a thousand convicts and left many injured real bad. The cause of the riot is unknown. There are a lot of "official" theories, but we knew at the time that most of them were bulls***. Racial and gang attitudes were factors, but no way were they the ultimate cause.

The riot started in the large upper yard. The media at the time spoke in terms of "organized group violence", but again that was bulls***. The sheer numbers of inmates in the yard, combined with the fact that the violence escalated so quickly made "organization" impossible. It was total chaos. The atmosphere was terrifying, confusing. Adrenaline was running high, and it seemed like a cloud of fear and anger—which to be fair had been bubbling up for weeks—descended over the entire prison. Jostling became pushing, and little, personal fights were started. Friends and nearby gang members quickly joined in, and soon there were brawls all over the yard. In turn these scuffles became the spark which fanned into a flame, and within the course of what seemed like a quarter hour the entire prison was total anarchy. It was crazy.

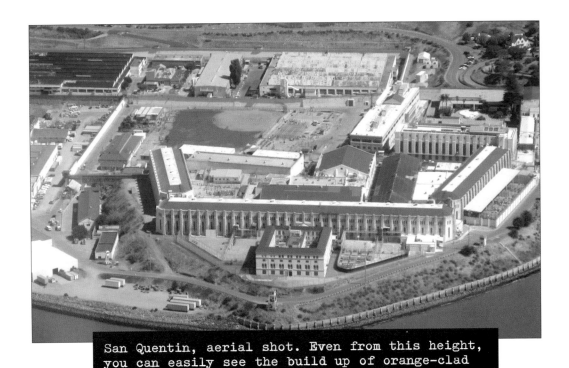

San Quentin, aerial shot. Even from this height, you can easily see the build up of orange-clad inmates. Trouble's brewin'.

I had nothing to do with the start of the riot, and I really had no interest in it. But like a lot of convicts I became involved, got sucked in, just because I was out in the yard when things went down. A lot of guys were wounded in the fights that broke out. Inspections have become much tougher since the seventies and eighties, and shanks and basic knives and stilettos made out of pens and toothbrushes were much more common in the joint then than they are now. For some, the riot was a perfect opportunity to facelessly act out little vendettas that had been brewing for years. One guy I knew was unlucky enough to receive a permanent razorblade smile. He was held down by two big gang members, while the third slashed him from ear to ear with a short shiv—a razorblade wound into the shaft of a split pencil.

I guess I was lucky that I didn't receive any injuries like that. But I *did* get injured. At some point into the most intense part of the riot, I got the idea into my head that some of my boys were in the north part of the yard, a place where they usually chilled during recreation breaks. I formulated the dumb notion of making my way towards them, fighting through the mass of orange-boilersuited brawlers. And this I did—at least for a few minutes. But eventually the crowd got real dense, and I found myself surrounded by panic-fuelled combat on every side. I began to get nervous as I was pressed and pushed around by the sprawling bodies. I knew that I had made a mistake venturing away from the periphery of the yard where I had started out. Icy fear gripped my insides—I had visions of myself being crushed or trampled to death if things got much worse. I thought about trying to fight my way back out of the riot, but by now I had no idea where I was going.

At this point I was sent sprawling assways as several guys slammed into me, back first. In retrospect, it's pretty obvious that this wasn't deliberate. I guess they were just at the tail end of a wave of pressure that started further up the crowd. But at the time I was about thirty pounds of beef lighter than I am now, and I got sent flying into the chest of a weasel-faced little con a few feet behind me. He didn't like this, and shoved me hard in the shoulder blades, sending me hurtling forwards. By now the blood was rising in my temples, and I made the mistake of turning round and smacking him square in his mean little jaw with a right cross. I've no idea whether he went down or not because a split-second later a larger guy—presumably a buddy of Mr Weasel—shoulder barged me from my left. I was quick enough to grab him and turn, so his own momentum slammed him onto the concrete. At some point he had snagged onto my boilersuit though, and I followed him down. I slung my leg over the dude to try and find the purchase to get up, but right at that moment something nasty happened.

I guess there had been more pushing around us, because suddenly, out of nowhere, this hugely fat, bald S.O.B. tripped back and landed right on top of the both of us. It wasn't his fault, and he landed pretty much flat on his back, but he must have weighed three-hundred pounds and he came down like a Harley or something. I was twisted up badly when he fell on me, and I heard a great big SNAP, even over the shouts of the crowd. I screamed as what felt like a bolt of lightning shot down my left leg. For a split second I got the impression that the chaotic swell packed tightly around us were all going to lose balance and topple down as well, killing us, but luckily no-one else followed him. I scrambled out from under King Kong and hobbled away.

In moments I was in a different part of the yard, but I knew I was hurt. I had no feeling at all in my left leg. It was like a useless chunk of wood.

Injured in San Quentin

The riot seemed to last forever, and luckily I survived. But into the night—as the adrenaline and endorphins began to wear off—the pain set in. I realized I had done something very, very bad to myself. The muscles at the rear of my thigh felt like they had been stripped off the bone, blowtorched, then sewn back in. I stupidly tried to walk it off, but the agony was off the scale. The next day my entire lower back had seized up. It was a struggle just to stand up, and I could barely walk even with support. I was convinced I had broken my back or something, and the fear of it made me talk to a hack.

The guards could see I was badly screwed up and I was sent to the prison hospital. Following the big riot, the place was completely packed full of casualties. Limping inside, my hands up against the wall, I remember thinking that it looked like something out of the TV show M*A*S*H. It was that bad. As it turns out, the 1982 riot still holds the dubious record of being the biggest and worst riot in the history of San Quentin, so it's a pretty safe bet that the hospital hasn't been so busy either before or since.

Eventually I got to see a couple of doctors who, although competent, were clearly being pretty much pushed beyond their limits by the conditions and workload they had to deal with. After giving my description of what happened, I was prodded, manipulated and had my leg moved round for about fifteen minutes. It was excruciating, and it was a major relief when the examination was over. Even though I'd barely moved, I lay back on the gurney I'd been placed on, soaking in sweat. After consulting with his fellow medic, the older doctor came and spoke to me. "Well," he said in a southern drawl, "it's pretty clear what you've done sir." I awaited the verdict in silence. "You've torn a ligament in your hip, probably the sacroiliac ligament. Judging by the amount of swelling, you've probably tore it clean away."

"When will it heal?" I asked. The doctor looked at me with raised eyebrows.

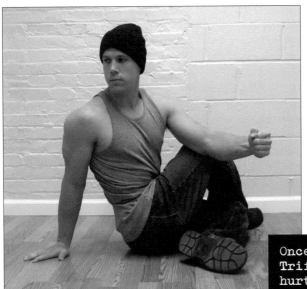

"Ruptured ligaments don't heal, sir. Once they're gone, they're gone. There's really not much we can do for you. I'll sign your sheet here, and make sure you get a break from your work details for the foreseeable future." And with that he turned on his heel to see whoever was next in line.

> Once you can perform the Trifecta movements without hurting yourself, recovery is not far away.

To my horror, I was given aluminum crutches to help me get back to my block. I could feel the eyes of the inmates burning into me as I slowly, pathetically, clicked and clacked the long, long walk back to my cell. I had felt scared and vulnerable in prison before—everybody does, no matter what they say. But for perhaps the first time in the joint, I had felt the way prey must feel when being eyed up by predators. My tottering trip along the gangways seemed to go on forever, and my thoughts became blacker and blacker with every step. What if this injury was permanent? The doctor had told me that torn ligaments don't grow back. Would I be limping around with a bum leg forever?

The thought of being a cripple in a hellhole like San Quentin filled me with dread. I knew I would have to get fighting fit again—freakin' quick—or be perceived as weak. This would mean a whole heap of trouble for me in the future, and I was looking at a lot more time inside at that point. I wasn't dumb. I knew that recovering from an injury like the one I had would require a lot of physical therapy. I also knew that my chances of getting any such specialist health care inside SQ were between slim and none. I was gonna have to fix this thing myself.

Healing through suppleness

I spent the rest of the week pretty much flat on my back on my bunk, except for mealtimes. I'm a big reader—it's a valuable hobby to have inside—and when I next got the chance, I tottered to the shabby prison library to look for books on injury rehab. I found two, and they both emphasized the same point about soft tissue injury; namely that it isn't the actual wound which limits motion after healing—it's *scar tissue*. Scar tissue is inevitable following almost any injury, and in many ways it's a good thing; it knits together damaged anatomical structures, replaces lost function and can even prevent the onset of infection. It is usually stronger than normal tissue, but there is a major downside to this strength—scar tissue is less flexible. This inflexibility makes injured areas tighter than they should be. Scar tissue pulls against surrounding muscle, reducing speed and function and causing joint pain. The only way to make scar tissue more supple is—you guessed it—by proper stretching.

I soon developed a few stretches I was able to do without pain, and I practiced them daily; hourly if I was up to it. This really helped my back and thigh, and in a couple of weeks I was able to resume some upper body calisthenics. After a month I was walking normally, and within six weeks I was able to resume my bodyweight training for legs. This really made my healing speed up. The fresh blood flow and tissue stimulation brought nutrients directly into the injured area so fast I could actually feel myself getting stronger every day. I kept stretching the area, and during my convalescence I read up on the topic, devouring every book I could on flexibility and yoga. After three months my hip was totally back to normal, and I've never had a single problem with it since—in fact it is now stronger than it was when I was in my twenties. Being a devotee of calisthenics before the accident definitely gave me a leg up on healing; my muscles were healthy and fit and my metabolism was quicker and more athletic than it would have been otherwise. But the constant stretching out of the injured hip without doubt played a massive part in my recovery.

Like I said, we only really learn something about our bodies when they get injured. When everything's runnin' smooth, we don't pay any attention. The experience of getting hurt in prison was horrible at the time, but I now see it as a blessing; it kick started my study of flexibility.

Prison Masters

After this incident I got into stretching more seriously, and began to search out guys inside who could teach me advanced stretching techniques. Prison athletes who stretch are hard to come by, and usually bring their techniques in from the outside. Eventually I hung out with several wrestlers who did a lot of stretching, and quite a few guys who knew a lot of yoga (if that sounds bizarre, remember that San Quentin is in California!). But early on I mostly got to speak to martial artists. I knew several martial artists in prison, and most of them were students of kenpo—a hybrid art similar to karate—which was very big on the West Coast at the time. It's a little known fact that James Mitose, the guy who actually brought kenpo to America, was imprisoned in Folsom in 1974 after being convicted of murder. Years later, he was moved to San Quentin. He was still there when I arrived, although he died not long afterwards. Sadly, I never even got the chance to meet him; he died just months after I got sent there. I didn't even discover that he had been incarcerated there until a couple of years after his death.

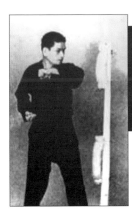
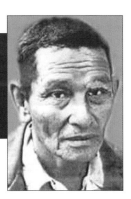

Left: A young James Mitose works on a striking board. Right: A mugshot of a much older Mitose, after years of imprisonment in California.

Ironically, I continued passive stretching (see chapter thirteen) after I got back into calisthenics, and guess what? I actually found I got injured *more often* when I stretched. You don't need to do passive stretching forever—just as rehab until your body relaxes, heals a little, and gets back to the point where you can do active stretching again without risk. When that time comes, drop passive stretching with a smile on your face. Get back to active stretching, and build up to some calisthenics to build supple strength and blood flow in the joints. This will make you heal at maximum speed.

Lights out!

Talking about healing isn't sexy. But it's an absolutely *crucial* part of any athlete's experience. Getting big, strong, fast, agile—or whatever you want to be—takes lots of training. It can take a long time. This is only possible if your body is functioning as it should. More athletes quit training due to nagging aches and pains than you would ever believe. The tragedy is that usually quitting is unnecessary—if you have the right knowledge, you can come back from an injury bigger and badder than ever before.

Unfortunately, knowledge about healing the body generally only comes with time and experience—and that translates into a lot of pain. I can't put my old head on your shoulders, but I can at least try to distill all the tricks I've learned in my years of coping with physical wounds behind bars into something you can take away. This is the point of the eight laws. Learn them, take them to heart and you'll save yourself *years* of healing time over a lifetime of working out.

21: THE MIND

ESCAPING THE TRUE PRISON

We are all alone in the dark.

To the best of my recollection, these were my grandfather's last words to me before he died. I was about ten at the time, and my grandfather—a widower for more than thirty years—was living by himself in a small, old, dirty house in Clayton, where my family hails from. He was in his eighties at the time, and not a particularly healthy or happy old man. My mom and I used to go and see him two or three times a week to do some chores for him. Well, my mom did the chores, I just used to sit with him and listen to him talk. I think when people get to a certain age they just love to be listened to.

That last time I saw him before his death, there'd been a spate of burglaries in the area, and my mom had made a big fuss about reminding him to lock his door before he went to bed. As we were leaving I asked him if he'd be scared in the house by himself all night, and it was then that he said it: *we are all alone in the dark.* I had never heard the phrase before, and it stuck with me with a long time after. I distinctly remember wondering what it meant at the old man's funeral, as his casket was lowered into the ground. *Why do we need to be alone in the dark? What if you have your mom or your wife or even a dog in the house?* The saying didn't make any sense to me as a child. Eventually I forgot about it.

I remembered it bitterly, years later, when I spent my first night in San Quentin after lights out. I don't think I slept at all that night, and although I had a cellmate I was more alone than I had ever been in my life. Surrounded by the terrifying shouts and screams of other convicts, I understood all too well what my grandfather had meant.

Sometimes during my first few months in prison, when I couldn't sleep, I set to thinking about my grandpa, and the other things he had told me. It's common to think back on family and happier times after the lights go out behind the bars. In his younger days, my grandfather had been something of a preacher back in the Bay. He was a very strict, traditional Lutheran; real fire-and-brimstone stuff. When I was a kid, he would sometimes tell me things that scared me, when my mother wasn't in the room. He never did it while she was around—she chided him if he did. One of the things he told me more than once was that if I was a bad boy, I would always get punished for it somehow, when I wasn't expecting. Not by him, but by the Devil himself. (To a Lutheran, the Devil is pretty much the boogieman—or at least, it was to my grandfather.) I was a gullible rube even back in those days, and I asked him once—all wide-eyed and breathless—how the Devil would be able to know if I had done wrong. What my grandfather told me chilled me to the bone and gave me the shivers for weeks afterwards. He leaned in close, and with an earnest expression on his weathered old face he confided to me that a multitude of invisible demons hang silently over every man's shoulders, just a-waiting for him to make a single slip up so's they could carry him straight down to Hell.

Inner negativity

Now, I don't know whether that's *literally* true; maybe it is, maybe it isn't. I was never too gifted when it came to religion. If I had been, I probably wouldn't have lived the life I ended up living. But after spending thousands of nights trapped inside different concrete fortresses alone with my own thoughts, I've come to realize that what my grandfather tried to teach me—which all the old time prophets before him preached—is *symbolically* true. There *is* some kind of army of negative forces lurking around every man and woman, constantly waiting on the periphery of our lives, ready to manifest the second we let our guard down.

These negative forces which have the power to drag us down to the lowest depths aren't devils with little wings and pitchforks. They are inner voices, personal criticisms, psychological barriers, doubts, destructive ideas, as well as the worst kind of emotions. They are all the things within us which drag us down rather than lifting us up. These things might start entirely within our own skulls, but trust me, just like grandpa's demons, these negative forces are always there; always a-waiting. As soon as we allow them to they will dominate us; overwhelm us. There's no doubt in me at all about this.

You get plenty of practice wrestling with your demons in the joint. When you're outside, there's always something to distract you from the bad voices we make for ourselves. You can turn on the TV, go for a walk, take in a movie, call up a friend. But when you are by yourself at night, locked away from the world, you can hear these demons loud and clear. That's why the majority of prison suicide attempts happen at night. It's probably also why so many convicts become turned towards religious ways when they're on the inside. The idea of demons suddenly becomes more real.

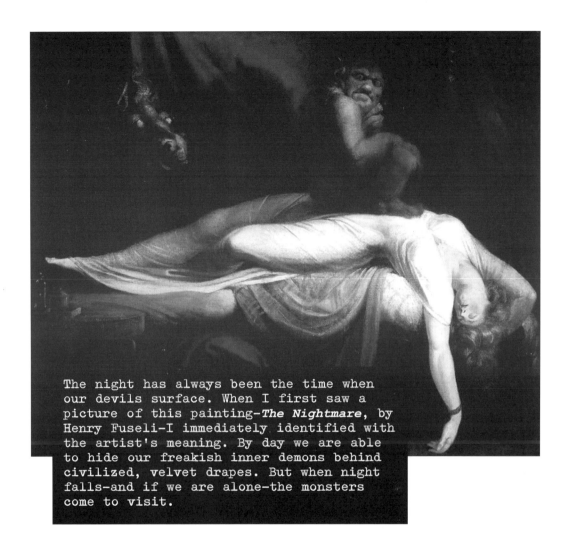

The night has always been the time when our devils surface. When I first saw a picture of this painting—*The Nightmare*, by Henry Fuseli—I immediately identified with the artist's meaning. By day we are able to hide our freakish inner demons behind civilized, velvet drapes. But when night falls—and if we are alone—the monsters come to visit.

Six training demons

These "demons"—our own negative inner states—are always with us. They are the products of our thinking, so we can't escape them any more than we can escape our own minds. They follow us around when we eat, when we have to deal with others, when we work, when we play. They are even with us during sleep, manifesting as nightmares, anxiety dreams and night terrors. It follows that since they are with us constantly, they affect everything we do. Our physical training is no exception.

The mind controls the body. No matter how physically fit we may be, or how much we should be gaining from consistent training, if our minds are not in the right place training falls by the wayside. Who cares if your *muscles* are strong? If your *mind* is weak, corrupted by destructive self-talk, you won't be breaking any personal records. You'll be lucky if you're able to drag your self off your bunk to do your daily pushups. What should be a constant part of our lives, full of pleasure, health and excitement can be easily ruined by this nasty internal chatter. Training seems painful, fruitless, boring—it's seen as a dry wasteland that eats away our time and erodes the energy.

Our "demons" are largely the result of wrong ideas. We acquire many of these ideas tacitly, almost by accident. It's certainly not deliberate. But once a bad idea gets lodged in your brain—maybe from something you've been told by somebody who should have known better—it's virtually impossible to shift. Good thoughts practically fly out of the mind, but bad thoughts dig their heels in. They want to stay forever.

Don't let them. Confront your demons and challenge them—every day, every night if you have to. If you let your negative ideas and destructive self-talk have free reign, the darker sections of your mind will grow larger and larger until they take control of your spirit and destroy you entirely. The only way to battle the negative ideas that attack your training life is to become conscious of them, and challenge them.

What follows is a list of six of the most common "demons" that assault our training drive and generally mess with our heads as we struggle to get stronger and fitter.

Let's tackle them, together.

DEMON #1:...INFERIORITY

"All the other guys I meet are bigger and stronger than me...
...I'm just not cut out for physical training."

In any worthwhile human endeavor that demands big changes, long stretches of time are required. No matter who you are. As a result, qualities like consistency and commitment are vastly more important than what we *imagine* our genetic potential to be.

Physical training is not an exception to this truth—if anything, it exemplifies it. I've met guys who had *phenomenal* genetics for strength—men who should have become the world's best at calisthenics—who never got past the beginner's level, because their minds were weak. They allowed their demons to control them, and they quickly quit their training. Likewise, I've met men inside who started their careers with all the muscular potential of Pee-wee Herman, who wound up as monsters that could snap redwood nightsticks in half with their bare hands, all because they took charge of themselves and confronted their negative inner talk.

Screw "potential". In anything meaningful, it doesn't matter where you start—it matters where you finish. None of us can see into the future to predict where that will be, so you'll never know unless you train. So train!

DEMON #2: ...DISCOURAGEMENT

"I'm not making progress."

The loss of motivation for training, in perhaps nine out of ten cases, can be traced back to this evil little idea. *I'm not getting stronger* and *my muscles are shrinking* are its ugly sisters. These are the kind of nagging thoughts that make people quit.

If you are thinking along these lines, it means something has gone wrong with your training. Usually the problem begins when a program is badly designed, or has become too intense or overcomplicated. Don't get stressed. Strip your bodyweight work back to basics. Work on the Big Six, with just two work sets per exercise, training each exercise only once per week. Start slow. Soon you'll be adding reps. If you are adding reps, you are building momentum. This means you'll start to advance from exercise to exercise. If you advance from exercise to exercise, you *are* getting stronger. And, if you are adding strength to your body, quality muscle *will* follow.

Rest assured, you'll get there. It's as certain as tomorrow's sunrise.

DEMON #3: ...PAIN

"I have aches and pains...if I continue training hard, I'll wind up with arthritis. It's just not worth it."

A lot of men get paranoid about experiencing pain. They don't often talk about it—it's a macho thing—but it interferes with training motivation more often than you might think.

Pain and training go hand in hand. There is the brief, intense ache you experience struggling to improve your performance in your exercises, the general discomfort and distress that comes from working your body hard, and the soreness deep in your muscles over the next day or two.

But this is *good* pain. It is the heat from the fire that transforms you daily into a bigger, stronger, tougher, better version of yourself. Embrace it. This kind of good pain is different from *injury* pain; the pain that comes from asking the muscles to do something they can't do. This is *bad* pain. It causes internal trauma to the body which builds up over time, leading to longer-term joint irritation and acute injuries. With experience, you will begin to learn the difference; good pain is largely in the muscles, and follows definite time scales relative to exercise. Bad pain lies largely in the joints and connective tissues, and lingers or appears in an unpredictable manner.

Calisthenics is the safest form of muscular training known to man. It works the body precisely as nature intended. Far from making you a cripple in years to come, it will keep you strong and lithe as a panther well into your Golden Years. We all get aches and pains I'm afraid—that's part of life. Quitting your training won't stop you getting the odd sore joint—it will actually *increase* your pain levels in the long run. Proper bodyweight training fends off extra pain and injuries and keeps the joints healthier and more supple than they ever could be otherwise.

As for acute injuries? We *all* get them from time to time. Strength training certainly isn't the culprit. People throw out their backs picking up pens, blow out their knees tripping over coffee tables, and get hernias from shoveling snow. Performed correctly, calisthenics training strengthens your body in a harmonious way, helping to prevent these sudden injuries. And when they do happen—and they will—far from being a burden, injuries are often a time to learn something really valuable about your body and mind.

Pain? *Pah*. It's just weakness leaving the body is all.

BODYWEIGHT—WITHOUT LIMITS

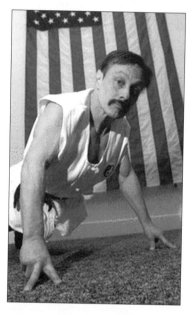

When you need a kick in the butt, it helps to get inspired by superior athletes. If you are looking for the best around, you could do a lot worse than Sifu John Morrow.

Morrow is a seventh degree Shaolin black belt whose humble demeanor belies the fact that he knows how to kick serious ass. Not only is he a champion fighter, Morrow is also one of the world's greatest calisthenics masters. He's not as famous as many (more publicized) American athletes, but trust me—when it comes to bodyweight, the man is a true legend.

Morrow is living proof that—despite what you read in magazines—optimal performance depends on *mental strength*, not steroids or expensive supplements. Morrow fasts every Spring, and has done since the '70s. In 2004 Morrow fasted for 41 days, surviving (and thriving) on nothing but fruit juices, water and soy drinks for protein. During this time he wasn't slacking off, either. He was performing hundreds of pushups daily, as well as practicing and teaching martial arts full time. Did he lose strength? On the last day of the fast he unofficially shattered the Guinness World Record for pushups—139 in one minute. (Yeah, you read that right.) He was 52 years old at the time. He later broke his own record under official conditions.

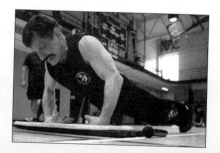

In 2011, at age 59, Morrow performed 2000 pushups on the back of his hands in a single hour. It wasn't done for glory—it was fundraising for *Kids Against Hunger*. Pay attention, people. This is what athletes without self-imposed limits look like.

DEMON #4: ...AGING

"I'm getting too old for all this."

Ah, this is a biggie—although you may not realize it. Yet.

If you are in your teens, you probably don't think about aging at all. Training is new, and so are you. In your twenties, you have a dim awareness that aging exists, but you don't truly believe it'll happen to you the way it happens to others; almost all the great athletes are in their twenties anyway. Suddenly you are thirty and your attitude changes. The pros are looking younger. Hey—where are all the champs in their mid-thirties? Guys you played football with in high school with are fat and bald. A few years pass and that big milestone— forty—is around the corner. You become aware that less and less of the people you see in fitness magazines, or working in the gym are your age. Then you are fifty. Old. Before long you will be sixty, and by then it's positively foolish to be seen training seriously. The big 7-0 comes next. By now—if you have been paying attention—you understand just how quickly time slips through your fingers.

This is how the average person thinks. You know what? It's all total bulls***!

The guy who originally trained me was in his seventies when I was in my twenties. He could still do five out of the six Master Steps of the Big Six exercises—and I couldn't do a single one. Most young athletes can't do any of the Master Steps either. He made me feel like a total weakling.

A lot of "authorities" push the idea that the *teens* are the best years for training—if you try gaining muscle and strength after this, results will be lousier. This is nonsense. In reality, the best age for strength training gains is from *thirty to forty*. Have you even noticed that skinny guys get a little huskier, more brawny as they hit the big 3-0? This is because their metabolisms slow down, allowing their bodies to accumulate the natural muscle that was always supposed to be on their frames—the tissue that got burned away by their fast metabolisms. Most teenagers are hopeless at building any real muscles, because at that age their body systems are like furnaces—all the energy that would go into the process of building muscle gets eaten up, no matter how hard they train or how heavily they eat. The only reason some teenagers progress so fast at bodybuilding these days is because vast amounts of performance drugs are readily available. You can bet the current crop of big teen bodybuilders won't be super-strong at seventy. They won't even be healthy. Hell, most will be lucky to be alive. It's tragic, really—the majority of guys experiment with bodybuilding in their teens, but give up because they get no results. Then by thirty or forty, they think they are too old!

Gaining pure, *genuine* strength takes *time*. Years, not months. True—*drug-free*—strength athletes of the past (like Thomas Inch, or Alexander "Iron Samson" Zass) sometimes didn't even reach their peak until their *fifties*. The body is more than capable of generating and retaining high levels of strength into its seventies. The Mighty Atom was still performing in his eighties! Scientists are only now coming to understand what Victorian strongmen knew only too well; that much of the decline seen in elderly people isn't down to aging—it's down to *disuse*. Sure, the ability of the body to adapt and recover slows down as you head into your Golden Years. I'm not denying that. But this is offset by the gifts that only aging can bestow; qualities such as training experience, body wisdom and discipline.

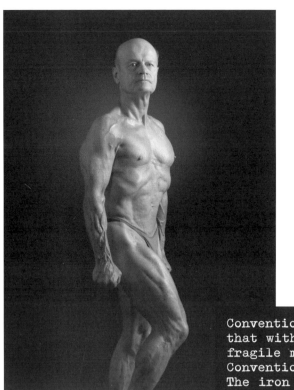

Far from being dangerous, strength training is positively *essential* to health as you get older (past seventy-five). Osteoporosis, arthritis and immobility can't be cured by chemical drugs—the best way to combat them is by resistance training. You *gotta* move that bodyweight.

Keep training as long as you live. You never really appreciate how quick the years pass until you are standing at the end of them. Please don't waste any more precious time. Go do your exercises right now!

Conventional wisdom tells us that with age comes flabby, fragile muscles and a paunch. Conventional wisdom is wrong. The iron six-pack you see above belongs to a seventy year-old athlete; the amazing Clarence Bass. A lifelong fitness enthusiast, Bass became a bodybuilding champion at the tender age of 40. In his fifties he became a nationally-ranked indoor rower. In his sixties, he could pump out a set of twenty pullups-more than the average advanced bodybuilder half his age. Now, in his seventies, he possesses the physique of a twenty-five year-old decathlete and is still stronger than you.

DEMON #5:...APATHY

"Working out is boring."

This is the perfect example of what I mean when I say that training problems have their source in the *mind*—not in the real world.

One guy can do pullups till the cows come home, and get nothing but pleasure and excitement out of them. He revels in the physical challenge, and goes to sleep practically *aching* for the next workout to roll around so he can go for it again. The act of exercising is electrifying to him; seeing improvement, beating his previous bests is a constant encouragement and source of inspiration. The knowledge that he will be more muscular and more powerful tomorrow than he was yesterday is a secret thrill. And yet his cellmate can try pullups and immediately hate them—see them as nothing but a drag that makes his arms sore.

What's the difference? It's not in what the two guys are doing—they are doing the same thing. The difference is in what they are *thinking*.

There will probably be times when you get bored and listless with your training. All athletes experience fluctuations in interest from time to time, no matter how committed they are. This doesn't mean you're fickle—it means you're human. When you get bored with training, the key to overcoming the problem is to understand that *boredom is a quality of the mind.* To find new inspiration, you need to change the way you are *thinking* about training. Here are a few surefire ideas that'll help:

- Keep in mind that boredom is a temporary state. Eventually you'll get your training enthusiasm back, and when you do you'll be real pissed at yourself if you allowed yourself to quit and lose all that precious time.

- Remember why you began training in the first place. Review your original goals, and reflect on how far you've come. Training made that happen.

- Set new, future goals. These should be challenging but achievable—such as moving up in exercises in all of the Big Six movements over the next month.

- Training shouldn't be monotonous. Prison is bad enough without adding even more forced labor. Training should be an act of rebellion, of freedom and personal expression. If you have gotten too locked into one type of workout, shake up your routine. Mix up the volume, the training days, the exercises. Throw in variants, cross-train. Get creative and excited about your workouts again!

- Remember that you will keep changing and getting better into the future. Visualize your ideal strength level and physique. Imagine how it would feel to get to that level, and remind yourself that only training can get you there.

- If your training sessions are too hard or too long, the subconscious mind will rebel. There are times to push hard, even very hard, but you should follow those periods with easier training periods to let your spirit breathe. Redesign your workouts with more breaks, and fewer work sets. Work hard, sure, but go easy on your body and mind from time to time.

- If the above ideas don't work, try dirty tricks. Reward yourself for training. Set a goal of training three days a week for the next two months, and get yourself a gift if you meet that goal.

Reflecting and acting on these ideas should put some fuel back in the motivational tank. If not, you might just be burnt out. Take two weeks off and don't think about training at all. Turn your attention to something else, another hobby. Come back refreshed, and begin again, gently. Before long the fire will be burning once more, I promise ya.

DEMON #6:...TIME

"I just don't have time to train."

Okay, I'll admit it—this *isn't* a demon I've really had to face in my own training career. During my long stretches in prisons and correctional facilities, I've had far *too much* time on my hands. When I was in Marion during lockdown—which was the vast majority of my stay—I pretty much had twenty-three hours to fill, every single day. And those hours stretched out long, let me tell you. For myself and many fellow inmates, working out was a desperate way to kill the endless monotony of lockdown. Time was the only thing I had too much of, in prison.

But it's not like this for everybody. On the outside, younger guys might have school or college, as well as homework and the other leisure commitments that youth delivers so readily. It rarely seems like you have enough hours in the day to fit life into. Trust me, as you get older it only gets worse. I know a lot of guys have families and responsibilities. Maybe you have to work eight hours a day. You need to shower and shave for work, then drive there and back—that's another hour or two. You need to spend time with your woman and perhaps your kids, plus you have other domestic duties; fix the sink, paint the back fence. You need a little downtime watching the tube to stay sane, followed by seven or eight hours in the sack (if you are lucky). Hell, where does all this leave time for working out?

Okay, that's all the negative stuff given a voice. Now time for the democratic response.

Calisthenics doesn't require any special equipment. Get a chinning bar for your doorframe or (even better) hang a couple of roped rings off a tree or your staircase, and you can do all your workouts at home, any time you have a few free minutes. If you have built up to two or three hour workouts, I can relate—I've done that too, and more. But you really don't *need* that kind of investment to improve your strength and fitness. Cut back. If you must, you can always go back to drawn-out workouts when you have more time. If you are into endurance, save longer workouts for your weekend, and focus on strength during the working week. Strength is built by *intensity*, not *volume*, so focus on quality over quality. A good, solid calisthenics workout can be achieved with only two working sets of a single exercise. It can take as little as five minutes. Who can't spare five minutes?

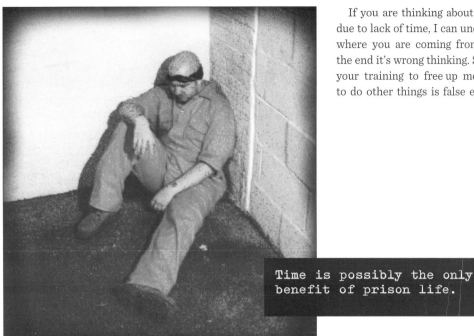

If you are thinking about quitting due to lack of time, I can understand where you are coming from but in the end it's wrong thinking. Stopping your training to free up more time to do other things is false economy.

Time is possibly the only benefit of prison life.

Training *produces* energy; being fit and strong allows you to get through your daily tasks much more quickly and efficiently than you could if you were a stressed workaholic or a couch potato. This is not to mention the years it can add to your life!

Training doesn't steal your time—it *gives* you time in the long run.

These six ideas are just a few of the demons I and others have encountered on the journey towards bettering our bodies and becoming stronger men. Perhaps you have encountered some of them also. Maybe you have your own demons to cope with. Whatever they might be, my thoughts and best wishes go out to you.

We are all alone in the dark.

Lights out!

Hey...The final section of the final chapter. I guess this really is *lights out*, huh? At least for now.

When I decided to write this book, I did it with one goal in mind; to record and publish all the hard-earned knowledge of prison conditioning methods I obsessively acquired through my long, long years in jail. Even though this book is all about training the body, it's fitting that the final chapter is dedicated to the *mind*.

I say that because there is something I've gained that from my training that goes well beyond physical strength. It's something internal, something psychological. Perhaps almost spiritual. Exactly what this benefit is, I find hard to put my finger on. The closest thing I can say is that it's something like *hope*. It's the slow-dawning faith in a future that can be good; that despite whatever mistakes a man makes, whatever terrible errors land him at the lowest ebb of human life, there is something we can learn, something we can change in ourselves. But to embrace this change, we need to let go of former mistakes, however big and bad. We need to look towards the best things inside us, the things we have the power to improve on, however small they may be.

I've said elsewhere that I'm not really a religious person, and I'm painfully aware of my inadequacies as a writer. Fortunately the sentiment I'm trying to get at has been expressed by a better man, the preacher Reinhold Niebuhr, in his *Serenity Prayer*. I heard these words so many times on the inside—it's the adopted prayer of Alcoholics and Narcotics Anonymous—that I guess some of the message sank in. I'd like to close this book with the first verse of Niehbuhr's prayer:

> *God grant me the serenity*
> *To accept the things I cannot change;*
> *The courage to change the things I can;*
> *And the wisdom to know the difference.*

Now go do your pushups.

— BONUS —
CHAPTER

!BONUS CHAPTER!

PUMPIN' IRON
IN PRISON

Myths, Muscle and Misconceptions

Shortly after my last stint inside, I had the misfortune to wind up watching a daytime talk show. (I'm still not sure how this happened.) The topic was *GYMS IN JAIL: The Ultimate Danger!* or some similar crap. Amongst the contributors was the leader of some mother's group who thought that lifting weights in prison turned men into super-strong sex-charged rapists, and a fat conservative congressman who said that if criminals need exercise they should bring back the rock-bashing chain gangs. Well, he might be right about that; but some of the other ideas the panel seemed to voice about prison gyms were way, way off. In fact, the image that the public seems to have about prison gyms is something like this:

Dangerous, antisocial scumbags go into prison and have nothing to do all day but lift heavy weights and pump iron in gangs out in the prison yard. As a result, when these guys finish their stretch, they're still dangerous, antisocial scumbags but they're bigger, stronger scumbags than when they went in.

This seems to be the common view, held mostly by people who've never been to prison. It's total bull.

It's true that prison is largely full of scumbags, sure. But in reality, weight-training in prison hardly ever gets anybody any bigger or stronger. This might sound ridiculous, but that's how it is. Everybody knows that prisoners get hugely strong and beefy from training inside, right? Wrong! This is a common misconception people on the outside have. It's based on a complex set of errors and confused ideas, which can be broken down into four basic myths. Let's look at these myths one by one.

MYTH #1

All prisons have gyms.

This is a basic myth. According to federal law, all prisons have to offer recreation areas for health and fitness—but in some cases this can mean no more than a yard to walk around. Prison gymnasiums with weights began cropping up in the fifties, and probably reached their peak in the eighties. These days there are fewer every year.

It makes me laugh when people think that all prisons have huge, well-equipped gyms. Read the papers— watch news reports when prisons and penitentiaries are mentioned. They're as overcrowded as hell. There's just no room in most prisons for the extensive floor space gyms require. As a result, where gyms do exist, they are constantly under threat of losing space. In some Californian jails, bunks are stacked three high, because there's just nowhere else to put the inmates. If you think prisons are like big health clubs, think again.

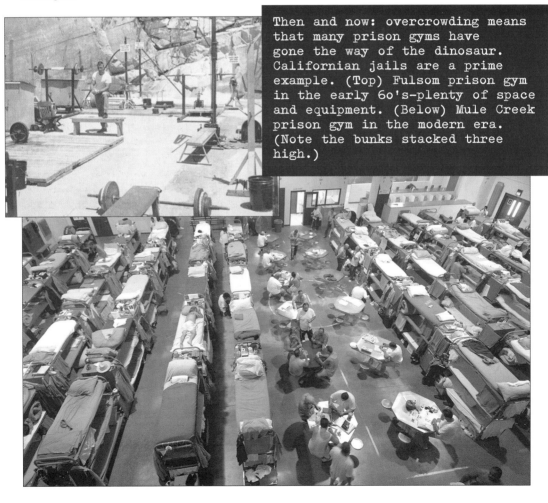

Then and now: overcrowding means that many prison gyms have gone the way of the dinosaur. Californian jails are a prime example. (Top) Fulsom prison gym in the early 60's-plenty of space and equipment. (Below) Mule Creek prison gym in the modern era. (Note the bunks stacked three high.)

It is true there are some large correctional facilities with really excellent, well-equipped gyms; Rikers Island springs to mind. But these are exceptions, not the rule—and they probably won't last too much longer, anyway. Due to media hype and public outcry, politicians are constantly under pressure to slash prison gym funding. Whenever Uncle Sam's purse begins to feel the pinch, public spending on prisons is always the first government budget to come under attack. As a result, the growth in the number of prison gyms—which exploded in the feel-good 1980's—has ground to a halt, and is even reversing in some places as equipment is sold off by recently privatized penitentiaries.

Some powerful people want to get rid of prison gyms completely. As recently as '99, New Jersey Congressman Bob Franks proposed a bill effectively banning all bodybuilding and weight-training in federal and state correctional institutions. The bill wasn't passed, but while convicts are being shown in movies and on TV as a bunch of steroid-crazy psychos who do nothing but lift weights all day, it probably won't be long before prison gyms in America get dirt poured on them.

MYTH #2

Prison gyms are ideal for getting guys stronger and more muscular.

Something most people don't realize is that prison gyms are nothing like regular gyms on the outside. To get big and strong using equipment you really need to handle free weights. To bodybuilders, weightlifters and powerlifters, free weights are king. On the outside, virtually all commercial or college gyms are based on free weights. This means plenty of dumbbells and barbells. The dumbbells are usually welded and range from 5lbs 'bells to 120lbs or more, going up in 5lbs increments. Standard Olympic barbells are equally versatile; going up from 45lbs (the empty bar) to over 800lbs—enough to crush most strong guys. You can regulate the weight of the bar to any level you like with some simple math. All you have to do is add or subtract the loose plates provided, which typically come in 45lbs, 25lbs, 10lbs, 5lbs and 2.5lbs varieties. This is important, because it means that can make any adjustable barbell on the outside the weight you need, to within five pounds.

Prison gyms aren't like this. Although some prison gyms have dumbbells, most prison gyms don't. Of the six gyms in the prisons I've seen, at the time only *one* had dumbbells—and they only had identical sets that weighed 35lbs. (They were chained to the rack.) And as for the barbells? Yes, most prison gyms *do* have heavy barbells, as you may have seen on TV or in movies. But these barbells aren't like the variable, plate-loading barbells in commercial gyms—the big old weight plates are *permanently welded* onto the bar. Fully equipped prison gyms do exist, but despite what you may have heard they are few and far between and are usually found only in lower security facilities, except on rare occasions.

Why are most of the tougher prison gyms like this? Any hack will tell you straight away—so that the inmates can't use weights as weapons! A heavy dumbbell (particularly the nice cast-iron hexagonal kind) makes for a fantastic cudgel and could cave in a human skull very easily. The large weight plates used on Olympic barbells are just as dangerous. In Rikers Island (NJ) back in 1994 there was a mini-riot in the gym, in which ten inmates and fifteen guards were pretty badly injured. Some of the guards where hit on the head with the 45lbs weight plates that go on the barbells and were nearly killed. Even the empty bars make pretty dangerous quarter-staffs. During the 1993 Easter riot in Lucasville Prison, several guards hid in an ante-room to the gymnasium. A gang of inmates used the empty iron barbell bars to batter down the concrete wall protecting the guards, one of whom was killed. Several inmates were killed during the riot, also.

Inmates have a terrifically strong sense of territory (particularly the gang members) and heated fights break out in the weights pit regularly. If free dumbbells and weights plates were left loose, you'd have dead bodies strewn about the gym floor before the hacks could even react. This is the reason why true free weights are rarer inside than most members of the public think, and the reason why they will probably become increasingly rare in the future.

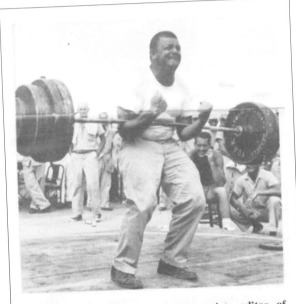

Bill Clark, the author, and an associate editor of Lifting News, is shown making a 405 Zercher lift. This was named after the famed old time Missouri strong man who developed and practiced it. A full squat is done while holding the weight in the elbows, as shown, and if you think this isn't rough, just try it. Bill has done 455 in this manner. He is shown performing before the Leavenworth prison in July at a contest he helped to promote there. Bill has also performed a 505 squat, 550 dead lift and 590 in the hack lift.

Liftin' in Leavenworth. In the early sixties, prison gyms were few and far between; but at least the ones that existed were stocked with bars and loose plates, and productive old school weight-training was possible. That changed forever in the eighties, when the plates were welded up.

The point I'm making is that virtually no inmates have access to barbells and dumbbells that get progressively heavier in small increments. People who don't regularly weight-train just don't understand what a huge, practically *insurmountable* problem this is for somebody who is trying to get stronger through lifting.

What happens when you lift a heavy weight is a phenomenon called *hyperadaptation*. The body gets really stressed out by all that unpleasant effort. Your cells think it's a life-or-death scenario. The body thinks to itself; *that was tough—better get a bit stronger in case this happens again.* And, dutifully, the body gets a little bit stronger for a week or so, in case the same thing happens again. But it only gets stronger by a tiny amount—let's say 1% (most of the time it will be much, much less). This means that next time you train, you will be able to lift a little bit more—but only 1% more! If you could bench press 250lbs before you got stronger, you'll

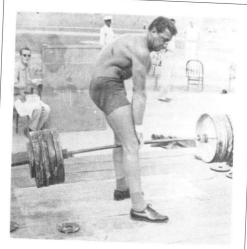

Joe Nanney, a 24 year old 198 pounder, inmate of Leavenworth Prison, making a one hand dead lift with 455 on October 6. This takes a fabulous grip when doing it with an Olympic bar.

only be able to bench press another 2.5 pounds more the next week. The only way people get stronger when lifting weights is by taking advantage of this tiny, less than 1% increase week in, week out, month after month after month, for years. It's how the body gets stronger. There simply is no other way.

If you don't have variable weights with plenty of different weight levels, you can't take advantage of this relatively small phenomenon of hyperadaptation. Let's take the bench press as an example. Maybe you are a rank beginner who has been stuck at 100lbs for the last month or two. Your muscles have hyperadapted and got a little bit stronger, and now you are ready to try 105lbs. On the outside, lifters have access to those 2.5 lbs plates to add to either side of the bar to make it up to 105lbs. (Many lifters use even smaller plates—1lbs and even .5 lbs discs.) In a prison gym, taking advantage of the hyperadaptation phenomena is next to impossible. The bars weigh 45lbs, and the weight plates on them each weigh 45lbs. This means that in most prison gyms, the lightest bar you can bench press is the bar with one big plate per side, weighing 135lbs—which is more than the average beginner can bench press anyway. The next weight up is the bar with two plates per side, weighing 225lbs. The third bar (and the heaviest most prison gyms have) has three plates per side and weighs 315lbs. Once you can bench 135lbs, the next weight up is a whopping *ninety pounds* heavier. There's *no way* you can get strong enough to handle 225lbs just by using the 135lbs bar. The same goes for going to 315lbs from 225lbs. The only guys that can bench these two big bars in the joint are guys who could bench press them coming in. Nobody becomes able to do it while in prison—or at least very few; and in these cases steroids are inevitably the cause. (See *myth #3*.)

There *is* a way to get massively stronger in prison—but it involves the old school calisthenics I described in *Convict Conditioning*. In calisthenics, the resistance—your bodyweight—stays the same, but you learn techniques of shifting your gravity or leverage to make that weight seem progressively heavier. The guys who become monstrously strong *in prison*—without steroids—do it using calisthenics in their cells, not by visiting the prison gym. The human body is way more versatile than welded prison weights.

"Weights only" training—behind bars or on the outside—is a relatively new mindset. Back in the day, all the great strength athletes understood the essential value of bodyweight work. In the sixties, Pat Casey was known as "the King of Powerlifters", and was the first man to officially bench press 6oo lbs. But despite his awesome strength and dedication to the weights, he still found it useful to move his bodyweight.

MYTH #3

All prisoners do all day is lift weights; it gets them huge and freaky.

I can understand how this myth got started. It certainly is true that if you get a chance to see a workout in the weights pit in one of the larger institutions of this nation, you'll inevitably see some huge guys working out; guys with nineteen-inch arms who can bench press a truck. But hardly any of those guys gained their strength and mass by training in prison. Virtually all of them got huge from a lifetime of training on the outside, and are desperately trying to maintain their intimidating muscle on the inside. Big muscles are inevitably a gang thing. Usually the big guys inside are in on assault or gang-related crimes and will be doing a stretch ranging from a few months to three years.

I've seen this time and time again. Often a big bodybuilder (occasionally a national level competitor) will come into the joint and strut around for a few weeks before they start to shrink through lack of steroids. I've never once seen a really muscular guy come into the joint and actually improve his physique. The best they can hope for is to get their hands on a supply of contraband steroids and maintain their body with the sub-standard weights pit in the joint until they can get back out again.

Despite all this, there is a grain of truth to the idea that some guys get bigger in prison. But in 99 cases out of 100, that has jack to do with weight-training. It's steroids. Steroids—like pretty much all drugs—are freely available in the American prison system, and trust me, they are very widely used. A lot of guys who come inside want to get huge and intimidating pretty damn quick, and the drugs combined with gym work gets them there.

But there's a drawback to the steroids. Steroids mimic your body's own muscle-building hormone, testosterone. Your body is intelligent. When you dump a load of stuff that's either testosterone (or a lot like it) into your system, your body figures that it doesn't need to make any of its own testosterone any more. To save energy, your body starts shutting down its own production. (Testosterone is made by the testicles—hence their similar names. This is why the balls of steroid users shrivel up. Their testicles slowly stop working.) This isn't a problem while you're taking steroids—except for the shrunken balls thing—but it is a *big* problem when prisoners stop taking steroids, usually when they get back to the outside world. Perhaps they don't have access to the drugs on the outside, or perhaps they just get sick from taking the steroids, but everyone has to stop eventually. And when they do, their body has no testosterone for a looooong time. This basically means that ex-steroid users rapidly lose all the muscle they built on the drugs, and then some. Due to lack of male hormone, they often become fat and sluggish too. I discuss this effect in more depth starting on page 235.

So much for gyms making guys intimidating muscle monsters for when they get outside. But people see the freaky guys working out in prisons and totally miss the bigger picture.

MYTH #4

There's nothing to do in prison but lift heavy weights all day, every day.

No wonder prisoners get huge and strong.

Another untruth. In all correctional institutes—with weight pits or not—recreation time is strictly limited. Where prison gyms do exist, access to those gyms is limited as well and is by no means automatic. Often cons have to fill out prison forms to be allowed time-slots to use the gymnasium and these periods are restricted to two per week (or less where demand is high). Sure, in *some* facilities, prisoners can spend a substantial amount of time during the day, nearly every day, working in the weights pit of the yard. But does this make inmates stronger? Nope.

What many novices and non-athletes fail to understand about heavy free weights work is the enormous toll it takes on the body. Barbell work wears down the joints (a type of damage scientists call *microtrauma*), inflaming the soft tissue and, over time, whittling down the more delicate structures like the shoulders, knees, elbows, lower back and wrists. Joint pain and muscular injury are constant companions of serious weight-trainers. Perhaps more gravely, heavy barbell and dumbbell work really puts a lot of stress on the hormonal system; the adrenal and endocrine glands in particular. This kind of training releases catabolic stress hormones like *cortisol* into the body, hormones that break down tissues and literally eat away the body from the inside if they are allowed to build up due to excessive training.

This is why I laugh when people say that long daily weights workouts will build up convicts. Just the opposite...it'll wear them down! If most guys—even people with natural athletic gifts—tried working out this way, they'd end up sick and injured. Some guys can stand it, but only if they've got a long history of training before they get to jail, and even then weight-training every day won't make them progress much in size and strength on such a brutal regimen. Only steroids can do that for them.

So why is it that in some institutions guys like to hang around the weights pit lifting whenever they can, if it doesn't do much for them? The answer: *status*. Many gang members and hard-cases are desperately insecure and vulnerable inside, and want to cultivate a dangerous, macho image very badly. You'll find them in the weights pit come recreation period, every chance they get.

Typical prison weights programs

The above myths are unbelievably prevalent amongst people on the outside—and even some green guys on the inside, who don't know much about training. These myths will probably still be alive and kicking long after I'm dead and gone. All the same, I still try to dispel them wherever I can. I'm all about old school calisthenics, baby! But despite my stance on the matter, it is true that a lot of guys on the outside have asked me about the weight-training routines of convicts. There seems to be an interest.

I have picked up weights a few times—I even entered a national prison powerlifting meet, on a bet (I came third). Although weights were never my thing, I've witnessed thousands of weight-training sessions done in the yards of half-a-dozen major prisons. I've talked to a lot of big guys who were really into it, as well as some semi-pro bodybuilders and powerlifters who found themselves behind bars. As a result of all this I can give you some of the inside dirt on the kind of training routines generally done in prison gyms.

In prisons you find a wide range of individuals, all with different backgrounds and at differing levels of athletic development. For this reason, you will find that individual inmates follow distinctly different types of training routines. Despite this, there do seem to be a few training guidelines the bigger guys seem to follow—the guys who manage to maintain the most mass and strength over the longest periods inside.

The Prison King

Certain exercises are favored over others, but bench press is king. If you want respect in the weights pit, it's largely based on how much you can bench. As I mentioned above, usually there are three barbell weights available; 135lbs, 225lbs and 315lbs. That 315lbs bar is a symbol in a lot of prisons; it's seen as pretty iconic—the symbol of true strength. In more than one prison, the big ol' 315lbs barbell has its own nickname. When I was in SQ, they called it the *Big Daddy*. The big lifters are always visible in the weights pit, so it's easy to assume that all prisoners are huge and strong. But it's not true. Not every convict is interested in working out, and of those who do only a handful are head and shoulders above the average guy on the street. As a rule of thumb, I'd say about 40% of the prison population can usually handle 135lbs for at least one rep, and perhaps 5% of guys can bench 225lbs. It's difficult to estimate how many men can bench 315lbs for reps, but it's not many. Given the whole prison population it's certainly much less than 1%. Those who can bench the Big Daddy get a lot of respect in the joint.

Because the perception of strength is so important inside, "forced reps" are a commonly used technique. A "forced rep" is supposed to occur at the end of the set, when exhausted muscles can't push the weight any more, and your partner grabs the bar just to guide its path, taking a few pounds of pressure off so you can complete the set safely. In reality forced reps are totally abused in prison workouts. This can be seen on a lot of exercises, but especially the bench press. You see guys trying to press way more weight than they can handle alone; the bar only moves because a friend (sometimes two people!) are lifting the bar to make their buddy appear mega strong. I call these "fake reps", not "forced reps". Afterwards the guys giving the assist make a big deal about saying stuff like "hey, I barely touched it! It was all you!" and other back slapping bull. It's total nonsense nine times out of ten. Often the guys helping are straining more than the guy on the bench. But to be fair this is largely because there are usually only the big three big barbells in many prisons and it's unlikely that a lifter's strength level will perfectly match one of these three.

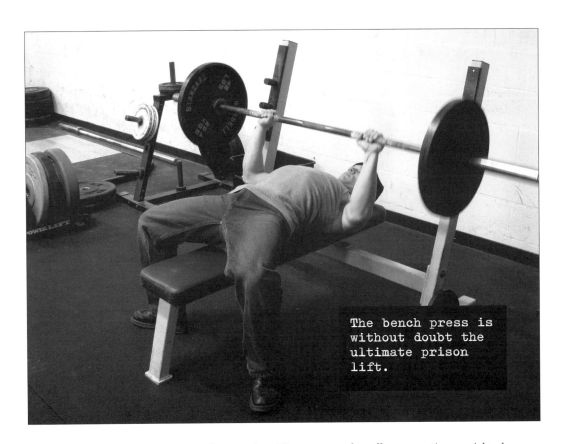

The bench press is without doubt the ultimate prison lift.

   The next favorite exercise amongst the top prison lifters seems to be pullups; sometimes weighted, sometimes not. You might expect curls to come second, as they do in the outside world; but there's an important reason why prison guys do pullups—it's seen as a "must do" exercise to improve the bench press. This might sound strange, since the bench press is a chest/triceps movement, with pullups hitting the back and biceps, but the reason has to do with prison gyms. Most prison gyms don't have the padded metal benches you see in commercial gyms. These are expensive and can be picked up and thrown. For this reason, the majority of prison benches over the past two decades have been made from concrete cinderblocks, cemented together. Just *lying* on these prison benches can be hard on the spine—imagine what it feels like while you're benching 225lbs of iron! This is why pullups are so popular. Pullups hit the lats and add beef to the muscles of the midback. More muscle on your back essentially acts as a cushion against the mercilessly hard benches when you're pressing, protecting your spine. If you don't have a thick, muscular back, you can forget about doing heavy bench presses on prison benches.

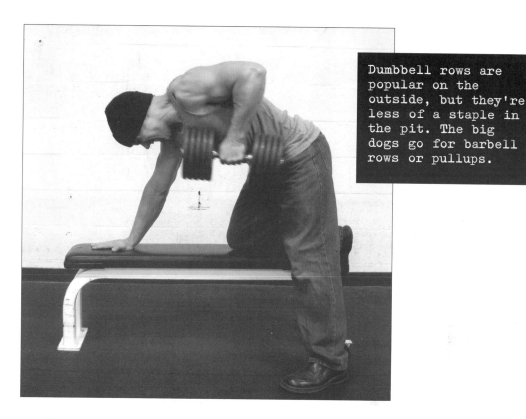

Dumbbell rows are popular on the outside, but they're less of a staple in the pit. The big dogs go for barbell rows or pullups.

Pullups tend to favor guys at lighter bodyweights. Because of this, even some of the really strong power-lifters have trouble due to their bulky bodies. Fat guys don't have a chance. For those lifters who can't do pullups, barbell rows are popular for back training. Since the back is bigger and stronger than the chest, *in theory* a trained athlete should be able to row more than he can bench press. This isn't always true, however. More guys are able to row the Big Daddy than can bench press it, but this is only because while rowing you can really cheat the weight up. Another favorite for the back is reverse grip rows, where the trainee uses a curl grip rather than an overhand grip on the bar. The guys I've spoken to believe it's a better exercise for building the lats than conventional rowing. I don't know if this is true though.

The obsession with arms

After the bench press, the next obsession in the prison weights pit tends to be big arms. Most convicts seem to spend half their gym time training their guns. They love 'em! In reality, the arms are one of the weak-est areas of the body; they have very little horsepower compared to the real muscle engines of the legs, hips, back and chest. But because they are usually the most visible muscle group, arms are a very apparent signi-fier of all-over musculature and fitness. A lot of this has to do with the psychology of intimidation. Big arms to an inmate are like tusks to a bull elephant—an important image of strength and masculinity. Guys hike up their sleeves to the shoulders, and wear T-shirts and tank tops wherever they can. There's a real culture of arms in the joint. One trick I've seen a lot of guys use is to pump up their arms in their cells before the rec-reation period, with a couple of sets of rapid close pushups. This forces all the blood into their arm muscles, temporarily making them look much larger and more vascular—and more impressive to the other inmates.

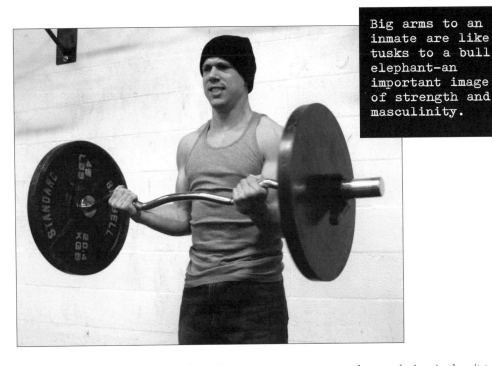

This need to look bigger, pumped up—is a major reason guys spend so much time in the pit training their arms. Supersets are popular—biceps exercises immediately followed by triceps exercises, repeated over and over. Supersets are common in prison gyms because they are probably the best way that exists to quickly engorge the arms with blood. This endless pumping up doesn't make lifters bigger or stronger in the long-term, it only makes the arms *appear* bigger while they're doing it, but that doesn't matter. It's an image thing. As any heavy duty bodybuilder will tell you, endlessly filling your arms up with blood will not make them grow—only short, sharp sessions with progressively heavier weights will make you grow. Just repeatedly filling your arms with blood, for very little in the way of long-term training results, may all sound vain and pointless, but remember that prisons are dangerous places. Reputation and your perceived place in the prison hierarchy are at least as important as genuine athletic ability. If the guy next to you in the yard has big guns, you have to pump yours up until they are bigger. It's an all-out arms race!

Supersets are often done with a relatively light weight. This is so that the arm workout (and the pump) can be prolonged. Depending on recovery levels and what day of the week it is, the guys who favor supersets will begin their time in the pit with straight sets of some heavier arm exercises. This is usually straight bar curls with 135lbs. That's quite a lot to curl, so expect to see a lot of cheating from the smaller guys. Only the real big dogs even *attempt* to curl 225lbs, and even here you'll see plenty of "forced reps" and "fake reps". As well as the big three barbells, some of the better-equipped gyms also have a few lighter cambered bars. These are useful for curling, as well as doing triceps presses when the 135lbs bar is just too heavy. Another common sight is guys doing towel work on arms day. This involves the trainee pulling or pushing on a towel to do an exercise, whilst his buddy holds onto the other end, applying resistance. Sometimes a thick old rope is used instead, where this is available (which is not very often due to the suicide risk). Various exercises can be done this way; curls, reverse curls, front raises, and French presses being the most common. Usually the two-arm exercises are preferred, but I've seen guys doing one-arm variations on these also. Towel or rope work is popular because the resistance can be tailored perfectly to allow the pump to be maintained—enough to pump up, but not too heavy that the workout starts to falter before the end of the rec period.

Some of the attention to arm training is functional however. In order to be able to ace huge bench presses, strong triceps or "back arms" are required. This means that some of the more serious powerlifters eschew the supersets style of training in favor of slower paced sets built around low reps with heavy iron. The exercise the really strong guys love for powerful tris is known by the sinister name "skullcrushers". Lifters do skullcrushers by lying back on a bench with the bar held up with arms locked or slightly bent. Using pure arm power, the forearms are bent back until the bar touches the forehead. The upper arms shouldn't move—only the forearms. This isolates the triceps muscles and places a massive amount of stress on the elbows. A guy has to be *hugely* strong to do skullcrushers with the 135lbs bar. I've heard legends of guys who can do this exercise with 225lbs but I've never seen it myself. The powerlifters inside do a lot of heavy triceps lifting as ancillary work for the bench press and their arms are cock diesel as a result. If you ask a guy to show you his muscles, most guys will roll up their sleeve and flex their biceps. In fact, the triceps are a far bigger, more powerful muscle than the biceps. Most guys in the weights pit spend hours pumping up their biceps in a vain attempt to get big arms, but remember the triceps muscle at the back of the arm makes up about two thirds of the size of the upper arm. There are lessons here for all bodybuilders.

Boulder shoulders

In classic bodybuilding, broad shoulders are the hallmark of a quality physique; combined with a lean waist, they create the illusion of perfect mass, the Holy Grail of aesthetics. But in prisons shoulder training tends to be little more than an afterthought following arm training. Preferred exercises seem to be upright rows, standing military presses, cleans and presses, seated presses, standing shrugs and the press-behind-neck, in that order. Upright rows are the favorite, because you can use momentum and cheat—this means that a lot of guys can handle the 135lbs bar for reps. The bigger and stronger the lifter, the more they seem to prefer seated presses. This might be for reasons of exercise technique, or it might just be because it's harder than the cheating upright row and only the strong guys can handle the heavier weights on this lift.

Lower body lifts

Two big exercises are favored for legs; barbell squats and deadlifts. Both exercises are done in powerlifting form; meaning that the squats are done to approximately parallel, and the deadlifts are full-range, bent-legged style. Leg training is nowhere near as popular as upper body work. A lot of guys will work upper body six or even seven days a week; squats only get a few sets as an appendix lift, usually no more than one day a week. Oddly—despite the fact that the average lifter can handle more weight on the deadlift than the squat—squats are way more popular than deadlifts.

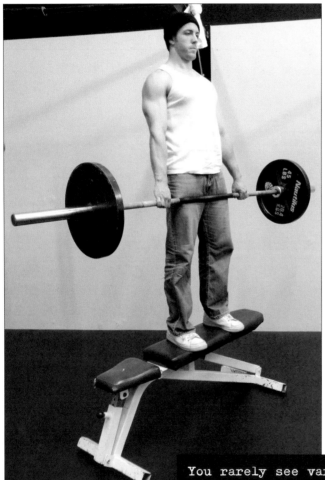

Virtually all hardcore gyms have power racks to aid squatting. There aren't many of these in prison gyms, although there are a few free standing squat racks chained together so it's harder to use them as cudgels. In many places even these are missing, and lifters have to lift the bar off the racks that form part of the bench used for bench pressing. Bench press racks aren't really designed for this purpose, and the big guys have to practically squash themselves under the bar to lever it up on the back of their necks. Ouch. Maybe this explains why squats aren't so popular as on the outside.

You rarely see variations like Romanian deadlifts or stretch deadlifts in jail. They require more coordinated technique, and less weight. Behind bars you're more likely to see variations that allow for *less* technique and *more* weight—like partials off the bench press rack, if there is one.

Abs usually get worked sporadically—often in-between upper body work to stretch the session out longer. They tend to get worked with knee raises and leg raises done from the chinning bar, although some prison gyms have Roman chairs for sit-ups. I've also seen tag team style ab training, where one guy stands on another's feet so he can do sit-ups, then they switch ends. Abs get moderately high reps, and don't seem to be worked out all that hard. On the outside, ab work is important to get that six-pack the ladies love. In prison, a rippling midsection isn't that much of a priority—unless you are someone's twink.

Calf training is an important part of bodybuilding—certainly competitive bodybuilding—because onstage a bodybuilder is judged as much by his weak areas as his strong ones. But in the joint I've seen exactly *three* people train calves in the weights pit over a period of about two decades. Two of those individuals were nationally-ranked bodybuilders trying to hold onto as much of their physiques as possible during their stints inside. On all three of these occasions, the exercise of choice was barbell calf raises for high reps. A reader who knows bodybuilding might assume that given the scarcity of calf machines and dumbbells in most prisons, the obvious choice for calf training would probably be donkey calf raises—where the trainee bends over and has someone straddle his back as he does calf raises off a block.

This would not be a wise choice for an exercise in a prison environment.

Lights out!

There are a lot of great athletes in prisons all over the US. These guys are big, and they are intimidating. But although these "big dogs" are highly visible, they actually only make up a relatively small group of the prison population. And of those guys who are strong or in great shape, hardly any of them got that way from pumping iron in jail. They were part of that culture of size and intimidation before they even got inside. Steroid use is rampant in jails—as is all drug use—but the effects steroids have on lifters is transient and usually negative in the long run.

There's a small group of guys who have got monstrously strong and reached the pinnacle of fitness while in prison—some even becoming world record holders. These are the guys who have been trained properly, not in the weights pit, but in traditional, old school calisthenics. With the correct instruction, you can learn these skills just as easily on the outside as you can in prison.

If you've never been inside, it's easy to be intimidated by the stereotype of the macho, beefed-up convict. A lot of this is smoke and mirrors. I'm a big believer in the philosophy of DTA—Don't Trust Anybody—but this applies on the *outside* just as much as in jail. There's one famous theory that says that guys in prison tend to have more testosterone than the average guy on the street—this is what makes men more aggressive and more likely to commit crimes, particularly violent crimes. I think this is bull. Your average guy buying stocks on Wall Street or sweeping up trash has as much testosterone as the regular guy in the joint. The difference between these guys is the environment they've been raised in and the decisions they make, not some chemical coursing through their veins. That's my ten cents worth. But I'm no psychologist; just someone who's spent more time in jails than walking the streets. In my experience there are as many sharks and predators on the outside as the inside. The ones on the outside are just not dumb enough to get caught.

ACKNOWLEDGEMENTS

I'd like to thank John Du Cane, who had the guts to go out on a limb and think about publishing the jottings of a weird old warhorse. A million thanks for all your advice, guidance and support. You're the best, Boss.

My thanks also go to Pavel Tsatsouline. Without the Evil Russian's pioneering efforts to bring true bodyweight work into the public consciousness, I'm not sure this book would've happened. When I first wrote *Convict Conditioning 2*, I very nearly included advanced methods of bodyweight strength specialization. In the end, I didn't. I realized that they would be redundant... because there's no way I could write anything better than Pavel's classic book *The Naked Warrior*. Athletes who want to take their training to the next level should all pick up this masterwork. Today, son!.

I owe a huge gratitude to Brooks Kubik for penning the foreword to this book. Brooks is a mentor and hero to many thousands of men and women in the world of strength training, and it's an unbelievable honor to have him write something to introduce this volume. His book *Dinosaur Bodyweight Training* should be considered the *bible* of strength calisthenics. Want to know how a guy with a 400 lbs bench press does his pushups? Go to *www.brookskubik.com* and demand that he re-issues this classic.

I want to send out my genuine and lasting thanks to all the athletes who modeled for this book. These men are my bodyweight brothers, and it's been a real honor to include some of the finest bodyweight athletes of this generation and the next.

The incredible Jim Bathurst—the model who made the first book such a sensation—has returned for some material in this sequel. Jim is amazing, and I wanted to use him a lot more for this book, but he was just too busy with his *Beastskills* project and training. That's no bad thing. I was lucky as hell to get him while I could. Thanks bro.

What an experience it has been working with Max Shank! It's not often you can honestly call an athlete a *physical genius.* John Grimek is one example of such a phenomenon. Max is another. He can do it all; heavy lifting, bodyweight, acrobatics. You did your first ever press flag on what? Your second attempt?! Jeez, you're making the rest of us look bad, kid. You've got some awesome ideas, and I look forwards to working with you in the future.

The stars must've been aligned when we got the chance to shoot with Al Kavadlo. Al is one of the greatest personal trainers in the whole world—legit. The man has forgotten more about bodyweight training than most coaches will ever know. More than just a brilliant athlete, Al was the consultant for the flag section of this book. His ideas have made *Convict Conditioning 2* far better than it could've been without him. His book *We're Working Out! A Zen Approach to Everyday Fitness* is a phenomenal catalog of techniques, ideas and tactics for achieving peak physical ability. *Possibly the best book on fitness ever—* if you enjoyed my book, go buy his. You won't regret it.

Al's brother, Danny Kavadlo, was kind enough to donate some flag shots for this book. He's on the cover, too! What do I think of this guy? Let's just say that when people ask me to point them to a personal trainer who can teach them authentic old school calisthenics, I point them straight to Danny. I was really hoping to show you what this kid could do in the pages of this book, but our schedules were out of whack, so it didn't happen. If you are in NYC and need a trainer, visit the dude's site: *www.dannythetrainer.com.*

This book, like its forerunner, is only made possible thanks to the editing contributions of Master RKC, Brett Jones. I said about the last book that anything that looks clever and true came from Brett, and the screw-ups come from me...and this is twice as true in this book! Brett can be found at *www.appliedstrength.com.*

A special thanks goes to the real creative power behind this book: the amazing Big D, Derek Brigham. To quote John Du Cane; "that man is gold." John—as usual, you are right on the money. Thanks for your endless patience and deciation, D. Check out Derek's site: *www.dbrigham.com.*

It's been a real honor to be able to include John Morrow in this book (page 276). John is the unsung hero of American calisthenics. While he's still out there breaking records and pushing the limits of human ability, the world can't be all that bad. John's still teaching kung fu to students who don't know how lucky they are. Check his site: *www.morrowsacademy.com.*

My thanks go out to the mighty Clarence Bass, who was kind enough to donate a photo to this project (page 278). Clarence is one of the most intelligent fitness writers of any generation. His website, *www.cbass.com,* is a treasure trove of useful information for the open-minded athlete.
The photographer was Pat Berrett.

Some of the photos in *Convict Conditioning 2* were shot in and around Balance Gym, which is located in the Kalorama neighborhood of Washington DC.
Balance gym is a phenomenal facility, and I'm incredibly grateful for the team's help. Thanks guys!

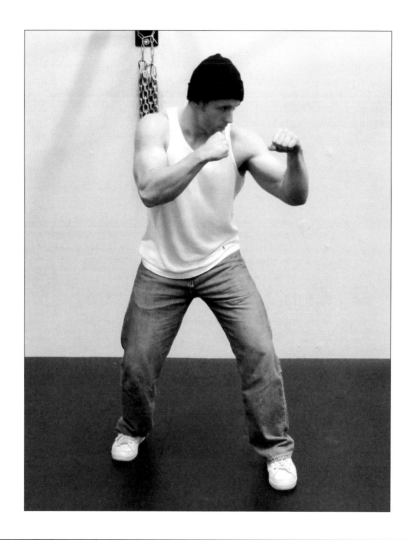

The main athlete featured in this book is Max Shank. Max is a strength coach, RKC instructor, and corrective exercise specialist based in Encinitas, CA. He uses a wide variety of tools to build an elite level of strength and conditioning, everything from kettlebells to natural stones at the beach. As well as being a highly talented bodyweight athlete, Max is also a martial artist who has competed in the Highland Games. Max has also received an Official Commendation from the United States Marine Corps for services rendered in the course of enhancing the athletic readiness of the 1st Anglico at Camp Pendleton. Max is the owner of Ambition Athletics and can be reached through his website at: *www. ambitionathletics.com*. Go visit the guy!

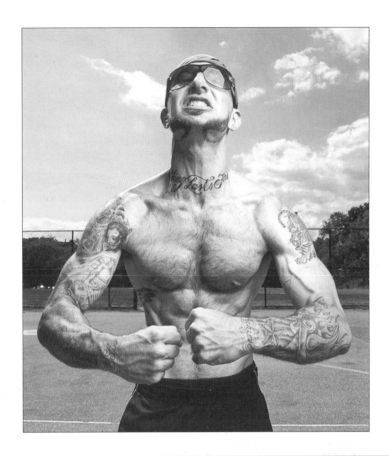

Al Kavadlo, CSCS is one of New York City's most passionate and successful personal trainers. A fixture in the ever changing fitness scene, Al has worked with all types of clients, including athletes, models and even an Olympic medalist. Al is recognized worldwide for his amazing bodyweight feats of strength, and his blog (*www.AlKavadlo. com*) has become one of the most popular online resources for information about strength training and calisthenics. Al also shares his unique perspective and exercise philosophy in his book, *We're Working Out! A Zen Approach to Everyday Fitness.*

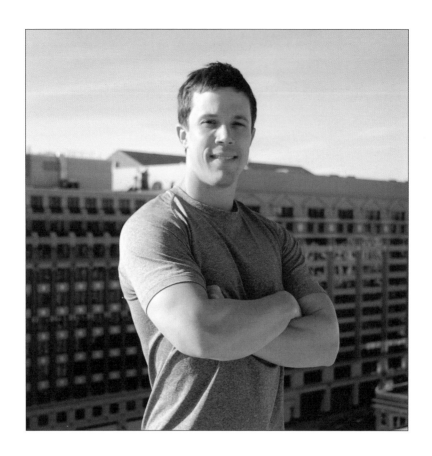

Many of the photos in this book feature the award-winning athlete Jim Bathurst. Jim has been studying acrobatics for well over a decade. He has taken that passion and experience and started *BeastSkills.com*, a website that teaches bodyweight feats of strength. BeastSkills.com has been well-received by the fitness community and Jim has been invited to host seminars internationally. He holds a CSCS from the NSCA, is a CrossFit Level 1 Trainer, and currently resides in Washington DC, where he works as a personal trainer.

PHOTO CREDITS

I'm incredibly grateful to Justin P for his donation of the one-arm fingertip pushups and handstand fingertip pushups in chapter five. He can be found at his site *www. thebodyweightfiles.blogspot.com*. This brother understands what true bodyweight training is about. If we're lucky, this guy is the future of fitness.

The Indian pole and rope images came courtesy of *www.mallkhambindia.com*. Thank you.

The perfect press flag on page 68 was donated by the amazing bodyweight master Vassili. This guy will make it really big one day—watch this space. Check his vids at: *www.youtube.com/user/VassTheSupersaiyan*. You the man, Vass!

The twisting flag was donated by phenomenal parkour athlete Anthony Ruiz. Bro, you are as generous as you are talented.

The shots of Danny Kavadlo were taken by Al Kavadlo, except the awesome flag shot in Mexico (the one over the lawn on page 93) which was taken by Danny's wife Jennifer. It's one of the best shots in the book. Thank you!

Most of the fantastic photos of Al Kavadlo were taken by the highly talented photographer Colleen Leung. Find her at *www.ColleenLeung.com*. I'm grateful for your eye, Colleen.

Big thanks to Tamar Kaye for the amazing pic of the Kavadlo men on page 99. Wow!.

The astonishing images of inverse neck bridges were kindly given to me by my pal Plato— one of this world's true Renaissance men. Hope you like the chapter on diet, Plato. *www.testosteroneprophet.com*.

The image of the cat stretching in chapter twelve is attributed to Hisashi of Japan.

The image of the pretty ballet dancer at the barre in chapter thirteen is attributed to Lambtron.

The truly awe-inspiring kick in chapter thirteen was kindly donated by Paul at *elasticsteel.com*. Paul is world famous for his vast knowledge on flexibility training. You wanna learn to kick like that? Go visit the site.

The advanced yoga position in chapter fourteen was donated by Dr Ronald Steiner. Dr Steiner is the perfect example of a man who has taken a bodyweight discipline beyond the physical level and into the spiritual level. A fascinating man—and many of our ideas overlap, believe it or not. If you are interested in finding out more about real yoga, visit his site at: *www.ashtangayoga.info.*

The ubercool image of Ric Drasin's many injuries is used with special permission from The Equalizer himself. I wouldn't have included it otherwise—don't wanna wind up on the wrong end of a sunset flip! Go pick up some words of wisdom from the great man at ricdrasin.com and *ricscorner.com.*

The image of the contortionist in chapter seventeen is attributed to Keith Allison of Baltimore, US.

The image of the bull in chapter nineteen is attributed to *Forum concoursvaches.fr.*

The image of meds in chapter twenty is attributed to Tom Varco.

The image of San Quentin in chapter twenty is attributed to Staunited.

Big thanks to Andy E for the donation of his beefy forearms.

Several images in this book were created by the US Government. All public domain images are used with my gratitude.

INDEX

F

Failure, training to point of, 19, 54, 57, 142, 185, 191

False grip, 9. *See also* Hang/Hanging grip

Finger holds, 41–43

Fingertip pushups, 47–55

    as basic movement/skill, 6, 47, 57

    before grip work, 17, 51, 58

    correct positioning for, 49, 50

    devices/gadgets for, 48

    effectiveness of, 6, 48, 55

    and progressive strength, 51–52

    and sample workout, 59

    series for, 53

    sets/reps for, 51, 54, 58, 59, 59

    variations of, 52, 54

    warming up for, 52, 58

Flag, 65–69

    effectiveness of, 65–66

    origins of, 67

    types/variations of, 65, 68–69, 71–88. *See also* Clutch flag; Press flag

Flexibility. *See also* Tension-Flexibility

    and calisthenics, 164

    vs. mobility, 164

    modern approach to training, 149, 155

    and neck, 125–127

    vs. relaxation, 149–151

    and strength, 163, 164, 165

Fluid intake, 242–243

Foot exercises, 133. *See also* Calves

Forced reps, 293–294

Forearms, 3.5–4, 7. *See also* Hands/Forearms

Front bridges. *See also* Neck

    effectiveness of, 114–115

    flexibility stages for, 125–127

    and range of motion, 128–129

    strength needed for, 117, 127

    versions of, 120–124

Full twist hold, 218

Functional triad, 176–181

    and active stretching, 179–180

    anatomy of, 176, 181

    elements/nature of, 175–177

    and joint training, 176–177

G

Goal setting, in training, 279

"Greek ideal," for physique, 71

Grip-and-switch, 60, 61

Grip work, 39–45. *See also* Hang/Hanging grip

H

Half twist hold, 216

Hands/Forearms, 1–13

    anatomy of, 3, 4–5, 7, 41, 47–48

    devices/gadgets for training, 45, 58

    modern approach to training, 3, 7, 8

    and overall strength, 1, 3, 61

    sample workout for, 58–59

    and strength athletes, 2

    training to develop, 5–6, 8–13, 20–38, 39–45, 57–55, 59–61

Hang/Hanging grip, 8–13. *See also* Grip work

    as basic movement/skill, 4–5, 6, 47, 57

    effectiveness of, 11–12

    grip positions for, 8–11

Hang progression, 15–38

    difficulty of, 38

    eight steps in, 20–37. *See also* specific steps

    injury prevention in, 19

    and sample workout, 59

    sets/times for, 59

    techniques for, 15–17

    tips for, 17–19

Hanging, as basic physical movement/skill, 5, 61–62

Hanging leg raises, vs. L-holds, 200

Head bridge hold, 192

Heat, as injury treatment, 261–262, 264

Hips

    injuries of, 199, 209, 219

    strength of, 199, 207, 211

    training to develop, 207, 211

Hook grip, 9. *See also* Hang/Hanging grip

Horizontal hang, 20–21, 36. *See also* Hang progression

Horizontal lever, 65. *See also* Flag

Horizontal press flag, 94. *See also* Press flag

Horizontal split clutch, 83, 87. *See also* Clutch flag

Horizontal tuck clutch, 82, 87. *See also* Clutch flag

I

Ice, for treating injury, 257

Illness, and training, 256. *See also* Injury/Injuries

Index finger pullups, 60, 61

Inferiority, as training demon, 274

Inflammation/Swelling, as response to injury, 256, 260, 261–262, 264

Injury/Injuries, 253–264

    of back, 189–190, 207, 209, 219

    from barbells, 159, 253, 292

    and calisthenics, xi, 153, 275

    of feet/ankles/shins, 132, 144

    and fingertip pushups, 49

    and hang progression, 19

    healing from, 254–264

    heat as treatment for, 261–262, 264

    of hips, 199, 207, 219

    immediate treatment of, 256–257, 264

    inevitability of, 253, 270, 275

    and joints, xi–xii, 148, 153, 177

    learning from, 263, 264

    from machine training, 159, 212, 253, 257

    and mindset, 262–263, 264. *See also* Attitude

    and modern approach to training, 211

    and relaxation/flexibility, 157, 158–159

    of neck, 117

    prevention of, xi–xii, 254–256, 264

    progression after, 262, 264

    of shoulders, 197, 211, 219

    and stretching, 157, 170, 172, 260

    as training demon, 275–276

    training throughout, 258–259, 264

Intensity variables, 134Iron Gauntlet, 59–61

Isometric exercise/techniques

    and bridges/bridging, 190

    clutch flag as, 73

    counting seconds for, 17

    definition of, 6

J

Japanese martial arts, 199–200

Joint circling, 169

Joints, 148–161

    and active stretching, 168–171, 172

    anatomy of, 177, 178

    and calisthenics, 153–155, 161

    and flexibility, 165

    as focus of training, xi–xii, 148

    injuries of/pain from, xi–xii, 148, 153, 157, 170, 172, 177

    modern approach to training, 153–155

    and muscle building, 148

    and tension-flexibility, 149–153, 159. *See also* Tension-Flexibility

    training to develop, 159, 160, 165, 169, 175–181, 211–221

Jones, Arthur, 132

Jumping, as explosive calf training, 143

Kick press, 102, 108. *See also* Press flag

Kipping, while hanging, 43

Knee flexion, and calf training, 134, 135. *See also* Calves

K

Kick press, 102, 108. *See also* Press flag

Kipping, while hanging, 43

Knee flexion, and calf training, 134, 135. *See also* Calves

L

L-hold, 199–209

    and abdominal muscles/training, 199–200

    as basic movement of Trifecta, 182, 185, 200, 201

    benefits of, 207

    effectiveness of, 201, 207

    vs. hanging leg raises, 200

    progression for, 201–206

Lateral chain, 63–69

    anatomy of, 66, 176, 181

    and functional triad, 176

    and joint training, 176–177

    modern approach to training, 63

    principles for training, 63

    purpose of training, 64–65

    and strength 71–72, 110–111

    training to develop, 65–69, 71–88, 89–112, 182, 221

Leg raise hold. *See* L-hold

Leg raises, for developing abdomen/lateral chain, 65, 110. *See also* L-hold

Leverage, and grip work, 41

Lifestyle, 225–236

    and activity level, 228

    and alcohol, 232–233

    and anabolic steroids, 234–236, 291

    and discipline, 226

    and drug use, 233–234

GET Dynamic, Chiselled, Power-Jack Legs and Develop Explosive Lower-Body Strength—With Paul "Coach" Wade's Ultimate

BODYWEIGHT SQUAT COURSE

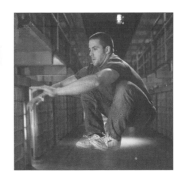

Paul Wade's *Convict Conditioning Ultimate Bodyweight Squat Course* explodes out of the cellblock to teach you in absolute detail how to progress from the ease of a simple shoulderstand squat—to the stunning "1-in-10,000" achievement of the prison-style one-leg squat. Ten progressive steps guide you to bodyweight squat mastery. Do it—and become a Bodyweight Squat Immortal.

This home-study course in ultimate survival strength comes replete with bonus material not available in **Paul Wade's** original **Convict Conditioning** book—and numerous key training tips that refine and expand on the original program.

A heavily and gorgeously-illustrated 80-plus-page manual gives you the entire film script to study at your leisure, with brilliant, precise photographs to remind you of the essential movements you absorbed in the DVD itself.

Paul Wade adds a bonus **Ten Commandments for Perfect Bodyweight Squats**—which is worth the price of admission alone. And there's the additional bonus of **5 major Variant drills** to add explosivity, fun and super-strength to your core practice.

Whatever you are looking for from your bodyweight squats—be it supreme functional strength, monstrous muscle growth or explosive leg power—it's yours for the progressive taking with *Convict Conditioning, Volume 2: The Ultimate Bodyweight Squat Course.*

Why every self-respecting man will be religious about his squats…

Leg training is vital for every athlete. A well-trained, muscular upper body teetering around on skinny stick legs is a joke. Don't be that joke! The mighty squat is the answer to your prayers. Here's why:

- Squats train virtually every muscle in the lower body, from quads and glutes to hips, lower back and even hamstrings.

- Squat deep—as we'll teach you—and you will seriously increase your flexibility and ankle strength.

- All functional power is transmitted through the legs, so without strong, powerful legs you are *nothing*—that goes for running, jumping and combat sports as much as it does for lifting heavy stuff.

Are you failing to build monstrous legs from

squats—because of these mistakes?

Most trainees learn how to squat on two legs, and then make the exercise harder by slapping a barbell across their back. In prison, this way of adding strength wasn't always available, so cell trainees developed ways of progressing using only bodyweight versus gravity. The best way to do this is to learn how to squat all the way down to the ground and back up on just one leg.

Not everybody who explores prison training will have the dedication and drive to achieve strength feats like the one-arm pullup, but the legs are much stronger than the arms. If you put in the time and work hard, the one-leg squat will be within the reach of almost every athlete who pays their dues.

But the one-leg squat still requires very powerful muscles and tendons, so you don't want to jump into one-leg squatting right away. You need to build the joint strength and muscle to safely attempt this great exercise. Discover how to do that safely, using ten steps, ten progressively harder squat exercises.

In the strength game, fools rush in where

angels fear to tread

The wise old Chinese man shouted to his rickshaw driver: "Slow down, young man, I'm in a hurry!" If ever a warning needed to be shouted to our nation of compulsive strength-addicts, this would be it. You see them everywhere: the halt, the lame, the jacked-up, the torn, the pain-ridden—the former glory-seekers who have been reduced to sad husks of their former selves by rushing helter-skelter into heavy lifting without having first built a firm foundation.

Paul Wade reveals the ten key points of perfect squat form. The aspects of proper form apply to all your squats, and they'll not only unlock the muscle and power-building potential of each rep you do, but they'll also keep you as safe as you can be.

Bodyweight training is all about improving strength and health, not building up a list of injuries or aches and pains. They are so fundamental, we call them the Ten Commandments of good squat form.

Obey the Ten Commandments, follow the brilliantly laid out progressions religiously and you simply CANNOT fail to get stronger and stronger and stronger and stronger and stronger—surely, safely and for as long as you live…

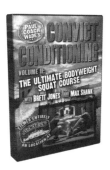

Convict Conditioning
Volume 2: The Ultimate Bodyweight Squat Course
By Paul "Coach" Wade featuring Brett Jones and Max Shank

#DV084 $29.95 DVD 59 minutes

COMPLEX MADE SIMPLE

Having read both *Convict Conditioning* and *Convict Conditioning 2*, the complementary DVD series is an excellent translation of the big six movement progressions into a simple to follow DVD. The demonstration of movement progression through the 10 levels is well described and easy to follow.

As a Physical Therapist it is a very useful way to teach safe progressions to patients/clients and other professionals.

NAVY SEAL ON THE ROAD

"My whole team uses it. We can work out effectively anywhere and I mean anywhere!"
—**Tyler Archer, Navy**

I have already used Volume I (the push up progression) to teach high school strength coaches how to safely progress athletes with pressing activity and look forward to using volume 2 with these same coaches. I think anyone who studies movement realizes very few athletes can properly squat with two legs, let alone one.

You will not find an easier way to teach the squat. Well done again Paul. Look forward to the rest of the series."
—**Andrew Marchesi PT/MPT, FAFS, Scottsdale, AZ**

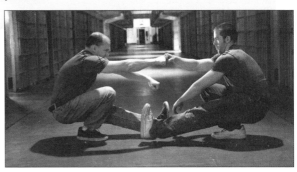

Demonic Abs Are a Man's Best Friend— Discover How to Seize a Six-Pack from Hell and OWN the World…

LEG RAISES

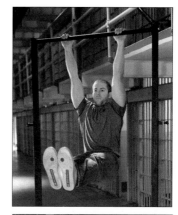

Paul Wade's *Convict Conditioning 3, Leg Raises: Six Pack from Hell* teaches you in absolute detail how to progress from the ease of a simple Knee Tuck—to the magnificent, "1-in-1,000" achievement of the Hanging Straight Leg Raise. Ten progressive steps guide you to inevitable mastery of this ultimate abs exercise. Do it, seize the knowledge—but beware—the Gods will be jealous!

This home-study course in ultimate survival strength comes replete with bonus material not available in **Paul Wade's** original *Convict Conditioning* book—and numerous key training tips that refine and expand on the original program.

Prowl through the heavily and gorgeously-illustrated 80-plus-page manual and devour the entire film script at your animal leisure. Digest the brilliant, precise photographs and reinforce the raw benefits you absorbed from the DVD.

Paul Wade adds a bonus **Ten Commandments for Perfect Bodyweight Squats**—which is worth the price of admission alone. And there's the additional bonus of **4 major Variant drills** to add explosivity, fun and super-strength to your core practice.

Whatever you are looking for when murdering your abs—be it a fist-breaking, rock-like shield of impenetrable muscle, an uglier-is-more-beautiful set of rippling abdominal ridges, or a monstrous injection of lifting power—it's yours for the progressive taking with *Convict Conditioning, Volume 3, Leg Raises: Six Pack from Hell*

Prison-style midsection training—for an all show AND all go physique

When convicts train their waists, they want real, noticeable results—and by "results" we don't mean that they want cute, tight little defined abs. We mean that they want thick, strong, muscular midsections. They want *functionally* powerful abs and hips they can use for heavy lifting, kicking, and brawling. They want guts so strong from their training that it actually hurts an attacker to punch them in the belly. Prison abs aren't about all show, no go—a prison-built physique has to be all show and all go. Those guys don't just want six-packs—they want six-packs from Hell.

And, for the first time, we're going to show you how these guys get what they want. We're not going to be using sissy machines or easy isolation exercises—we're going straight for the old school secret weapon for gut training; progressive leg raises.

If you want a six-pack from Hell, the first thing you need to do is focus your efforts. If a weightlifter wanted a very thick, powerful chest in a hurry, he wouldn't spread his efforts out over a dozen exercises and perform them gently all day long. No—he'd pick just one exercise, probably the bench press, and just focus on getting stronger and stronger on that lift until he was monstrously strong. When he reached this level, and his pecs were thick slabs of meat, only then would he maybe begin sculpting them with minor exercises and higher reps.

It's no different if you want a mind-blowing midsection. Just pick one exercise that hits all the muscles in the midsection—the hip flexors, the abs, the intercostals, the obliques—then blast it.

And the one exercise we're going to discover is the best midsection exercise known to man, and the most popular amongst soldiers, warriors, martial artists and prison athletes since men started working out—the leg raise.

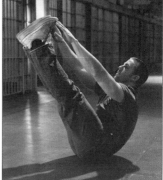

You'll discover ten different leg raise movements, each one a little harder than the last. You'll learn how to get the most out of each of these techniques, each of these ten steps, before moving up to the next step. By the time you get through all ten steps and you're working with the final Master Step of the leg raise series, you'll have a solid, athletic, stomach made of steel, as well as powerful hips and a ribcage armored with dense muscle. You'll have abs that would've made Bruce Lee take notice!

The Ten Commandments You Must Obey to Earn a Real Monster of an Athletic Core

Paul Wade gives you ten key points, the "Ten Commandments" of leg raises, that will take your prison-style core training from just "okay" to absolutely phenomenal. We want the results to be so effective that they'll literally shock you. This kind of accelerated progress can be achieved, but if you want to achieve it you better listen carefully to these ten key pointers you'll discover with the DVD.

Bodyweight mastery is a lot like high-level martial arts. It's more about principles than individual techniques. Really study and absorb these principles, and you'll be on your way to a six-pack from Hell in no time.

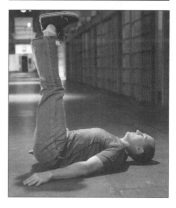

The hanging straight leg raise, performed strictly and for reps, is the Gold Standard of abdominal strength techniques. Once you're at the level where you can throw out sets of twenty to thirty rock solid reps of this exercise, your abs will be thick and strong, but more importantly, they'll be functional—not just a pretty six-pack, but a real monster of an athletic core, which is capable of developing high levels of force.

Hanging will work your serratus and intercostals, making these muscles stand out like fingers, and your obliques and flank muscles will be tight and strong from holding your hips in place. Your lumbar spine will achieve a gymnastic level of flexibility, like fluid steel, and your chances of back pain will be greatly reduced.

The bottom line: If you want to be stronger and more athletic than the next guy, you need the edge that straight leg raises can give you.

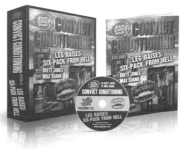

Convict Conditioning
Volume 3: Leg Raises
Six Pack from Hell
By Paul "Coach" Wade featuring Brett Jones and Max Shank

#DV085 $29.95
DVD 57 minutes with full color Companion Manual, 82 pages

Erect Twin Pythons of Coiled Beef Up Your Spine and Develop Extreme, Explosive Resilience— With the Dynamic Power and Flexible Strength of

ADVANCED BRIDGING

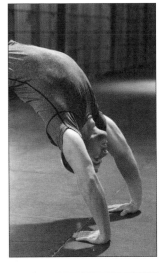

Paul Wade's *Convict Conditioning* system represents the ultimate distillation of hardcore prison body-weight training's most powerful methods. What works was kept. What didn't, was slashed away. When your life is on the line, you're not going to mess with less than the absolute best. Many of these older, very potent solitary training systems have been on the verge of dying, as convicts begin to gain access to weights, and modern "body-building thinking" floods into the prisons. Thanks to Paul Wade, these ultimate strength survival secrets have been saved for posterity. And for you...

Filmed entirely—and so appropriately— on **"The Rock"**, Wade's *Convict Conditioning Volume 4, Advanced Bridging: Forging an Iron Spine* explodes out of the cellblock to teach you in absolute detail how to progress from the relative ease of a Short Bridge—to the stunning, "1-in-1,000" achievement of the Stand-to-Stand Bridge. Ten progressive steps guide you to inevitable mastery of this ultimate exercise for an unbreakable back.

This home-study course in ultimate survival strength comes replete with bonus material not available in **Paul Wade's** original *Convict Conditioning* book—and numerous key training tips that refine and expand on the original program.

Prowl through the heavily and gorgeously-illustrated 80-plus-page manual and devour the entire film script at your animal leisure. Digest the brilliant, precise photographs and reinforce the raw benefits you absorbed from the DVD.

Paul Wade adds a bonus **Ten Commandments for Perfect Bridges**—which is worth the price of admission alone. And there's the additional bonus of **4 major Variant drills** to add explosivity, fun and super-strength to your core practice.

Whatever you are looking for from your pushups—be it supreme functional strength, monstrous muscle growth or explosive upper-body power—it's yours for the progressive taking with *Convict Conditioning Volume 4: Advanced Bridging: Forging an Iron Spine.*

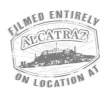

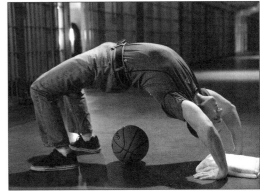

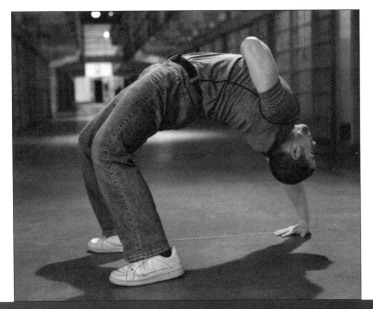

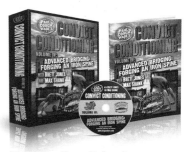

Convict Conditioning
Volume 4: Advanced Bridging: Forging an Iron Spine
By Paul "Coach" Wade featuring Brett Jones and Max Shank

#DV087 $29.95
DVD 59 minutes with full color Companion Manual, 88 pages

Tap into the Dormant Ancestral Power of the Mighty Pullup—to Develop a Massive Upper Back, Steel-Tendon Arms, and Etched Abs Mastering

THE ONE-ARM PULLUP

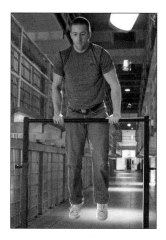

P aul Wade's *Convict Conditioning Volume 5, Maximum Strength: The One-Arm Pullup Series* explodes out of the cellblock to teach you in absolute detail how to progress from the relative ease of a Vertical Pull—to the stunning, "1-in-1,000" achievement of the One-Arm Pull-Up. Ten progressive steps guide you to inevitable mastery of this ultimate exercise for the upper back, steely, bulging biceps and etched abs.

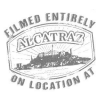

This home-study course in ultimate survival strength comes replete with bonus material not available in Paul Wade's original Convict Conditioning book—and numerous key training tips that refine and expand on the original program.

Filmed entirely—and so appropriately—on "The Rock", Wade's Convict Conditioning Volume 5, Maximum Strength: The One-Arm Pullup Series explodes out of the cellblock to teach you in absolute detail how to progress from the relative ease of a Vertical Pull—to the stunning, "1-in-1,000" achievement of the One-Arm Pullup. Ten progressive steps guide you to inevitable mastery of this ultimate exercise for supreme upper body survival strength.

This home-study course in ultimate survival strength comes replete with bonus material not available in Paul Wade's original Convict Conditioning book—and numerous key training tips that refine and expand on the original program.

Prowl through the heavily and gorgeously-illustrated 88-plus-page manual and devour the entire film script at your animal leisure. Digest the brilliant, precise photographs and reinforce the raw benefits you absorbed from the DVD.

Paul Wade adds a bonus Ten Commandments for Perfect Pullups—which is worth the price of admission alone. And there's the additional bonus of 4 major Variant drills to add explosivity, fun and super-strength to your core practice.

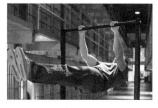

Whatever you are looking for from your pullups—be it agile survival strength, arms of steel, a massive upper back with flaring lats, Popeye Biceps or gape-inducing abs—it's yours for the progressive taking with Convict Conditioning Volume 5, Maximum Strength: The One-Arm Pullup Series.

These exercises have been broken up into a set of stages, which is sometimes called the "ten steps". This is a key feature of the Convict Conditioning system. Without following some kind of structured, progressive approach, it would be impossible for even the most naturally powerful athlete to achieve incredible feats like assisted pullups and one-arm pullups.

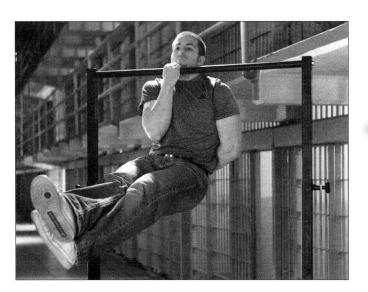

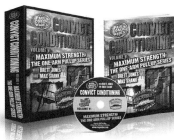

Convict Conditioning
Volume 5: Maximum Strength: The One-Arm Pullup Series
By Paul "Coach" Wade featuring Brett Jones and Max Shank

#DV088 $29.95
DVD 59 minutes with full color Companion Manual, 88 pages

GET a ROCK-Hard, Brutishly Powerful Upper Frame and Achieve Elite-Level Strength— With Paul "Coach" Wade's

PRISON-STYLE PUSHUP PROGRAM

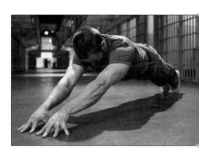

Paul Wade's *Convict Conditioning* system represents the ultimate distillation of hardcore prison bodyweight training's most powerful methods. What works was kept. What didn't, was slashed away. When your life is on the line, you're not going to mess with less than the absolute best. Many of these older, very potent solitary training systems have been on the verge of dying, as convicts begin to gain access to weights, and modern "bodybuilding thinking" floods into the prisons. Thanks to Paul Wade, these ultimate strength survival secrets have been saved for posterity. And for you...

Filmed entirely—and so appropriately— on **"The Rock"**, Wade's *Convict Conditioning Prison Pushup Series* explodes out of the cellblock to teach you in absolute detail how to progress from the ease of a simple wall pushup—to the stunning "1-in-10,000" achievement of the prison-style one-arm pushup. Ten progressive steps guide you to pushup mastery. Do it—and become a Pushup God.

This home-study course in ultimate survival strength comes replete with bonus material not available in **Paul Wade's** original *Convict Conditioning* book—and numerous key training tips that refine and expand on the original program.

A heavily and gorgeously-illustrated 80-plus-page manual gives you the entire film script to study at your leisure, with brilliant, precise photographs to remind you of the essential movements you absorbed in the DVD itself.

Paul Wade adds a bonus **Ten Commandments for Perfect Pushups**—which is worth the price of admission alone. And there's the additional bonus of **5 major Variant drills** to add explosivity, fun and super-strength to your core practice.

Whatever you are looking for from your pushups—be it supreme functional strength, monstrous muscle growth or explosive upper-body power—it's yours for the progressive taking with *Convict Conditioning, Volume 1: The Prison Pushup Series.*

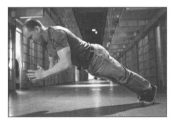

AWESOME RESOURCE FOR COACHES & STRENGTH DEVOTEES

"I am using this manual and DVD not just for my own training, but for the training of my athletes. It shocks and amazes me how varsity high school athletes can NOT perform a solid push up.... not even 1! Getting them to perform a perfect push up requires regressions, progressions, dialing in the little cues that teach them to generate tension and proper body alignment, ALL of which carry over to other exercises.

This manual is an awesome resource for Coaches. It can & should be used to educate those you train as well as shared with your staff. For those who have a love for strength, you will respect all the details given for each and every push up progression and you will use them and apply them.

As a Strength devotee for over 2 decades, I've been through the grinder with free weights and injuries, push ups are something I KNOW I'll be doing for the rest of my life which is why I RESPECT this course so much!

The lay out of this manual and DVD are also BIG time impressive, the old school look and feel fires me up and makes me wanna attack these push ups!"
—Zach Even-Esh, Manasquan, NJ

I RECOMMEND IT

"I fully expected to be disappointed with **Paul Wade's** *Convict Conditioning, Volume I: The Prison Pushup Series*. John Du Cane will tell you: I am not a fan of some of the stuff in these books. It's been said by others that this might be one of the most striking DVDs ever made. It's on location in Alcatraz and the graphics are pretty amazing. So, yes, stunning. This DVD from Wade is stunning and very cool.

The manual that supports the DVD is very helpful as much of the material is done too well in the DVD. Many of us need to take some time looking at the DVD then flipping the manual back and forth to 'get it.'

Once again, there are parts of this DVD and the series that rub me the wrong way. Having said that, I am frankly amazed at the insights of the product here. As a coach, I am better than when I popped the box open. I have a whole set of tools, and the progressions, that I can use tomorrow with my group. That to me is the testimony that people should hear from me: I watched it and I applied it instantly! This one 'gets it.' You can apply what you learn instantly and know where you are going from there. I highly recommend it."
—Dan John, Master RKC, Burlingame, CA

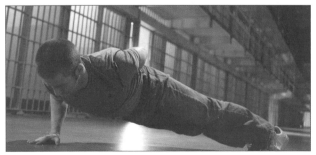

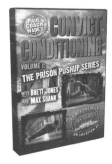

Convict Conditioning
Volume 1: The Prison Pushup Series
By Paul "Coach" Wade featuring Brett Jones and Max Shank

#DV083 $29.95
DVD 59 minutes

How Do YOU Stack Up Against These 6 Signs of a TRUE Physical Specimen?

According to Paul Wade's Convict Conditioning you earn the right to call yourself a 'true physical specimen' if you can perform the following:

1. AT LEAST one set of 5 one-arm pushups each side—with the ELITE goal of 100 sets each side

2. AT LEAST one set of 5 one-leg squats each side—with the ELITE goal of 2 sets of 50 each side

3. AT LEAST a single one-arm pullup each side—with the ELITE goal of 2 sets of 6 each side

4. AT LEAST one set of 5 hanging straight leg raises—with the ELITE goal of 2 sets of 30

5. AT LEAST one stand-to-stand bridge—with the ELITE goal of 2 sets of 30

Well, how DO you stack up?

Chances are that whatever athletic level you have achieved, there are some serious gaps in your OVERALL strength program. Gaps that stop you short of being able to claim status as a truly accomplished strength athlete.

The good news is that—in *Convict Conditioning*—Paul Wade has laid out a brilliant 6-set system of 10 progressions which allows you to master these elite levels.

And you could be starting at almost any age and in almost in any condition...

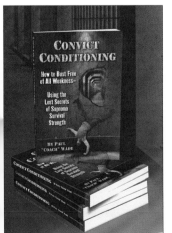

Paul Wade has given you the keys—ALL the keys you'll ever need— that will open door, after door, after door for you in your quest for supreme physical excellence. Yes, it will be the hardest work you'll ever have to do. And yes, 97% of those who pick up *Convict Conditioning*, frankly, won't have the guts and the fortitude to make it. But if you make it even half-way through **Paul's Progressions**, you'll be stronger than almost anyone you encounter. Ever.

Here's just a small taste of what you'll get with *Convict Conditioning*:

Dragon Door Customer Acclaim for Convict Conditioning

Fascinating Reading and Real Strength

"Coach Wade's system is a real eye opener if you've been a lifetime iron junkie. Wanna find out how really strong (or weak) you are? Get this book and begin working through the 10 levels of the 6 power exercises. I was pleasantly surprised by my ability on a few of the exercises...but some are downright humbling. If I were on a desert island with only one book on strength and conditioning this would be it. (Could I staple Pavel's "Naked Warrior" to the back and count them as one???!) Thanks Dragon Door for this innovative new author."—*Jon Schultheis, RKC (2005) - Keansburg, NJ*

Single best strength training book ever!

"I just turned 50 this year and I have tried a little bit of everything over the years: martial arts, swimming, soccer, cycling, free weights, weight machines, even yoga and Pilates. I started using *Convict Conditioning* right after it came out. I started from the beginning, like Coach Wade says, doing mostly step one or two for five out of the six exercises. I work out 3 to 5 times a week, usually for 30 to 45 minutes.

Long story short, my weight went up 14 pounds (I was not trying to gain weight) but my body fat percentage dropped two percent. That translates into approximately 19 pounds of lean muscle gained in two months! I've never gotten this kind of results with anything else I've ever done. Now I have pretty much stopped lifting weights for strength training. Instead, I lift once a week as a test to see how much stronger I'm getting without weight training. There are a lot of great strength training books in the world (most of them published by Dragon Door), but if I had to choose just one, this is the single best strength training book ever. BUY THIS BOOK. FOLLOW THE PLAN. GET AS STRONG AS YOU WANT. "—*Wayne - Decatur, GA*

Best bodyweight training book so far!

"I'm a martial artist and I've been training for years with a combination of weights and bodyweight training and had good results from both (but had the usual injuries from weight training). I prefer the bodyweight stuff though as it trains me to use my whole body as a unit, much more than weights do, and I notice the difference on the mat and in the ring. Since reading this book I have given the weights a break and focused purely on the bodyweight exercise progressions as described by 'Coach' Wade and my strength had increased more than ever before. So far I've built up to 12 strict one-leg squats each leg and 5 uneven pull ups each arm.

I've never achieved this kind of strength before - and this stuff builds solid muscle mass as well. It's very intense training. I am so confident in and happy with the results I'm getting that I've decided to train for a fitness/bodybuilding comp just using his techniques, no weights, just to show for real what kind of a physique these exercises can build. In sum, I cannot recommend 'Coach' Wade's book highly enough - it is by far the best of its kind ever!"—*Mark Robinson - Australia, currently living in South Korea*

A lifetime of lifting...and continued learning.

"I have been working out diligently since 1988 and played sports in high school and college before that. My stint in the Army saw me doing calisthenics, running, conditioning courses, forced marches, etc. There are many levels of strength and fitness. I have been as big as 240 in my powerlifting/strongman days and as low as 185-190 while in the Army. I think I have tried everything under the sun: the high intensity of Arthur Jones and Dr. Ken, the Super Slow of El Darden, and the brutality of Dinosaur Training Brooks Kubic made famous.

This is one of the BEST books I've ever read on real strength training which also covers other just as important aspects of health; like staying injury free, feeling healthy and becoming flexible. It's an excellent book. He tells you the why and the how with his progressive plan. This book is a GOLD MINE and worth 100 times what I paid for it!"
—*Horst - Woburn, MA*

This book sets the standard, ladies and gentlemen

"It's difficult to describe just how much this book means to me. I've been training hard since I was in the RAF nearly ten years ago, and to say this book is a breakthrough is an understatement. How often do you really read something so new, so fresh? This book contains a complete new system of calisthenics drawn from American prison training methods. When I say 'system' I mean it. It's complete (rank beginner to expert), it's comprehensive (all the exercises and photos are here), it's graded (progressions from exercise to exercise are smooth and pre-determined) and it's totally original. Whether you love or hate the author, you have to listen to him. And you will learn something. This book just makes SENSE. In twenty years people will still be buying it."—Andy McMann - Ponty, Wales, GB

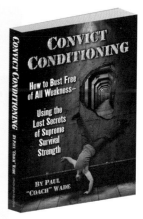

Convict Conditioning
How to Bust Free of All Weakness—
Using the Lost Secrets of Supreme Survival Strength
By Paul "Coach" Wade

Book #B41 $39.95
eBook #EB41 $19.95
Paperback 8.5 x 11
320 pages • 191 photos

WHY THE Bodyweight Master™
FREE STANDING PULL UP BAR
is the ultimate solution for your upper body build out...

The noble Pull Up and the mighty Muscle Up are two body-weight aristocrats that DO need a sturdy, indestructible piece of equipment to properly deliver their full, strength-enhancing benefits. Because to heap righteous slabs of etched meat on to your upper body—and get the military-industrial results you crave from your Pulls—you need the heavy-duty hardware to match your efforts…

But in the past, if you wanted to entertain bodyweight exercise royalty at home—and achieve the highest levels of Pull Up mastery—you would have been plain out of luck when it comes to a truly rugged, versatile and reliable free standing unit. Until now…

Enter the peerless *Bodyweight Master™ Free Standing Pull Up Bar,* designed by Dragon Door's calisthenics experts to specifically address the demands of the most hardcore bodyweight exercise fanatics. This unit looks tough and is tough—it reflects the inner and outer toughness of the user it is meant to serve…

We engineered our *Bodyweight Master™ Free Standing Pull Up Bar* to be the all-terrain, all-purpose battle tank of home exercise equipment… This thing does not take No for an answer—when it comes to rigorous abuse and a relentless quest for physical perfection…

And the *Bodyweight Master™* doubles up on your Dips, with detachable units and bars that allow all kinds of heights and challenges. Plus, at the top position, the Dip units let you set up for the more joint friendly neutral-grip Pull Up…

This is one investment in your health and strength that you can truly bank on—offering you year-upon-year of phenomenal physical gains and overall athletic enhancement!

Want to do low-bar work like Australian Pull Ups? Again, the *Bodyweight Master™* offers the perfect solution with its multiple low settings…

So: no more half-assed nonsense with jiggly rigs and ergonomically wretched devices that at best frustrate with weak, sub-par, inadequate results—and are usually doomed to become expensive coat hangers…

And no more door-frame wrecking, cheapo bars that limit your range of motion and cripple your athletic potential…

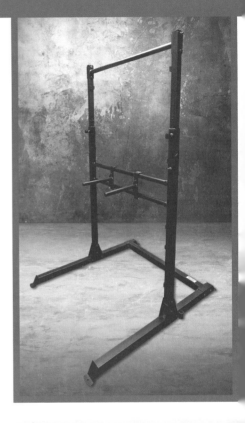

ADDITIONAL PRODUCT DETAILS:

- 2 detachable Dip units and bars which can be mounted at 7 different heights
- 1.5" diameter, 5" circumference Pull Up Bar
- 7 adjustable Pull Up bar heights: from 5' 2" to 8' 4"
- Easy assembly & disassembly
- 3' 11" wide x 4' 11.5" long base provides strong stability
- Wobble free
- Holes in the base allow unit to be screwed into the floor, for additional stability

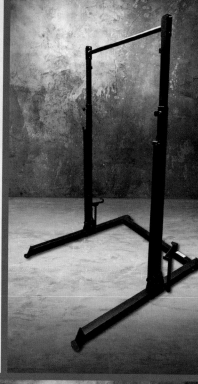
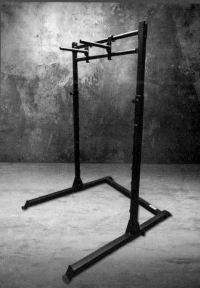

Teach your body to be the lightning-fast, explosive, acrobatic super-hunter your DNA is coded to make you...

With **Explosive Calisthenics**, Paul Wade challenges you to separate yourself from the herd of also-ran followers—to become a leader, survivor and winner in the physical game of life. But he doesn't just challenge and inspire you. He gives you the direct means, the secrets, the science, the wisdom, the blueprints, the proven methods and the progressions—that make success inevitable, when you supply your end in consistent, diligent, skillful application.

Now a legendary international bestseller, **Convict Conditioning** can lay claim to be the Great Instigator when it comes to the resurgence of interest in bodyweight exercise mastery.

And—while **Convict Conditioning 2** cemented Wade's position as the preeminent authority on bodyweight exercise—there is no doubt that his magisterial new accomplishment, **Explosive Calisthenics** is going to blow the doors off, all over again.

What makes **Explosive Calisthenics** so exciting—and so profound in its implications?

See, it goes back to the laws of brute survival. It's not "Only the strongest shall survive". No, it's more like: "Only the strongest, quickest, most agile, most powerful and most explosive shall survive." To be a leader and dominator and survivor in the pack, you need to be the complete package...

A vanishing percent of people who workout even attempt to unlock their body's inherent power and speed—choose to be different: reclaim your pride and dignity as a fully-realized human being by fully unleashing your true athletic capacity...

Now—for those who have the balls and the will and the fortitude to take it on—comes the next stage: Explosive Calisthenics. The chance not only to be strong and healthy but to ascend to the Complete Package. If you want it, then here it is...

You don't have to achieve a full back flip or kip up to get HUGE benefit from mastering the early progressions. It doesn't matter if you are a 20-year old looking to push your power and agility to new heights or approaching middle age, trying to slow the hands time. Do yourself a favor and get this amazing work. This book wi be the gold standard for developing bodyweight power, skill, and agility." **–CHRIS HARDY**, D.O. MPH, CSCS, author, **Strong Medicine**

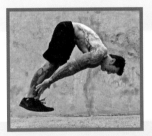 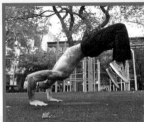

"**Explosive Calisthenics** is an absolute Treasure Map for anybody loo ing to tear down their body's athletic limitations. Who doesn't want be able to kip to their feet from their back like a Bruce Lee? Or make a backflip look easy? Paul makes you want to put down the barbells learn and practice these step-by-step progressions to mastering the most explosive and impressive bodyweight movements.

The best part? You can become an absolute Beast in under an hour of practice a week. Way to go, Paul! AROO!" **–JOE DISTEFANO, Sparta Race**, Director of Training & Creator of the **Spartan SGX Certification**

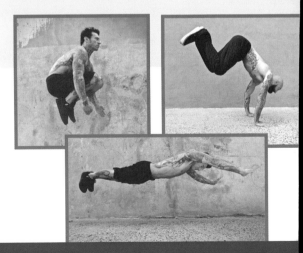

PART I: POWER, SPEED, AGILITY

Power Up! The Need for Speed

The difference between complex power and simple power—and what it means for athletic success…P 7

Discover how to enhance your reflexes to generate higher levels of power, speed and agility…P 9

Why most gym-trained athletes lack THESE qualities—and will therefore never attain true athleticism…P 10

Explosive Training: Five Key Principles

The 5 key principles for developing speed, power and agility… P 12

Why traditional box work, core training and Olympic lifting simply won't cut it—when your goal is high-level explosiveness…P 14

If you really want to build monstrous power, speed and agility in the shortest possible time—HERE is what you absolutely MUST stick with…P 18

The 6 movements you must master—for the ultimate in hardcore explosiveness…P 19

The true essence of calisthenics mastery lies here—and only here…P 19

PART II: THE EXPLOSIVE SIX

4: Power Jumps: Advanced L eg Spring

If you really want to become explosive, then the legs are the source of it all—and the best way to train the legs is with progressive power jumps. Here is the 10-step blueprint for achieving ultimate leg power…

Power Pushups: Strength Becomes Power

To round out a basic power training regime, you need to pair jumps with a movement chain which performs a similar job for the upper-body and arms. The best drills for these are power Pushups. Here is the 10-step blueprint for becoming an upper-body cyborg…

How to get arms like freaking jackhammers…P 73

How to skyrocket pour power levels, maximize your speed and add slabs of righteous beef to your torso and guns…P 73

How to develop upper-body survival-power—for more effective punching, blocking, throwing and pushing…P 73

How speed-power training trains the nervous system and joints to handle greater loads…P 73

The Kip-Up: Kung Fu Body Speed

The mesmerizing Kip-Up is the most explosive way of getting up off your back—and is a surprisingly useful skill to possess. Discover the secrets here…P 109

The Front Flip: Lightning Movement Skills

The Front Flip is THE explosive exercise par excellence—it is the "super-drill" for any athlete wanting more speed, agility and power.

Discover how to attain this iconic test of power and agility—requiring your entire body, from toes to neck, to be whip-like explosive…P 141

The Back Flip: Ultimate Agility

The Back Flip is the most archetypal acrobatic feat—displaying integrated mastery of some of the most fundamental traits required for total explosive strength.

If you want to be a contender for the power crown, then you have to get to own the Back Flip—which defines true agility…

Discover how to develop a super-quick jump, a massive hip snap, a powerful, agile waist and spine—and an upper body that can generate higher levels of responsive force like lightning…

Simply put, this is the single greatest test of explosive power, true speed and agility found in nature. Here is how to pass the test…

The Muscle-Up: Optimal Explosive Strength

If ever one popular strength exercise qualified as a "complete" feat, it would probably be the mighty Muscle-Up—one of the most jealously-admired skills in all of bodyweight training…

The Muscle-Up requires a very explosive pull, plus a push—so works almost the entire upper-body; the back and biceps pull, while the chest, triceps and shoulders push. Your grip needs to be insanely strong, your stomach crafted out of steel and you require a highly athletic posterior chain.

Discover the complete blueprint for achieving the planet's hottest bodyweight move…

Learn how to achieve the elusive, total-body-sync, X factor the Muscle-Up requires—and build insane explosive power in a highly compressed time frame…

PART III: PROGRAMMING: THEORY AND TACTICS

Making Progress: The PARC Principle

If you can work your way up to the ice-cold, bad-ass master Step for all Explosive Six—you will become the most explosively powerful athlete you know. No question…

So how DO you move safely and effectively upwards through these chains—and achieve bodyweight immortality? The answers are fully contained in these next sections…

Power and Skill: Twin Training Methodologies

How to express your power in a more sophisticated manner through skill-based movement training…P 274

Power Building: The Rule of Three and the Rule of Six

What is raw power?…P 275

The 3 main qualities you need to have established in order to successfully perform Kip-Ups and Flips…P 275

How to build enduring power and joint integrity throughout your whole athletic life…P 276

How to build a bigger and more turbo-charged "power vehicle"—fail to achieve this and you will be like a speedster running on empty…P 276

THIS is the bread-and-butter rule-of-thumb followed by most successful explosive athletes and coaches…P 280

Skill Development: Time Surfing and Consolidation Training

Sample Programs: Session Templates

Why you should focus on progressions, not templates…P 293

Some fundamental, applicable approaches to training plans that will fit different goals and objectives…P 294

How much and how should you warm up?…P 295

4 keys to an effective warm-up protocol…P 295

How to integrate explosive work with strength and bodybuilding programs…P 301

BONUS MATERIAL

Bonus Section 1: Advanced Speed Training: "Coach" Wade's Top Ten Tricks and Hacks

Bonus Section 2: Animal Agility Drills

10 major animal-type movements that can be your wild card/X-factor in your power and strength training…P 327

These animal agility drills increase strength and efficiency while reducing the chance of injury. The legs stay "springy" whatever your age and total-body coordination

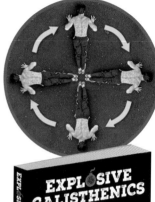

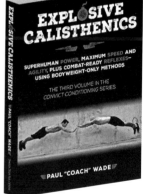

Explosive Calisthenics
Superhuman Power, Maximum Speed and Agility, Plus Combat-Ready Reflexes— Using Bodyweight-Only Methods
By Paul "Coach" Wade

Book #B80 $39.95
eBook #EB80 $19.95
Paperback 8.5 x 11 • 392 pages, 775 photos

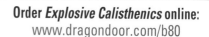

C-MASS

How To Maximize Muscle Growth Using Bodyweight-Only Training

Is it really possible to add significant extra muscle-bulk to your frame using bodyweight exercise only? The answer, according to calisthenics guru and bestselling *Convict Conditioning* author Paul Wade, is a resounding Yes. Legendary strongmen and savvy modern bodyweight bodybuilders both, have added stacks of righteous beef to their physiques—using just the secrets Paul Wade reveals in this bible-like guide to getting as strong AND as big as you could possibly want, using nothing but your own body.

Paul Wade's trenchant, visceral style blazes with hard-won body culture insight, tactics, strategies and tips for the ultimate blueprint for getting huge naturally without free weights, machine supplements or—God forbid—steroids. With *C-Mass*, Paul Wade further cements his position as the preeminent modern authority on how to build extraordinary power and strength with bodyweight exercise only.

1. Bodyweight Muscle? No Problem!

Build *phenomenal* amounts of natural muscle mass and discover how to:

- Add 20-30+ pounds of solid muscle—with perfect proportions
- Reshape your arms with 2-3 inches of gnarly beef
- Triple the size of your pecs and lats
- Thicken and harden your abdominal wall into a classic six-pack
- Generate hard, sculpted quads and hamstrings that would be the envy of an Olympic sprinter
- Stand head and shoulders above the next 99% of natural bodybuilders in looks, strength and power
- Boost your testosterone naturally to bull-like levels
- Understand the radically different advantages you'll get from the two major types of resistance work, nervous system training and muscular system training.
- If you really want to explode your muscle growth—if SIZE is your goal—you should train THIS way...

2. The Ten Commandments of Calisthenics Mass

Why reps are key when you want to build massive stacks of jacked up muscle.

- Want to turn from a twig into an ok tree? Why working demonically hard and employing brutal physical effort is essential to getting nasty big...
- These are the very best dynamic exercises—for bigger bang for your muscle buck.
- How to ratchet up the heat with THIS kick-ass strategy and sprout new muscle at an eye-popping rate.
- What it takes to trigger explosive muscle growth.
- Why so few wannabe athletes ever achieve a good level of strength and muscle—let alone a great level—and what it really takes to succeed.
- How to transform miniscule, incremental gains into long-range massive outcomes.
- 10 secrets to optimizing the magic rest-muscle growth formula...
- Discover the 3 main reasons why, sleep, the natural alternative to steroids, helps prison athletes grow so big...
- Why your mind is your most powerful supplement...
- How 6 major training demons can destroy your bodybuilding dreams—and where to find the antidote...
- Understanding the relationship between the nervous system and the muscular system—and how to take full advantage of that relationship.
- Why, if you wish to gain as much muscle as your genetic potential will allow, just training your muscles won't cut it—and what more you need to do...
- The secret to mixing and matching for both growth AND strength...

3. "Coach" Wade's Bodypart Tactics

Get the best bodyweight bodybuilding techniques for 11 major body areas.

1. QUADZILLA! (...AND QUADZOOKIE.)

- Why the Gold Standard quad developer is squatting—and why you absolutely need to master the Big Daddy, the *one-legged squat*...
- How to perform the Shrimp Squat, a wonderful quad and glute builder, which is comparable to the one-leg squat in terms of body-challenge.
- Why you should employ THESE 7 jumping methods to put your quad gains through the roof...

2. HAMSTRINGS: STAND SIDEWAYS WITH PRIDE

- Enter *Lombard's Paradox:* how and why you can successfully brutalize your hammies with calisthenics.
- Why bridging is a perfect exercise for strengthening the hamstrings.
- How to correctly work your hamstrings and activate your entire posterior chain.
- Why THIS workout of straight bridges and hill sprints could put muscle on a pencil.
- How to employ the little-known secret of the *bridge curl* to develop awesome strength and power in the your hammies.

3. SOFTBALL BICEPS

THIS is the best biceps exercise in the world *bar none*. Discover what you are missing out on and learn to do it right...

4. TITANIC TRICEPS

Paul Wade has *never* met a gym-trained bodybuilder who understands how the triceps work. Not one.

- Learn how the triceps REALLY work. This stuff is gold—pay attention. And discover the drills that are going to CRUCIFY those tris!

5. FARMER FOREARMS

The forearms are best built through THESE exercises, and you can build superhuman grip by utilizing intelligent THESE progressions.

6. IT's NOT "ABS", IT's "MIDSECTION"

The single greatest exercise for scorching your abs in the most effective manner possible is THIS...

- How to best train your obliques and lateral chain...
- Why crush-style grippers are a mistake and the better, safer alternative for a hand-pulping grip...

7. Maximum Chest

The roll call of classical bodyweight chest exercises is dynamic and impressive. It's an ancient, effective, tactical buffet of super-moves. Get the list here...

- THE best chest routine is THIS one...
- THIS could be the ultimate bodyweight drill to get thick, imposing pectoral muscles...

8. Powerful, Healthy Shoulders

If you want to give any of your shoulder heads an enhanced, specialist workout, a great tactic is THIS.

- If you *really* want to build your rear delts, THIS drill should be your number one exercise...
- THESE kinds of drills can result in shoulder injury, rotator cuff tears, frozen shoulder and chronic pain—what to stick with instead...
- THIS is a fantastic deltoid movement which will swell up those cannonballs fast...

9. Ah'll be Back

THIS exercise is the finest lat-widener in the bodybuilding world and should be the absolute mainstay of your back training. This one's a no-brainer—if adding maximum torso beef as fast and efficiently as possible appeals to you...

- Paul Wade demands that all his students begin their personal training with a brutal regime of THIS punishing drill. Why? Find out here...
- How bridging fully works all the deep tissues of the spine and bulletproofs the discs.
- The single most effective bridge technique for building massive back muscle...

10. Calving Season

THIS squat method will make your calves larger, way more supple, more powerful, and your ankles/Achilles' tendon will be bulletproofed like a steel cable...

- Whether you are an athlete, a strength trainer or a pure bodyweight bodybuilder, your first mission should be to gradually build to THIS. Until you get there, you don't need to waste time on any specialist calf exercises.
- If you DO want to add specific calf exercises to your program, then THESE are a good choice.

11. TNT: Total Neck and Traps

Do bodybuilders even need to do neck work? Here's the answer...

- The best neck exercises for beginners.
- HERE is an elite-level technique for developing the upper trapezius muscles between the neck and shoulders..

4. Okay. Now Gimme a Program

If you want to pack on muscle using bodyweight, it's no good training like a *gymnast* or a *martial artist* or a *dancer* or a *yoga expert*, no matter how impressive those skill-based practitioners might be at performing advanced calisthenics. You need a different mindset. You need to train like a bodybuilder!

- Learn the essential C-Mass Paul Wade *principles* behind programming, so you can master your own programming...
- The most important thing to understand about bodybuilding routines...
- When to Move up the Programming Line
- Fundamental Program Templates

6. The Democratic Alternative... how to get as powerful as possible without gaining a pound

There is a whole bunch of folks who either want (or need) massive strength and power, but without the attendant muscle bulk. Competitive athletes who compete in weight limits are one example; wrestlers, MMA athletes, boxers, etc. Females are another group who, as a rule, want to get stronger when they train, but without adding much (or any) size. Some men desire steely, whip-like power but see the sheer weight of mass as non-functional—many martial artists fall into this category; perhaps Bruce Lee was the archetype.

But bodybuilders should also fall under this banner. All athletes who want to become as huge as possible need to spend some portion of their time focusing on *pure strength*. Without a high (and increasing) level of strength, it's impossible to use enough load to stress your muscles into getting bigger. This is even truer once you get past a certain basic point.

So: You want to build power like a Humvee, with the sleek lines of a classic Porsche? The following Ten Commandments have got you covered. Follow them, and we promise you *cannot* fail, even if you had trouble getting stronger in the past. Your days of weakness are done, my friend...

Enter the "Bullzelle"

There are guys who train for pure mass and want to look like bulls, and guys who only train for athleticism without mass, and are more like gazelles. Al Kavadlo has been described as a "bullzelle"—someone who trains mainly for strength, and has some muscle too, but without looking like a bulked-up bodybuilder. And guess what? It seems like many of the new generation of athletes want to be bullzelles! With Paul Wade's C-Mass program, you'll have what you

need to achieve bullzelle looks and functionality should you want it...

- If you want to generate huge strength without building muscle, here is the precise formula...
- How pure strength training works, in a nutshell...
- Why frequency—how often you train—is often so radically different for pure strength trainers and for bodybuilders...
- Training recipe for the perfect bodybuilder—and for the perfect strength trainer...

If there is a "trick" to being supremely strong, THIS is it...

- As a bodybuilder, are you making this huge mistake? If you want to get super-powerful, unlearn these ideas and employ THIS strategy instead...

Another great way to learn muscular coordination and control is to explore THESE drills...

- If there is a single tactic that's guaranteed to maximize your body-power in short order, it's bracing. Bracing is both an art-form and a science. Here's how to do it and why it works so well.
- If there is an instant "trick" to increasing your strength, it's learning the art of the breath. Learn the details here...
- When the old-time strongmen talked about strength, they rarely talked about muscle power—they typically focused on the integrity of the tendons. THIS is why...
- The concept of "supple strength" and how to really train the tendons for optimal resilience and steely, real-life strength...
- Why focusing on "peak contraction" can be devastating to your long-term strength-health goals...

THIS is the essential difference between a mere *bodybuilder* and a *truly powerful* human being...

- Pay extra attention to your weakest areas by including THESE 4 sets of drills as a mandatory part of your monster strength program...
- The nervous system—like most sophisticated biological systems—possesses different sets of *gears*. Learn how to safely and effectively shift to high gear in a hurry using THESE strategies...
- Why it is fatal for a bodyweight master to focus only on tension-generating techniques and what to do instead...
- The difference between "voluntary" and "involuntary" strength—and how to work on both for greater gains...
- How to train the mind to make the body achieve incredible levels of strength and ferocity—as if it was tweaking on PCP...

- 5 fundamental ways to harness mental power and optimize your strength...

7. Supercharging Your Hormonal Profile

Why you should never, ever, ever take steroids to enhance your strength...

Hormones and Muscle Growth

Your *hormones* are what build your muscle. All your training is pretty secondary. You can work out hard as possible as often as possible, but if your hormonal levels aren't good, your gains will be close to nil. Learn what it takes to naturally optimize a cascade of powerful strength-generating hormones and to minimize the strength-sappers from sabotaging your gains...

Studies and simple experience have demonstrated that, far from being some esoteric practice, some men have increased their diminished total testosterone levels by *over a thousand percent!* How? Just by following a few basic rules.

What rules? Listen up. THIS is the most important bodybuilding advice anyone will ever give you.

The 6 Rules of Testosterone Building

THESE rules are the most powerful and long-lasting, for massive testosterone generation. Follow them if you want to get diesel.

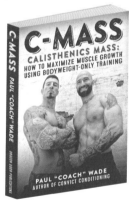

WEEKDAYS
:30AM–5:30PM CST

1•800•899•5111
www.dragondoor.com

Order *C-Mass* online:
www.dragondoor.com/b75

Reader Praise for *Convict Conditioning Ultimate Bodyweight Training Log*

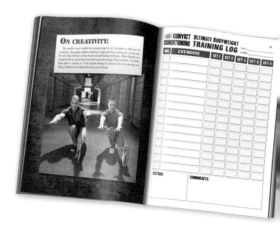

Above and Beyond!

"Not JUST a log book. TONS of great and actually useful info. I really like to over complicate programming and data entries at times. And honestly, All one has to do is fill in the blanks... Well that and DO THE WORK. Great product."
—**NOEL PRICE, Chicagoland, IL**

A unique training log

"This log book is one of a kind in the world. It is the only published body weight exclusive training log I have personally seen. It is well structured and provides everything for a log book in a primarily body weight oriented routine. The book is best integrated with the other books in the convict conditioning series however has enough information to act as a stand alone unit. It is a must have for anyone who is a fan of the convict conditioning series or is entering into calisthenics."
—**CARTER D., Cambridge, Canada**

Excellent Companion to *Convict Conditioning 1 & 2*

"This is an amazing book! If you are a fan of Convict Conditioning (1 & 2) you need to get this training log. If you are preparing for the Progressive Calisthenics Certification then it's a must-have!!! The spiral bound format is a huge improvement over the regular binding and it makes it that much more functional for use in the gym. Great design, amazing pictures and additional content! Once again - Great job Dragon Door!"
—**MICHAEL KRIVKA, RKC Team Leader, Gaithersburg, MD**

Excellent latest addition to the CC Program!

"A terrific book to keep you on track and beyond. Thank you again for this incredible series!"
—**JOSHUA HATCHER, Holyoke, MA**

Calling this a Log Book is Selling it Short

"I thought, what is the big deal about a logbook! Seriously mistaken. It is a work of art and with tips on each page that would be a great book all by itself. Get it. It goes way beyond a log book...the logging part of this book is just a bonus. You must have this!"—**JON ENGUM, Brainerd, MN**

The Ultimate Bodyweight Conditioning

"I have started to incorporate bodyweight training into my strength building when I am not going to the gym. At the age of 68, after 30 years in the gym the 'Convict Conditioning Log' is going to be a welcome new training challenge."
—**WILLIAM HAYDEN, Winter Park, FL**

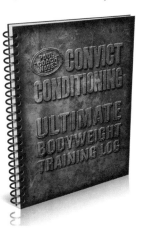

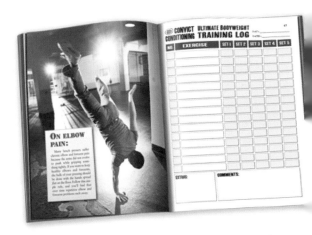

Convict Conditioning Ultimate Bodyweight Training Log
By Paul "Coach" Wade

Book #B67 $29.95
eBook #EB67 $19.95
Paperback (spiral bound) 6 x 9
290 pages • 175 photos

1·800·899·5111

FAX YOUR ORDER (866) 280-7619
ORDERING INFORMATION

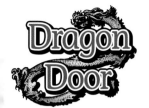

Telephone Orders. For faster service you may place your orders by calling 1-800-899-5111 between 9:30am-5:30pm CST, Monday to Friday. When you call, please have your credit card ready.

Customer Service Questions? Please call us at 1-800-899-5111 between 9:30am-5:30pm CST, Monday to Friday. Local and foreign customers call 651-487-2180 for orders and customer service. You may also email us at support@dragondoor.com.

100% One-Year Risk-Free Guarantee. If you are not completely satisfied with any product—we'll be happy to give you a prompt exchange, credit, or refund, as you wish. Simply return your purchase to us, and please let us know why you were dissatisfied--it will help us to provide better products and services in the future. Shipping and handling fees are non-refundable.

Complete and mail with full payment to: Dragon Door Publications, 5 County Road B East, Suite 3, Little Canada, MN 55117

Please print clearly

Sold To:
A

Name_____

Street_____

City_____

State _____ Zip _____

Day phone*_____

Please print clearly

Sold To: (Street address for delivery)   **B**

Name_____

Street_____

City_____

State _____ Zip _____

Email_____

Warning to foreign customers:

The Customs in your country may or may not tax or otherwise charge you an additional fee for goods you receive. Dragon Door Publications is charging you only for U.S. handling and international shipping. Dragon Door Publications is in no way responsible for any additional fees levied by Customs, the carrier or any other entity.

ITEM #	QTY.	ITEM DESCRIPTION	ITEM PRICE	A OR B	TOTAL

HANDLING AND SHIPPING CHARGES • NO CODS
Total Amount of Order Add (Excludes kettlebells and kettlebell kits):

$00.00 to 29.99	Add $7.00	$100.00 to 129.99	Add $14.00
$30.00 to 49.99	Add $6.00	$130.00 to 169.99	Add $16.00
$50.00 to 69.99	Add $8.00	$170.00 to 199.99	Add $18.00
$70.00 to 99.99	Add $11.00	$200.00 to 299.99	Add $20.00
		$300.00 and up	Add $24.00

Canada and Mexico add $6.00 to US charges. All other countries, flat rate, double US Charges. See Kettlebell section for Kettlebell Shipping and handling charges.

Total of Goods	
Shipping Charges	
Rush Charges	
Kettlebell Shipping Charges	
OH residents add 6.5% sales tax	
MN residents add 6.5%	

METHOD OF PAYMENT ___CHECK ___M.O. ___MASTERCARD ___VISA ___DISCOVER ___AMEX

Account No. (Please indicate all the numbers on your credit card)   EXPIRATION DATE

☐☐☐☐ ☐☐☐☐ ☐☐☐☐ ☐☐☐☐   ☐☐/☐☐

Day Phone: _____

Signature: _____ Date: _____

NOTE: We ship best method available for your delivery address. Foreign orders are sent by air. Credit card or International M.O. only. **For RUSH processing** of your order, add an additional $10.00 per address. Available on money order & charge card orders only.

Errors and omissions excepted. Prices subject to change without notice.